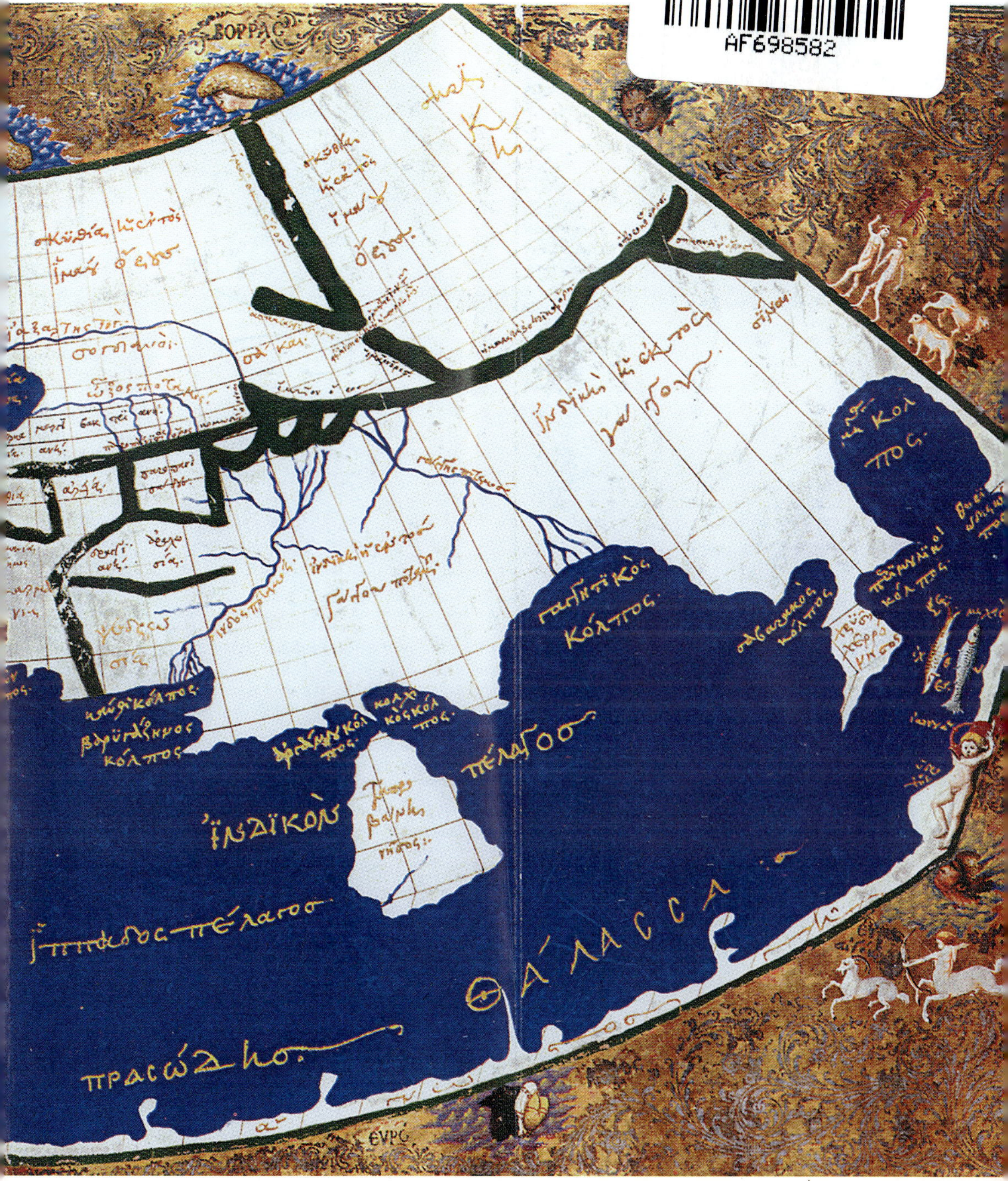

Bridging Hippocrates and Huang Ti

Inside cover:

One of Gerhard Kremer's (Mercator) (1512–1594) maps representing Europe, Asia and Africa (*Ptolemaeus*, *Geographia*, Greek code Z. 388 (= 333), pp. 50v – 51r, Venice, Biblioteca Marciana)

BRIDGING
HIPPOCRATES AND HUANG TI

Volume 1

A COMPARATIVE THESAURUS OF TRADITIONAL
CHINESE AND WESTERN
UROLOGY, ANDROLOGY AND SEXOLOGY

Editors:

Paolo Marandola
University of Pavia, Italy

Sergio Musitelli
University of Pavia, Italy

Wei Li Chen
Guyiang Medical College, Guyiang, Guizhou, P.R. China

2003

ELSEVIER

Amsterdam – Boston – Heidelberg – London – New York – Oxford
Paris – San Diego – San Francisco – Singapore – Sydney – Tokyo

ELSEVIER B.V.
Sara Burgerhartstraat 25
P.O. Box 211, 1000 AE Amsterdam, The Netherlands

First edition 2003

Library of Congress Cataloging in Publication Data
A catalog record from the Library of Congress has been applied for.

British Library Cataloguing in Publication Data
A catalogue record from the British Library has been applied for.

ISBN: 0-444-51520-8

∞ The paper used in this publication meets the requirements of ANSI/NISO Z39.48-1992 (Permanence of Paper).
Printed in The Netherlands.

CONTENTS

ACKNOWLEDGEMENTS

This volume has been planned and written at the Foundation A. Scarpa for the Advanced Research in Urology and Andrology, in Pavia, under the leadership and supervision of P. Marandola and S. Musitelli. A full time research grant for the project was given to Mrs Wei Li Chen.

The illustrations and layout could never have been realized without the generous collaboration of Dr. Hussein Jallous and Dr. Carlo Magnaghi, to whom we express our deepest gratitude.

Secretarial work was done, wonderfully, by Mrs. Claudia De Paoli.

The financial generosity and advice of the following Institutions and individuals was the feeder conveyor of all efforts, encountered during three years of research and traveling in Italy, China and on the Internet:

- Dr. R. Chatanay, *M.B.A. P.H.D. – EMS Electro Medical Systems*
- Dr. Cheng Huaijin, *The Traditional Peace and Maternity & Child Health Hospital of China Welfare, Shanghai*
- The Historical Committee of EAU
- Indena S.p.A., Milano

This Volume is published under the Patronage of

Historical Committee, European Association of Urology
Historical Committee, American Urological Association
I.R.C.C.S. Policlinico San Matteo, Pavia, Italy
School of Medicine, University of Pavia, Italy
Historical Committee, Chinese Association of Urology

CONTRIBUTORS

Ezio Bombardelli
Scientific Director
Indena S.p.A.
Milan
Italy

Wei Li Chen
Teaching Professor of English Language
Guyang Medical College
Guyiang, Guizhou
P.R. China

Hussein Jallous
Specialist Urologist
IRCCS Policlinico San Matteo
Pavia
Italy

Paolo Marandola
Professor of Urology
University of Pavia
Pavia
Italy

Paolo Morazzoni
Assistant Scientific Director
Indena S.p.A.
Milan
Italy

Sergio Musitelli
Professor of Philosophy of Science and of
History of Medicine,Consultant Historian
School of Urology
University of Pavia
Pavia
Italy

PREFACE I

After the sweeping political changes that occurred in the Countries of Eastern Europe, the Western Democracies have felt the need of aiding those peoples to reach their own political, economical and chiefly scientific level. Most recently China too has begun opening itself to the Western scientific world and establishing more and more intense intercourse with Western Medicine in general and Western Urology, Andrology and Sexology in particular.

Moreover the Third Millennium seems more and more likely to become the Millennium of economical, financial, political and social "globalisation".

Medicine in general, and Urology, Andrology and Sexology in particular cannot stop at the starting line and have nothing to do with.

But "globalisation" does not mean removal and annulment of the "other cultures" considered as "inferior" or even "void" cultures, only because of their being "different" from the "Western Culture".

It means reciprocal approach, dialogue and reciprocal contribution to create a "new" and "global" culture, to which each culture concurs with its original and particular experience and ideas, in which each culture can recognise itself and which it may feel as "its own culture".

In fact, the many and intense exchanges of views and experiences promoted by many European Scientific Associations, and chiefly by the European Association of Urology (EAU), which organises yearly refresher courses in Eastern Europe, have pointed out that on the one hand China feels more and more engaged in mastering the Western scientific methods and results; on the other hand, Western Medicine, and mainly Western Urology, Andrology and Sexology have realised the need first of all of acquiring and interpreting under their own point of view and method of research the immense pharmacological patrimony of Traditional Chinese Medicine; secondly of recovering the connection between the physician and the patient, rather than between the physician and the illness, that Traditional Chinese Medicine did never forget.

This being the case, the University of Peking and the Chinese Government have entrusted to the School of Urology of the University of Pavia a grantee (Dr. Wei Li Chen) who has worked under the guidance of Prof. Paolo Marandola – Chair of Urology – and his collaborator for the History of Urology (Prof. Sergio Musitelli) for one year in order to project and realise this book, the aim of which is just to put the necessary historical basis for such an enterprise.

Under this new perspective, the glorious St. Mathew Polyclinic Hospital of Pavia, born from the oldest University, that is our University of Pavia, established in the year 825 A.C., could not betray its centuries-old tradition of being one of the leading centers of universal culture in general and of medical research in particular, if one only remembers – to confine ourselves to some of the most significant examples – that Simon-André Tissot, from Switzerland, and Johann Peter Frank, from Germany, were teaching in Pavia side by side with Lazzaro Spallanzani and Antonio Scarpa and that

Giovanni Brambilla, who was the founder of the University Library of the city where he had graduated and practised Medicine for many years, also was one of the most active and prestigious promoters of the foundation of the Military Medical and Surgical Academy of Vienna, where he transplanted the scientific patrimony of Pavia.

If the School of Medicine and the inseparable St. Mathew Hospital have been one of the most important points of reference, and, at the same time, one of the greatest and most active champions of European medical culture for more than five centuries, no doubt it could not afford not to be in the front line to improve the medical studies in a "global" perspective by sponsoring this publication that is the result of an intense co-operation between the University of Pavia (Chair of Urology), the "A. Scarpa Foundation for Advanced Urological Research", the University of Peking and the Urological Association of Asia and has been promoted, supported and patronaged by the Historical Committee of the European Association of Urology.

It emphasises the correspondence and the close resemblance between Traditional Chinese and Western Medicine at least up to the beginning of the XVII century and proves that they have started from the same empirical and theoretical premises, have run the same way for a long series of centuries, have devised the same interpretative theories and the same doctrines, though in different languages. No doubt, for instance, the particular "Qi" of each organ of the human body is perfectly corresponding to the "virtue" of our hippocratic and galenic tradition.

This "going back to our common roots" is the premise to the dialogue and the following integration of Traditional Chinese and Modern Western Urology, Andrology and Sexology, which will give birth to the "New Urology, Andrology and Sexology" of the Third Millennium.

The University of Pavia School of Medicine and St. Mathew Hospital feel bound to take part to this dialogue and to this fundamental integration as one of the leading interlocutors and actors.

The second volume of this Opera ("Bridging Traditional Chinese and Western Medicine") will put the basis for this integration, and our two Institutions will be certainly as much involved as it has been in this first historical volume most of all because if History – according to Thukydides – is "a conquest for ever", this volume is surely a premise to this "conquest".

Prof. E. Solcia
Scientific Director
Policlinico S. Matteo Hospital – Pavia

Prof. C. Meloni
Dean School of Medicine
University of Pavia

PREFACE II

Western Medicine as we see it today has a strong scientific basis in its development. The pathogenesis of most diseases and their symptomatology and physical signs are well studied and understood. Our managements of patients are based on firm understanding of these disease processes. In contrast, Traditional Chinese Medicine came about through accumulation of experiences of many generations of practitioners over thousand of years. Undoubtedly, many of these treatments have shown to be effective in its own way. However, a firm scientific basis in therapy is still lacking.

While most Western Medicine advocates control of disease by eradication of pathogens and surgical removal of diseased organ as in the case of cancer, the Traditional Chinese Medicine seeks remedy to improve the host resistance against the disease. There is probably a great wealth of therapeutic value in Traditional Chinese Medicine, which has not been discovered or explored fully. Hence, by combining the knowledge of both Western and Traditional Chinese Medicine, one might be able to improve the results of efficacy of treatment and survival of patient. The integration of Medicine from East and West would of course take time to evolve and would need interested physicians from different parts of the world to come together and work closely to realize such possibility.

This book is a good attempt in bridging the medical world of two great and ancient civilizations in their approach in treatment of diseases. It is both informative and readable with detail account of history of medical development. It is highly recommended for those medical practitioners from both East and West who are interested to explore into alternative medicine and research into newer areas of medical frontier.

Dr. E. C. Tan
President
Urological Association of Asia

PREFACE III

For hundreds of years, Chinese and Western culture and science developed in almost complete isolation from each other.

For many centuries, Europeans saw Western Europe as the intellectual and political center of the world, but at the same time, the Chinese emperors ruled what they called their "middle empire" because China was to them the center of the world.

In 1492, when Christopher Columbus set sail from the “old continent” in the Santa Maria, a small 30-meter vessel, to explore the “new Americas” for the first time, the Chinese admiral Zheng He had already explored the African coasts of Somalia and Kenya in 1431 in an impressive 140-meter ship!

It is only since the last century of the second millennium that things have begun to change very quickly, and the Third Millennium is set to be the Millennium of economic, financial, political and social globalisation.

Medicine in general, and Urology, Andrology and Sexology in particular cannot afford to miss the boat of the new millennium.

But globalisation does not mean discarding or ignoring other cultures, or regarding them as inferior because they are different from Western ideas.

To create a new, global culture, we need a reciprocal approach, dialogue and cooperation. Each culture should contribute its own particular experience, philosophies and ideas, so that the members of all cultures will recognise the new global culture as their own.

It is from this perspective that the Historical Committee of the European Association of Urology has proposed, supported and encouraged this publication, which is the result of intense cooperation between the University of Pavia (Chair of Urology and the A. Scarpa Foundation for Advanced Urological Research), the University of Beijing and the Chinese Association of Urology.

The aim of this study is implicit in two words in the title: “*bridging*” and “*thesaurus*” – it is the bringing together of two treasuries.

There are 7 chapters: 1: A brief comparative history of Traditional Chinese Medicine (TCM) and Western Medicine (WM); 2: A brief introduction to TCM Urology – an entry for a medical dictionary; 3: The visceral manifestation of Urology, Andrology and Sexology; 4: Aetiology and Pathology; 5: Typical diseases; 6: External and other treatment; 7: Herbal medicine, both English and Chinese, compiled as a real and complete overview of the two traditions.

“Going back to our common roots” is the premise of a dialogue, which will culminate in the "new medicine" of the new millennium.

The European Association of Urology and its Historical Committee are honored to participate in this dialogue as the leading interlocutors.

If History is a "conquest forever" – as Thukydides tells us – then this book is a fundamental step towards achieving this conquest.

Prof. Dr. F. M. J. Debruyne
Secretary General
European Association of Urology

Dr. J. J. Mattelaer
Chairman Historical Committee
European Association of Urology

INTRODUCTION

A comparison between the History of TCM (Traditional Chinese Medicine) and that of WM (Western Medicine) reveals, on the one hand, a series of parallel elements, and, on the other, a no less abundant series of profoundly different, but, in the final analysis, absolutely complementary characteristics.

Originally, both TCM and WM (like all primitive medicines) were closely connected to magic, witchcraft, and, in the end, religion, as is demonstrated by the Chinese ideogram for «medicine», which is comprised of four signs that stand respectively for «quiver», «arrow», «to strike» and «potion», so that the complete ideogram reads «(to strike with an) *arrow* (taken from) *the quiver* (evil spirits) *and* (to give the patient) *a potion* (to cure him)». In the western world, on the other hand, this same connection can be seen by the number of those who practised medicine in the «Asclepièia» (the temples of Asclepios, the God of Medicine) and boasted that they were «Asclepiads», or «descendants of Aesculepios».

But it was not long before both TCM – starting roughly from the Third Millennium B.C – and WM – starting from the 7th century B.C – began to take on a more and more philosophical character, so that even in the oldest texts (the famous «Simple Questions of the Yellow Emperor» and the no less famous «Canonical Book of the Hub of the Soul», both attributed to the legendary Huang Ti, who lived around 2700 B.C, but whose works are known from versions published in circa 200 B.C and 1100 AD respectively) the former is clearly presented as «philosophical medicine» exactly like the most famous school of Western Medicine, the School of Cnidos, which was to be opposed by Hippocrates (a contemporary of Socrates, 469 – 399 B.C) and his School, the renowned School of Cos.

However, whereas TCM has introduced practically no changes to its theories or diagnostic and therapeutic methods in over four millennia, with the result that it is still very much alive to this day, WM has an extremely troubled history starting from the first half of the 5th century B.C, in other words, starting from Hippocrates, who marked a profound breach with «philosophical medicine» and ushered in a medicine based on the «observation» and the «rational analysis and evaluation» of observed data, in accordance with the principle of «observatio et ratio» and on the basis of a clear cut and radical rejection of all abstract theorizing.

And along the trail blazed by Hippocrates stand the first great Alexandrine physicians and anatomists (who lived from the 3rd century B.C to the end of the 1st century AD) and Galen. But the same Galen, profoundly influenced by Hippocrates, on the one hand, but also by the philosophy of Plato (428/27 – 348 B.C) and of Aristotle (384 – 322 B.C), on the other, refounded a «philosophical medicine» (his little treatise entitled «The Excellent Physician is also a Philosopher» is particularly important) that was to win a position of absolute dominance for over fifteen centuries.

As a matter of fact it is in the 17th century that we witness the second and, this time, definitive breach between all of Western Science and, in particular, Medicine (Urology included, obviously) and the Aristotelian-Platonic and Hippocratic-Galenic tradition, a breach that marks the dawn of modern and contemporary Western Science and Medicine.

But although this definitive breach offered an extraordinary series of positive aspects and attained undeniably valid goals, it was also characterized by some aspects that were so negative as to compromise not only a line of development suited to the requirements of today but also, and above all, one capable of responding adequately to the needs of the fledgling Third Millennium.

The History of Science in general and of Medicine in particular in the West – apart from the presumed Science and Medicine of Ancient Mesopotamia and Ancient Egypt, which, at most, were no more than generalizations of empirical data in an abstractly theoretical vein with religious, political and economic overtones, and apart from the admittedly great Hippocratic period – can be divided into two periods corresponding to two different and opposed postulates: the «qualitative» and the «quantitative».

From the beginnings to the 17th century there were only two attempts at a «quantitative» interpretation of phenomena: that of the «atomists» (Leucippus, 5th century B.C; his disciple Democritus, born in c. 470 B.C, and Epicurus, 343 – 270 B.C) and that of the Hellenistic scientists, in other words the Alexandrine physicians and anatomists mentioned earlier (particularly Herophilus, who lived in the first half of the 3rd century B.C, and his disciple Erasistratus) and by the great physicist and mathematician Archimedes (287 – 212 B.C). But both of these extremely bold attempts (it should suffice to remember Herophilus' statement, «the heart is a pump», or the discoveries made by Archimedes: the «relation of Archimedes» regarding the lever, the famous «Archimedes' principle», the «endless screw» and «specific weight», not to mention the studies on «infinitesimal calculus by exhaustion» etc.; or of the discovery of the «power of steam» on the part of Heron, who lived in the 1st century B.C) failed owing to the impossibility of demonstrating, on a rigorously «quantitative» basis, phenomena such as fermentation, digestion, fecundation, the motion of celestial bodies, or that of the blood in the veins and arteries.

These limitations determined the triumph of the «qualitative» concept, which in the doctrine and works of Galen (c. 129 – c. 199 AD) had its definitive and monumental organization into an edifice so complete and perfect that it reigned unchallenged until the 17th century.

Obviously the «qualitative» concept of phenomena is «animistic» (or «vitalistic») and as a consequence, «finalistic»: every phenomenon is «animated» by a «virtue» (or «quality») that is predisposed to realize itself completely, that is to attain its «end». Thus a stone plunges downward insofar as it is "animated" by the «virtue (or the "quality") of falling», which makes it fall downwards, «down» being seen as its own «natural place» and its own natural «end». Thus every organ of the human body possesses its own natural «virtues» that predispose it to the realization of its own «end»: the attractive, retentive, transformative and expulsive virtues by which, for example, the liver draws chyle from the intestine, retains it, transforms it into blood, and expels it by pushing it into the veins, and so on.

All these «virtues», which are specific to each organ (so, for example, the kidneys draw only the superfluous serum contained in the blood, before retaining it, transforming it into urine and discharging it into the bladder via the ureters), manage to explain everything, or, better, claim to explain everything, without explaining anything at all in reality: every new phenomenon or fact is attributable to an imaginary new «virtue» that has no correspondence and cannot be confirmed experimentally, but locates the phenomenon perfectly within the «system», in which, obviously, the virtues multiply and grow more complex until we have the creation of an authentic «algebra of the virtues» in which each of them is characterized by four «degrees» and combines with the others in accordance with a practically infinite series of possibilities.

But at the beginning of the 17th century the entire edifice collapsed under the «Galilean revolution», which replaced the «qualitative» and «finalistic» concept with the «quantitative» and, therefore, strictly «mechanical» concept of the universe and of all phenomena: a stone falls because «it can do nothing else but fall», insofar as its fall is strictly determined by the product of its mass and that of the earth, divided by the square of the distance, the whole thing multiplied by the «gravitational constant». As can be seen, the stone is not «animated» by any «virtue», it is not predisposed to any «end» and its fall is no more than a purely mechanical phenomenon determined exclusively by relationships of «quantity» (mass and distance).

This revolution was transferred and applied to the interpretation of anatomo-physiological phenomena by Giovanni Alfonso Borelli (1608 – 1679) and thereafter extended to all of Medicine and animal and vegetable Biology by the so-called «iatromechanical» or «iatrophysical» school, whose most illustrious representative was without doubt the great Marcello Malpighi (1628 – 1694).

«Iatromechanics» was joined (after initial disagreement gave way to a close alliance) by «iatrochemistry», which supported an equally «mechanical» concept of physiological phenomena: «chemical reactions» (interpreted fairly correctly until the foundation of modern chemistry by Antoine Laurent Lavoisier (1743 – 1794)) are purely mechanical phenomena, even though they take place on the level of «humours» and «fluids», like, for example, the «nervous fluid» of Malpighi and Albrecht von Haller (1708 – 1777); the very theory of «irritability» and «sensitivity» formulated by Francis Glisson (1597 – 1677) and perfected and completed by Haller was strictly and absolutely mechanistic.

However, while it is certain that this concept, on the one hand, permitted marvelous conquests in the field of anatomy and physiology and, later, in pathology, diagnostics, and therapeutics; and while, in other words, it beat the «disease», on the other hand it lost out in terms of the «patient», of the «quality of life», of people; it lost, in substance, the fundamental Hippocratic precept: «Where there is love of man, there is love of the Art», that is of Medicine. As knowledge of the mechanisms of disease became more and more detailed, more and more emphasis was laid on research into disease, but less and less consideration was given to the patient in his entirety, and above all in his human, social, cultural, spiritual and religious individuality.

For its part, TCM has never adopted the «quantitative» concept, consistently retaining the «qualitative» concept, and, as a consequence, it has never adopted the «experimental method», maintaining close ties with empiricism (vast and bountiful as it may be), and framing it in an *a priori* anatomo-physiological, prognostic, and therapeutic concept of a typically «qualitative» type, in which everything is explained by the various «virtues». Yin and Yang, the various *Qi*, etc., are «virtues» that correspond exactly – on a conceptual level as well as on the level of anatomo-physiological, prognostic, and therapeutic theory – with those of the Western Hippocratic-Galenic tradition. The concept of «disease» as the «imbalance of Yin and Yang» or of the *Qi* of this or that organ, corresponds exactly to the «humoral imbalance» of the Western tradition and the therapy that aims to restore the «balance» is the exact correspondent of the «evacuant therapy» of the Galenic tradition, inspired by two principles: «*contraria contrariis*» (for example, combating a cold with «calefacient» medicines) and «*similia similibus*» (combating a cold with ice cold baths).

But this is by no means a negative aspect; on the contrary it is the positive premise of a dialogue that is becoming steadily more fertile and constructive, in the discovery that we start off, substantially, from the same roots.

However, the most positive aspect of TCM and the most important contribution it has to make are constituted by the fact that man, the patient, and his «quality of life», have always been at the center of its attention and the primary goal of all its work. Therefore TCM has retained (even though it has never known Hippocratic doctrines) precisely that part of Hippocratism that is beyond doubt the most important and up to date; a part that, instead, we have lost and must at all costs re-conquer: the love of mankind, of the patient as an individual in all his complexity, seen as the key element underpinning the love of the Art.

There is no doubt that Western Medicine must recover the patient, if it wishes to employ suitable and efficacious instruments with which to meet the ever more pressing requirements of the «quality of life», which emerges at once as a practical, physical and spiritual problem. In the first place, in fact, we need a profoundly radical renewal of the «quality of services», bearing in mind however that «quality of services» does not necessarily correspond to an improvement in the «quality of life», something that services can at best only make a certain contribution to. In the second place «quality of service» is often confused with «efficiency of services», where, all too often, efficiency is a synonym for «non quality of life» insofar as it is realized in relation to services and not in relation to the patient. In the third place «physical well-being» cannot and must not be detached from «spiritual well-being». On the other hand «spiritual well-being» cannot come into being detached from «physical well-being», which, in its turn, does not coincide exclusively with «health» kept or recovered. In other words, Western Medicine must recover the Hippocratic vision.

Furthermore, the extraordinary patrimony of empirical data provided by TCM cannot be ignored by Western Medicine, especially in view of the extremely serious problems that are now arising, for example, from the indiscriminate abuse of antibiotics, sedatives, and stimulants, problems for which it is indispensable to find a solution, a solution that cannot ignore the fertile contribution made by alternative medicines.

On the other hand, the pharmacological assets of alternative medicines in general and of TCM in particular should be subjected to scientific investigation conducted in accordance with the experimental method, that is with the method of post-Galilean Western Medicine. This is for two fundamental reasons: in the first place because within the framework of the «globalization» that looks like becoming the distinguishing mark of the new Millennium, the notion that such assets may not become a «universal heritage», or the «heritage of all humanity» is unthinkable; in the second place, and precisely as a consequence of this, because it is unthinkable that methods for the preparation of drugs, whose frequently extraordinary efficacy is borne out by millennia of experience acquired in China, should remain at the level of mere empirical data complied with for over four thousand years: the identification of the active ingredients – realizable only through the experimental method, that is with the investigatory tools perfected by Western Science – is the only instrument that may permit Chinese pharmacology to become a fecund and beneficial asset for humanity as a whole. Hence the necessity for TCM to acquire Western methods of research and investigation not only for phytotherapy, but also and in particular for diagnostics.

Suffice it one example: consequent to the recognition of the efficacy of acupuncture, which has been adopted as a therapeutic practice in many Western hospitals, it is now necessary to investigate it and, so to speak, «explain» and «understand» it both in the light of pathological and anatomo-physiological and neuro-physiological knowledge, and on the basis of the methods of research and analysis proper to Western Science and Medicine. In other words it is indispensable first of all to «understand why» acupuncture works and to «understand why» it should be practised on the basis of what is abstractly defined and described as «meridians»; second, we need «to understand» the nature of the anatomo- and neuro-physiological mechanisms thanks to which acupuncture works. And there is no doubt that none of these can be effected if not by the experimental method.

For its part, in at least one sense Western Medicine cannot afford to fail to turn the «*humanitas*» of TCM to account regarding the indispensable and urgent need to cure the patient rather than the disease; in another sense it cannot afford to relegate thousands of years of Chinese experience to the level of mere «empirical fortuitousness»: it cannot but hold TCM in the highest consideration nor can it fail to carry out detailed and exhaustive research into the efficacy of the drugs typical of the Chinese herbal pharmacopoeia or into the efficacy of acupuncture. The first of these can be substituted for many synthetic drugs, which often involve collateral phenomena even more serious than the illness to be cured, while the second, in numerous cases, can stand in for what are often seriously invasive therapeutic methods. For Western doctors, therefore, acupuncture represents a particularly effective instrument that is, at the same time, capable of attaining that «quality of life» whose centrality is by this time a primary and fundamental component of Western medical science.

That same science, moreover, cannot and must not forget that some of the most extraordinary discoveries in the pathological and therapeutic field over the last two centuries have been the result of research into vegetable products: from *Botrytis bassiana* – which made such a fundamental contribution to the modernization and the safety of silkworm farming and, as a consequence to the silk industry itself – to penicillin (and the whole range of antibiotics that followed it), discovered by analysing the effects of *Penicillum notatum* on bacterial cultures and identifying the active ingredient applying the rigorously experimental methods of Western Science.

But a dialogue cannot even get underway without an initial possibility of mutual understanding, something that cannot, in its turn, be detached from – in the first place – a mutual understanding of the language, and therefore the creation of a kind of «*lingua franca*» that would render dialogue possible and fruitful; in the second place from a closely studied and clear critical awareness of the respective roots and respective histories; and in the third place by a reciprocal acquisition of the common elements, over and above the traditional language in which they have been expressed until now.

The Third Millennium looks set to become the Millennium of social, political, economic, and scientific globalization. Medicine in general and, in particular Urology, Andrology and Sexology cannot afford to ignore such a prospect.

The Third Millennium also looks likely to be the Millennium of «racial integration» and, as a consequence, of «cultural integration». Medicine cannot afford to shirk this and Urology, Andrology and Sexology certainly cannot afford to turn a blind eye to it.

However, «integration» does not mean «acculturation», it does not mean the deletion and elimination of cultures that are «other», absorbed by Western Culture in its presumptuous conviction that it is *the* Culture and not, more simply and more modestly, «one of the infinite number of possible Cultures».

Integration means:

1. recognition of the «other» in all his dignity;
2. understanding the «other»;
3. construction «with the other» of a new planetary culture, to which all cultures will contribute, on an equal footing.

These are the objectives that the new Culture and the new Science must strive for.

And it is right that we begin with a dialogue-confrontation between West and East, between the Mediterranean tradition and the Chinese tradition, which are (also owing to the intense exchanges that have taken place over the millennia between Chinese and Indian culture, whose roots are sunk in the same ground as Indo-European Mediterranean culture) the cradles of the world's greatest civilizations, of which all of today's civilized world is the descendant.

But such a dialogue cannot get underway if not on the basis of reciprocal knowledge and a reciprocal and clear understanding of the cultural and scientific history of the two worlds, in order to emphasize the convergences – as a solid and essential point of departure – but above all the divergences, the motivation for which and the critical comparison of which beyond any doubt constitute the most fertile element of the dialogue.

This book is intended to create the historical and critical basis for the whole-hearted promotion of this relationship – presently in the process of being established – which we can neither do without, slow down, nor postpone.

Paolo Marandola
Professor of Urology
University of Pavia

Sergio Musitelli
Consulting Professor of History of Urology
University of Pavia

FOREWORD

The columns of Chapter One and Chapter Seven represent Chinese History, Knowledge and Tradition (left) and Western History, Knowledge and Scientific Tradition (right). The white tracts of each column mean that either Chinese or Western History, Culture, Knowledge and Scientific Tradition are missing.

This has been done in order to facilitate the reader in realising immediately the differences and the parallels between Chinese and Western History and scientific contributions.

Chapter One

The Brief Comparative History of TCM and WM

Table of Successive Dynasties Of Chinese Countries (see Figure 1)	**Table of Successive Western Civilisations**
[nian dai]年代Years [chao dai] 朝代 Dynasties **2205-1766 B.C. [xia]夏Xia** **1766-1122 B.C. [shang]商Shang** **1066-221B.C. [zhou] 周Zhou** **221-206 B.C. [qin] 秦Qin** **206B.C.-23 AD [xi han] 西汉 Western Han** **25- 220 AD [dong han] 东汉 Eastern Han** **20-265 AD [wei] 魏Wei** **265-420 AD [jin] 晋Jin** **420-589 AD [nan chao] 南朝 Southern Dynasties** **386-581 AD [bai chao] 北朝 Northern Dynasties** **581-681 AD [sui] 隋Sui** **618-907 AD [tang] 唐Tang** **907-960 AD [wu dai] 五代 Five Dynasties** **960-1279 AD [song] 宋Song** **1279-1368 AD [yuan] 元Yuan** **1368-1644 AD [ming] 明Ming**	**5000-538 B.C. Assyro-Babylonian Civilisation** **538-351 B.C. Persian Empire** **3000-31 B.C. Egyptian Civilisation** **3000-2100B.C. Ancient Egyptian Reign** **2100-1580 B.C. Middle Reign** **1580-1550 B.C. Hyxos Invasion** **1550-525 B.C. New Reign** **525-323B.C. Persian domination** **323-31 B.C. Greek domination (Ptolemaic Dynasty) HELLENISTIC CIVILISATION AND CULTURE (Main centers Alexandria and Pergamum)** **3000-1400 B.C. Minoan civilisation** **1400-900 B.C. Mycenaean civilisation** **900-146 B.C. Greek civilisation** **753 B.C. Foundation of Rome** **753-509 B.C. The Seven Kings** (Romulus, Numa Pompilius, Ancus Martius, Tullus Hostilius, Tarquinius Priscus, Servius Tullius, Tarquinius, the Proud) **509-31 B.C. Roman Republic**

1644-1911 AD [qing] 清Qing	**31- B.C.- 395 Roman Empire**
Based on many important, historical events and discoveries , Chinese medical practice can be divided into four great periods: **The Ancient or Legendary Period (2697-1122B.C.)** **The Historical or Golden Period** **(1121B.C.-960 AD)** **The Mediaeval or Controversial Period** **(961-1800 AD)** **The Modern or Transitional Period (1801-1936 AD)** (see Figures 2 – 8).	**GRECO-ROMAN CIVILISATION AND CULTURE** **(Main centers Rome, Alexandria, Rhodes, Athens)** **395 The Emperor Theodosius divides the Empire between his two sons: Arcadius** becomes Emperor of the **Eastern Roman Empire; Honorius** of the **Western Roman Empire.** **395-476 Western Roman Empire** **ROMAN LATIN CIVILISATION AND CULTURE** **476-800 Romano-barbarian Reigns** (Visigothic, Gothic, Ostrogothic, Vandal, Longobard, Frank, etc.) **711-1492 Arabian Empire** **Arabian domination on Spain and spread of Arabian culture through Europe (Main centers Baghdad, Cairo, Alexandria, Corduba, Seville and Granada)** **800-843 Charles the Great and Holy Roman Empire** 843-1492 **Birth of the Great European Nations** (France, England, Germany, Spain, etc.) **395-1453 Eastern Roman Empire**

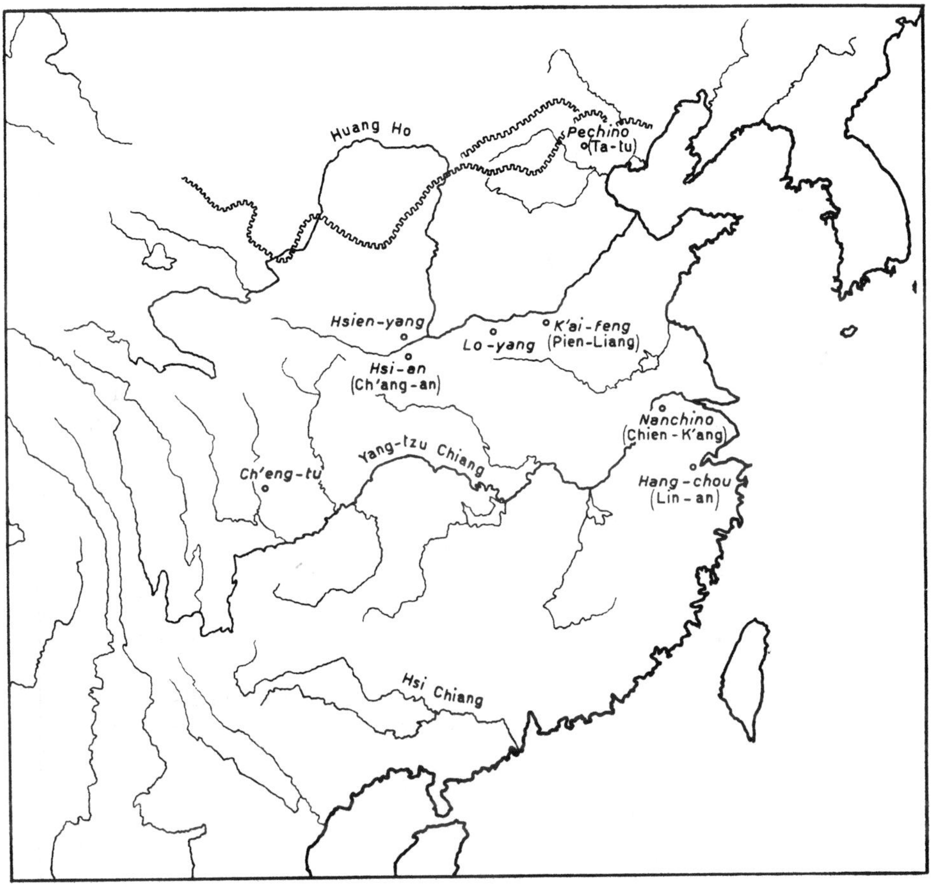

Figure 1: The historic capitals of China

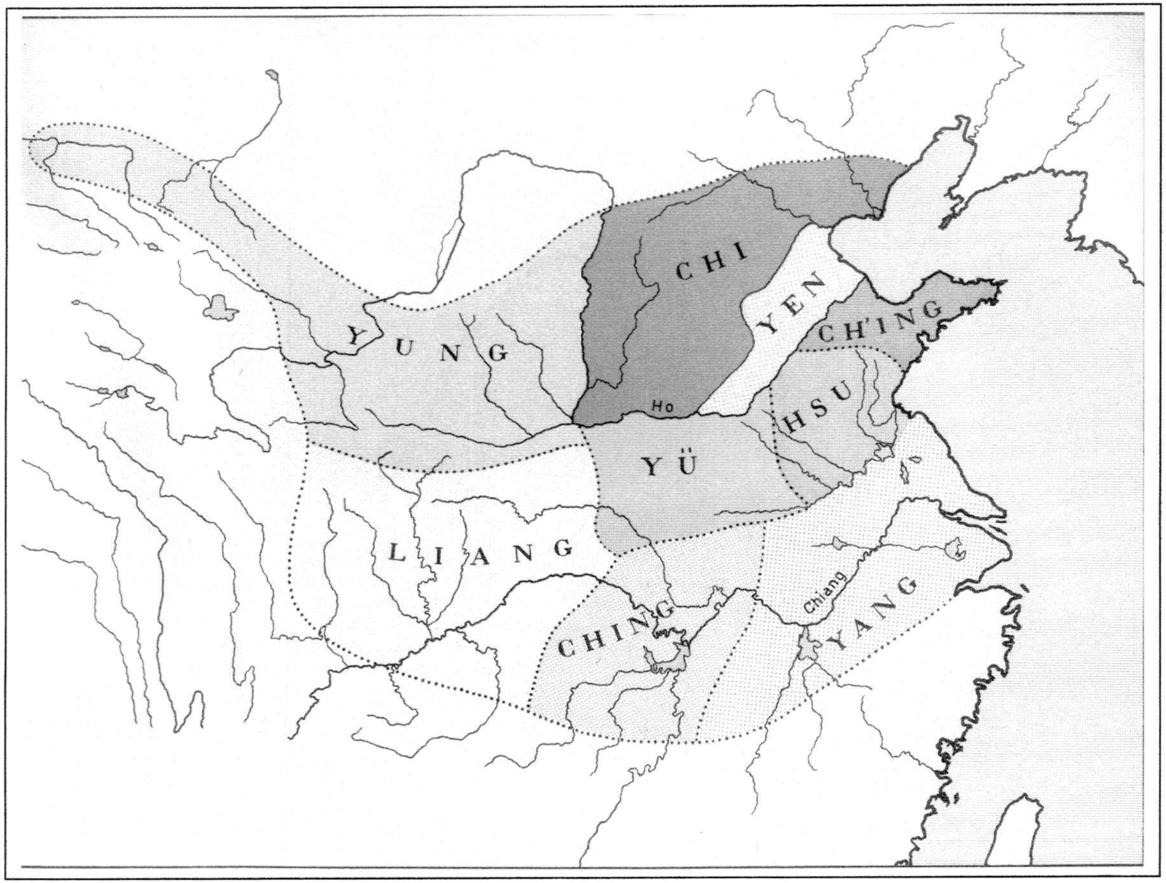

Figure 2: The nine Provinces (chu) of ancient China according to legendary tradition

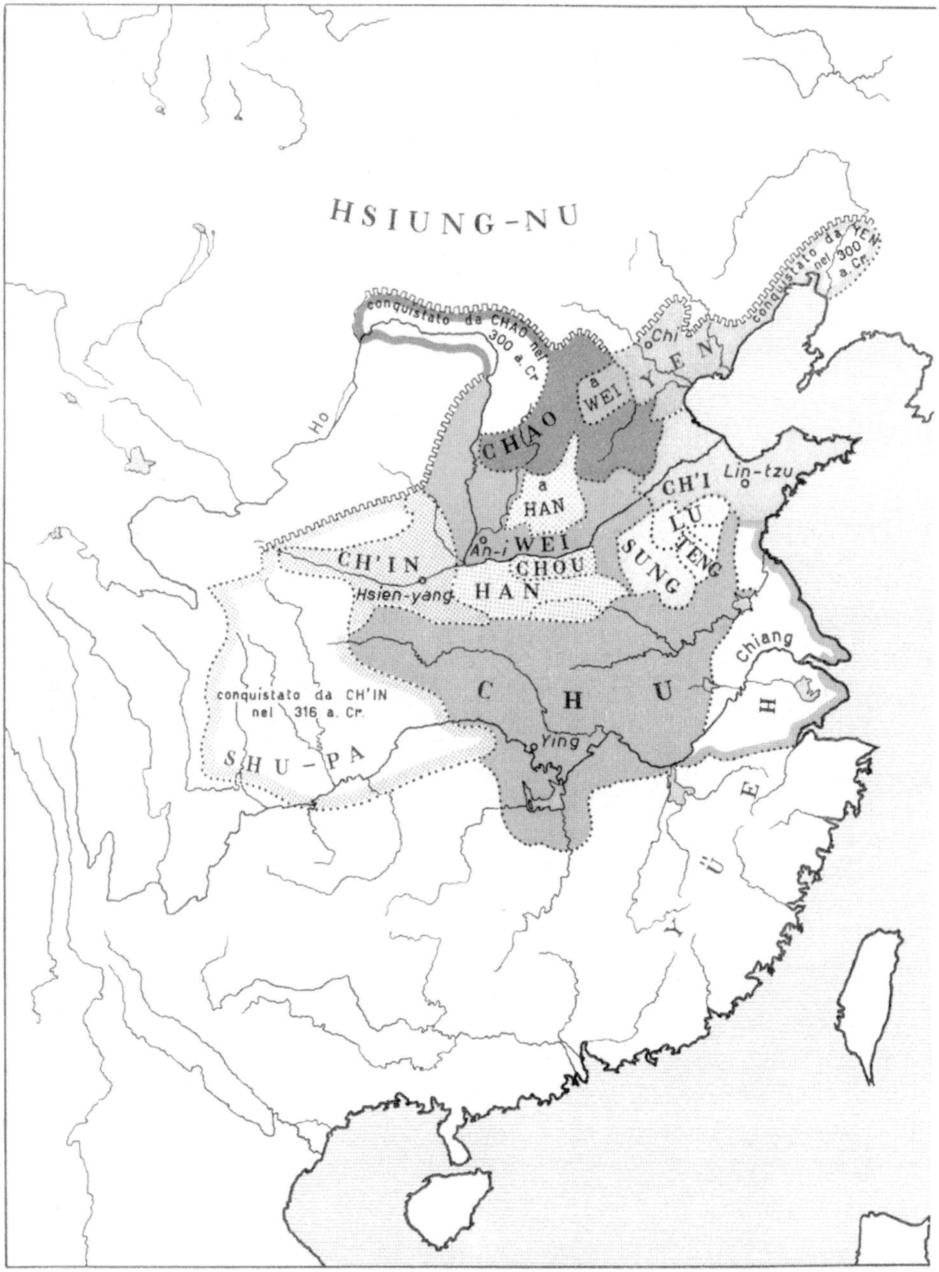

Figure 3: China in the 5th century B.C.: the so-called "Fighting States".

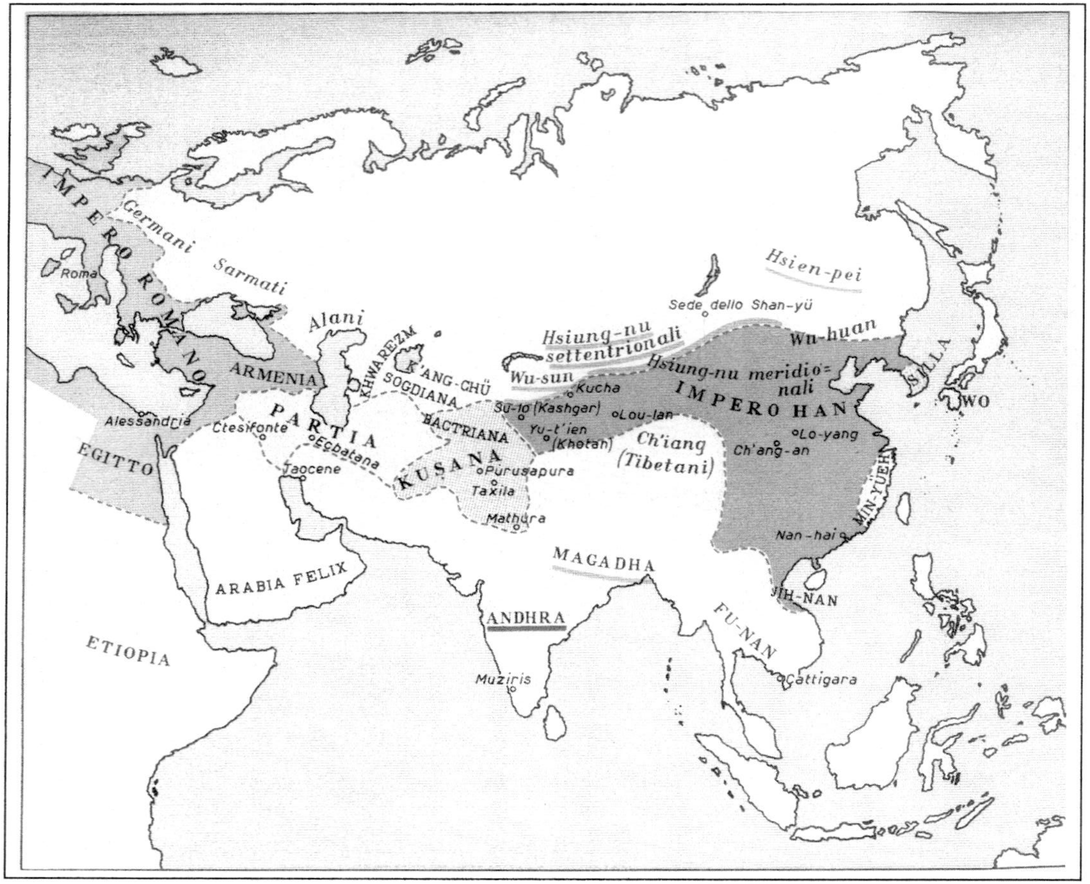

Figure 4: The Han Empire during the 1st century A.D.

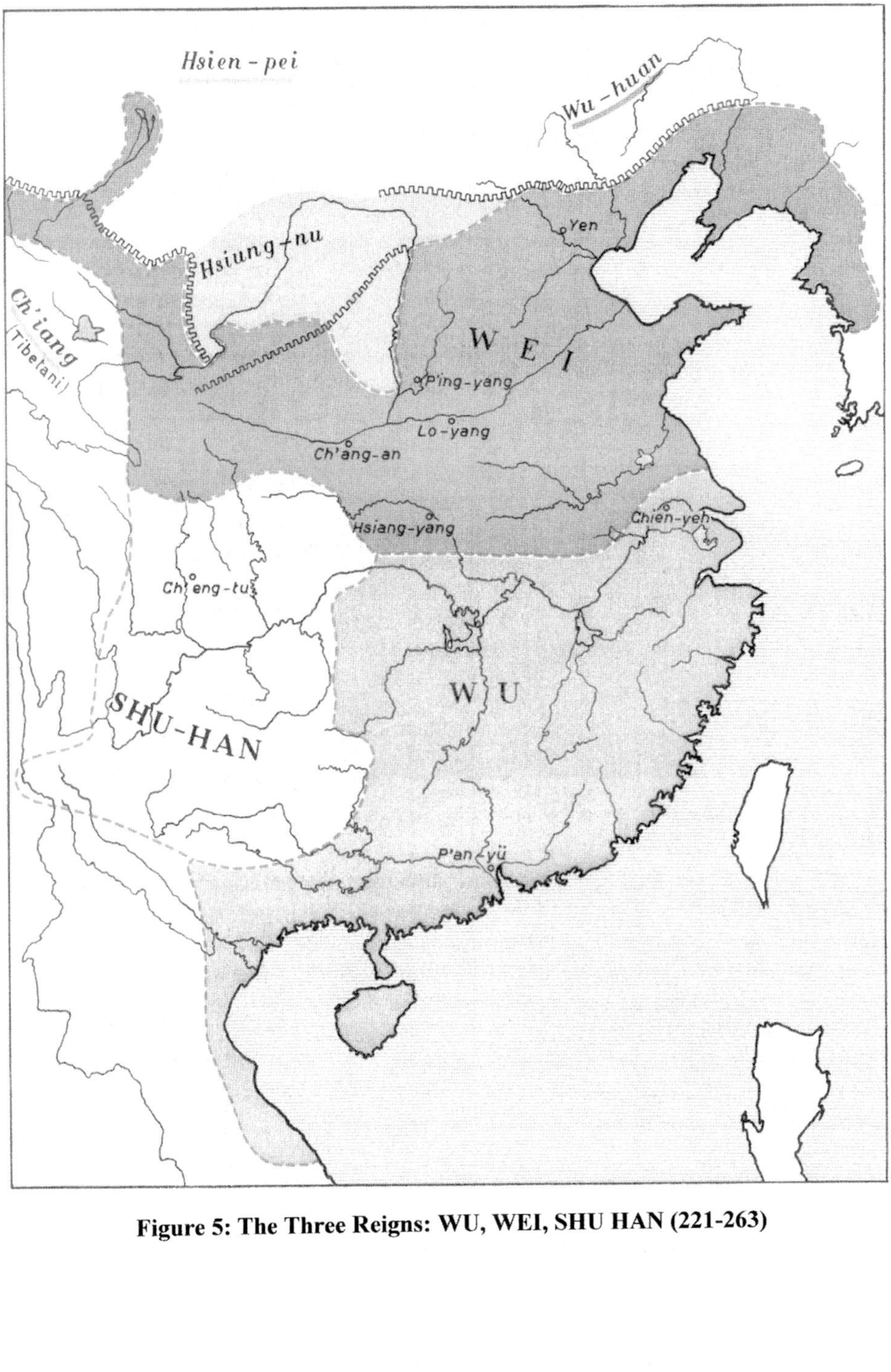

Figure 5: The Three Reigns: WU, WEI, SHU HAN (221-263)

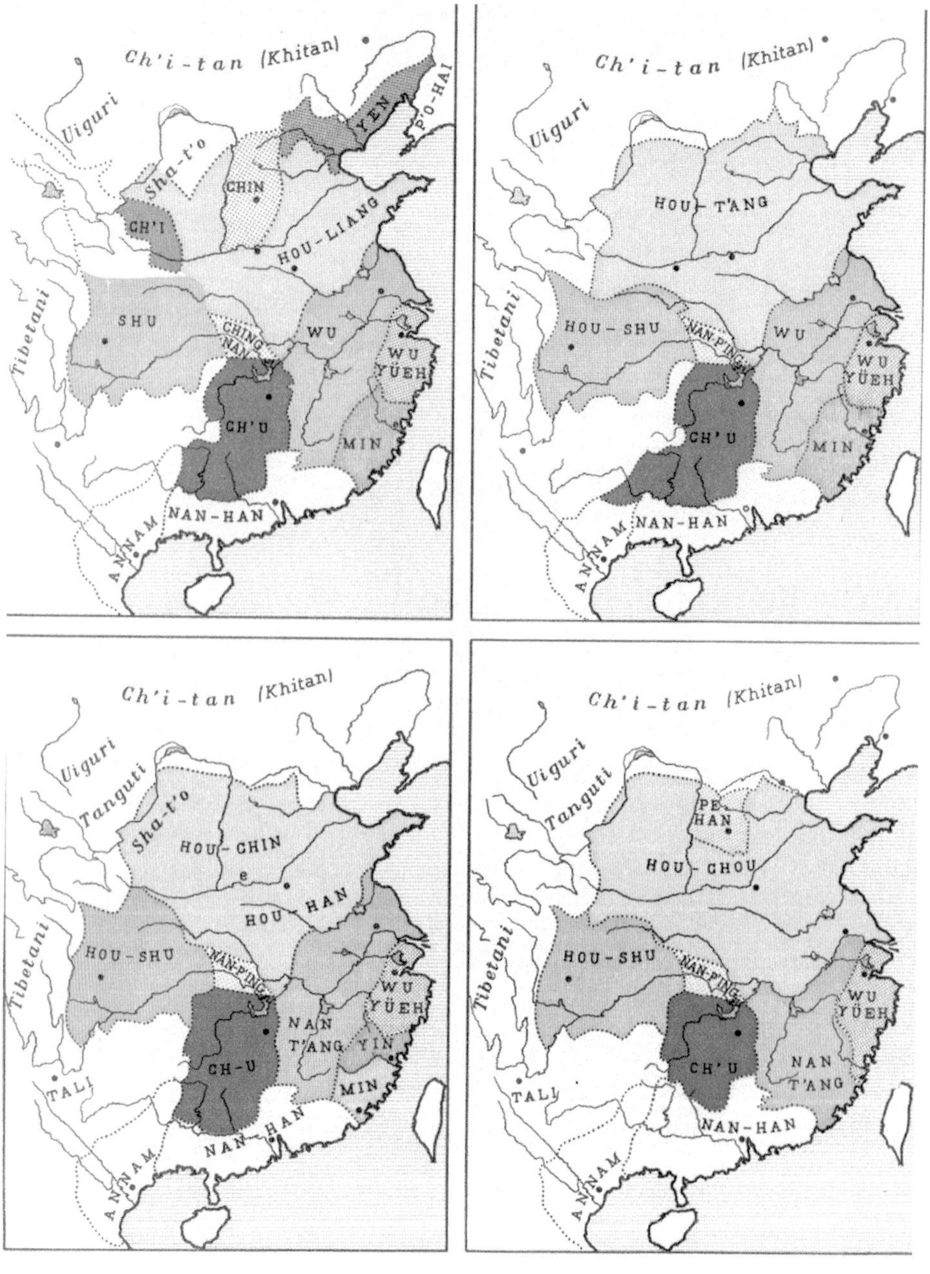

Figure 6: **Above (left): the later Liang dinasty (907-923)**
Above (right): the later T'ang dinasty (923-936)
Below (left): the later Chin dinasty (936-946) and the later Han dinasty (947-951)
Below (right): the later Chou dinasty (951-960)

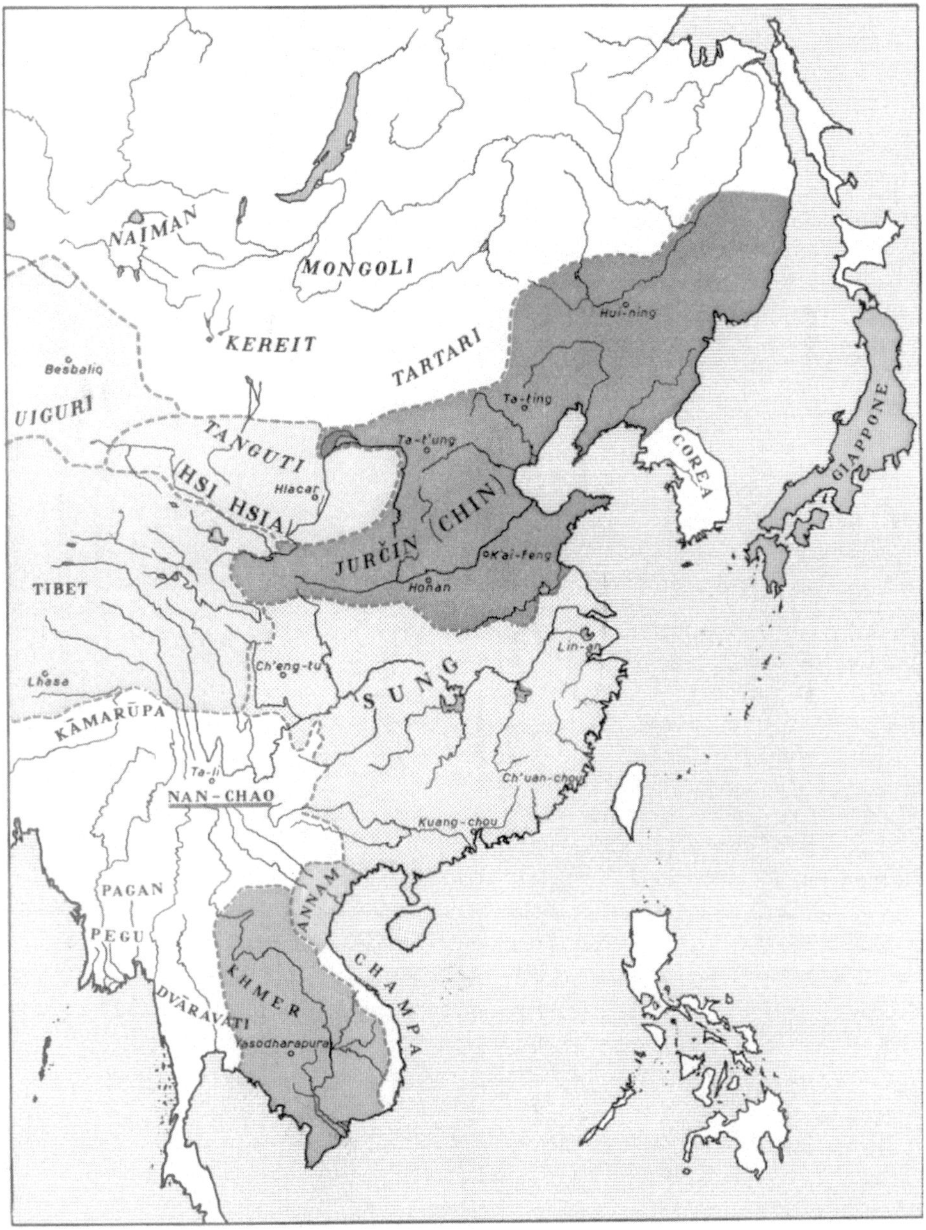

Figure 7: China around 1150 A.C.

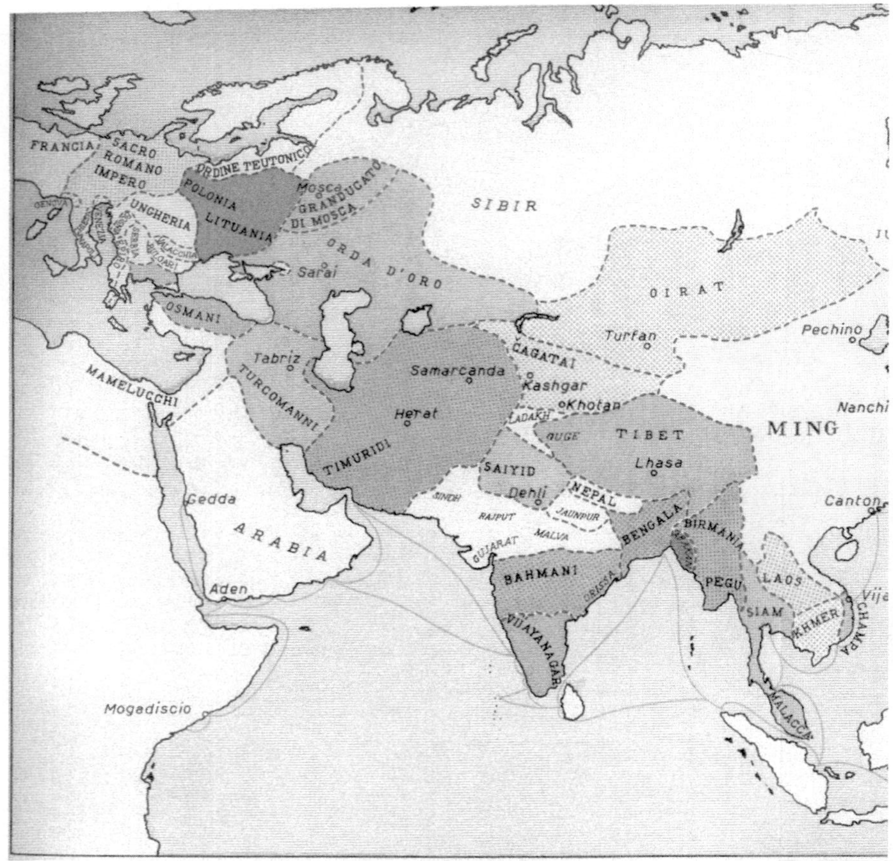

Figure 8: The Ming Empire (the line indicates the voyages of the Chinese Fleets during the 15th century)

BYZANTINE CIVIZATION AND CULTURE

1492 **Birth of the great European Nations: Spain, France, Germany, England, etc.**

End of Arabian domination on Spain

Discovery of America by Christopher Columbus

END OF THE Middle-AGES

1400-1500 HUMANISM

1500-1600 RENAISSANCE

PRE-HISTORICAL PERIOD

With its long and glorious history, China is one of the largest and greatest nations in the world. The real origin of the Chinese race remains an unsolved problem. When the natives in Europe and America were fighting against nature in half-naked condition, the Chinese were enjoying the higher stage of culture in silk dresses. Before Moses led the Israelites through the dark wilderness, there existed laws, literature, which were superior to those of Egypt. While Homer was travelling and singing the story of Iliad, China's minstrels were celebrating her ancient heroes, whose tombs had already been with them for nearly thirteen centuries. It is the Chinese who

PRE-GREEK MEDICINE

Though many scholars have emphasised and still emphasise Assyro-Babylonian and Egyptian medicine, surely physicians existed, or better existed a lot of people who gave themselves out to be physicians as well as surgeons, but they were simply empirical and practical men who mixed a sum of traditional and empirical, and chiefly magic pseudo-knowledge with a lot of superstitions and religious ideas, so that they were nothing but primitive wizards and sorcerers wearing the pretentious mask of scientific knowledge. Even the so much praised Assyro-Babylonian tablets dealing with Medicine and Surgery or the not less prised Egyptian

invented the firearms long before Schwartz, and the art of printing five hundred years before Caxton was born. The Chinese first discovered gunpowder, the mariner's compass and the making of porcelain. And the Great wall completed two hundred and twenty years before Christ is one of the great engineering feats of the world. The real origin of the Chinese race remains an unsolved problem. As far as reliable record shows, the Valley of the Yellow River was the cradle of the Chinese nation.

Like the primitive folks of the other races, prehistoric Chinese lived in caves, ate wild fruits, seeds, and roots, they drank the blood of the animals, covered their bodies with the skin of animals. They had to fight against the wild beasts and sometimes got hurt and wounded. Their food was coarse and uncooked, and their bodies exposed to all kinds of weather. What they suffered could provoke stomach trouble, vomiting, diarrhea, headache and even death. The most universal symptom of the diseases is pain. So to seek and to apply remedies is the most primitive of the primitive instincts. In order to liberate man himself from the pain, he began to use saliva, peat, plant-stalks, tree-bark, leaves and moss to dress a wound. Chance and empiricism led him to try various herbs and food as remedies, after innumerable and repeated experiments, primitive people gradually began to learn the property of the plants and began to learn to use them specially to deal with certain diseases. The Classics **[shu jing] 书经 "Books of History", [shi jing]诗经 "Book of Odes", [zhou li] 周礼 "Rituals of the Zhou Dynasty", [shan hai jing]山海经 "Mountains and Seas Classic",** contain man names of plants

medical texts - like Ebers' and Edwin-Smith papyrus - reveal a lot of abstract and pseudo-scientific theories about anatomo-physiology, moreover always interwoven with superstitions, prayers, magic and apotropaic formulas, spells and exorcisms that have nothing to do with science in general and medicine in particular. No doubt they knew some internal organs of man and many other animals, like brain, lungs, stomach, heart, liver, kidneys, urinary bladder, uterus and bowels, blood vessels (but didn't make any difference between veins and arteries); they knew blood and urine; they knew that a man like many other animals cannot live without breathing and eating and without having his blood; they knew that a man like every other animal is died when his heart has stopped beating; they knew that men like every other animal may be affected by many diseases, and they surely knew the pains caused by diseases, also by urological ones, like urine retention or kidney pains or stones in the bladder (which the Egyptians surely could observe on the occasion of embalming cadavers), but all this has nothing to do with science in general and medicine in particular. The famous Greek historian Herodotus (484 - 428 B. C.) tells us (cf. *Histories*, book II, ch. 84) that "*Egypt is full of physicians" and that "each physician is for one only and not for several diseases, that is some are physicians of the eyes, others of the head, others of the teeth, others of the belly and others of invisible diseases*", but it would be a very great historical mistake to take this statement for "*medical specialisation*" in the modern sense of the word. It is surely a "*specialisation*" but it is the same "*specialisation*" of the primitive wizards, one of whom has the

and animals used as medicine. E.g. More than eighty substances are enumerated, including various of fishes, fowl, flesh of animals, herbs, vegetables, barks, etc. "Stone used as needles", archaeological activity has brought to light a number of strangely-pointed stones (called [bian] 砭 in Chinese) as stone slivers for medical usage; they were used to make skin incision. It is virtually certain that the acupuncture originated with the use of these stone, and then the bone and bamboo, needles, which people later learnt to employ for therapeutic purpose.

The legendary period may be understood between the dawn of civilization and the end of **[shang] 商 "Shang" Dynasty** (1766-1122 B.C.). It is said that during this period, shamans were often asked to consult the ancestors on an imminent birth, what arouse a headache might take, or even the meaning of the dreams (maybe 3,000 years before Freud). But the most important factor in prehistoric healing is the belief in the supernatural: Human knowledge at this period was extremely limited for primitive man, knowing nothing whatever of physical laws, cause or effect, he was frightened by the flash of lighting, the eruption of an earthquake, the crash of thunder. The sun, moon, star, clouds, storm and fire were to him the outward manifestations of gods, demons, devils, spirits or other supernatural agencies. Consequently health and disease were thought to be controlled by them and diseases, particular, were regarded as the work of devils or were devils in temporary possession of the human body, which could be cured by the application of appropriate incantation, charms, and other superstitious practices. Divination by fire, human sacrifice and

"*specialisation*" of being the "*wind wizard*", another the "*rain wizard*" and so on, and has nothing to do with our present "*specialisation*", which is the result of accumulated scientific knowledge and of a highly complex technology. So we can conclude by saying that before the Greek civilisation of the VI century B. C. there has been a lot of men, and chiefly priests, that were called "*physicians*", but there has not been any "*medicine*", as well as since the IV millennium B. C. there has been a lot of priests that made astronomical observations, but there has not been any "*astronomy*": they were nothing but "*priests-astrologers*" who made simply "*astrology*" and to call them "*astronomers*" and their pseudo-science "*astronomy*" is to make the absurd mistake of projecting modern experiences into the past.

ritual worship of deceased kings were the most striking manifestations of these religious practices. The celebrated "oracle-bone inscription" (written on turtle-shells and shoulder-balders of cattle and other animals) have revealed numerous aspects .They refer to a number of activities, from a military campaign to a certain illness. Instead of using the crude herb-therapy, the beginning of superstitious primitive healing art became an affair of charms, spells, incantations and offerings. In fact the history of Chinese popular religion is accompanied with monks or Taoist priests who sold written talismans, charms and spells to the ordinary people. Even before the shaping of the medical principles more than 2000 years ago, the Chinese often appealed to faith-healing sorcerer. So witch doctor, faith and nature healers appeared and the medical practice was carried out by shaman-healers, because **[yi] 医 "Medicine"** contained the character **[wu] 巫 "Shaman"**. They combined drugs and incantations Ro cure diseases such as scabies and malaria, two afflictions that were current at the time. "It was incumbent upon the faith-healer to forge the link between man and powerful occult forces".

During the **[chun qiu] 春秋 "Spring and Autumn"** period (770-470), the Chinese medical world underwent fundamental change. The theories of the **[yin yang]** 阴阳 " Yin and Yang" and of the **[wu xing]** 五行 "Five Elements" made their appearance, providing the basis for newly-developing medicine and an answer to the question proposed by **[huang di] 黄帝 "the Yellow Emperor".** The Yellow Emperor asked his physician **[qi bo] 歧伯 Qi Bo**:" I have heard that in ancient times people lived 100 years, yet today they only live fifty years. Why?". **Qi Bo** replied that men in ancient times attached great importance to Yin and Yang, ensuring that the spirit (Yang) and the body (Yin) were in perfect harmony. Man could not escape, he had to continue, the universal law of Yin and Yang, and his health depended on the equilibrium of these two opposing forces. An excess of one or a deficiency of the other could bring about illness.

CHINESE-MEDICINE

(see Figures 9 – 10)

Long before the earliest records appeared, and long before the initial structure of Chinese civilization took shape, herbal medicine claimed a prominent place in the primitive cycle of Chinese tribal life. The birth of Traditional Chinese of Medicine can be supposed to be roughly established at around 3500 B.C.. The history of Yin and Yang seems to have 3000 years. But the confidence in the Chinese orthodox doctor is still kept alive due to the fact that Chinese medicine is known to have brought about enough successful cures. Dr.T.Nakayaman writes: "Is it possible to consider ancient Chinese medicine as a real science? This is a troublesome question. To the moderns, indeed, there seems nothing scientific about it. On the contrary, it is covered with a prehistoric mystic patina, and sometimes appears to be scarcely comprehensible. Nevertheless, when one is aware of its therapeutic efficacy, one can not deny its value".

The early phallicism of the ancient

GREEK/WESTERN MEDICINE

First period (from the origins up to the VI century B. C.)

During this period every disease was thought to be caused by Gods, and therefore Medicine was practiced by priests - like in all the other ancient civilisations - and was always strictly connected with Religion, religious and superstitious believes and practices with which also more or less efficacious slops were joined, that the priests told to be suggested by Asclepius (the God of Medicine) himself, chiefly by sending to the sleeping patient particular dreams, that the priest had to interpret in order to prepare the correct medicine for him. It is particularly significant that the two great physicians who - according to Homer (IX - VIII century B. C.) take part to the Troy War (perhaps in the XII century B. C.) to cure the Achean Heroes were Podalirius and Machaon, sons of the God Asclepius. And just into the *Asclepièia*, that is Asclepius' temples, medicine was practiced. At any rate, the Homeric poems - *Iliad* and *Odyssey* - and the objects and ex voto found on the occasion of archaeological excavations show

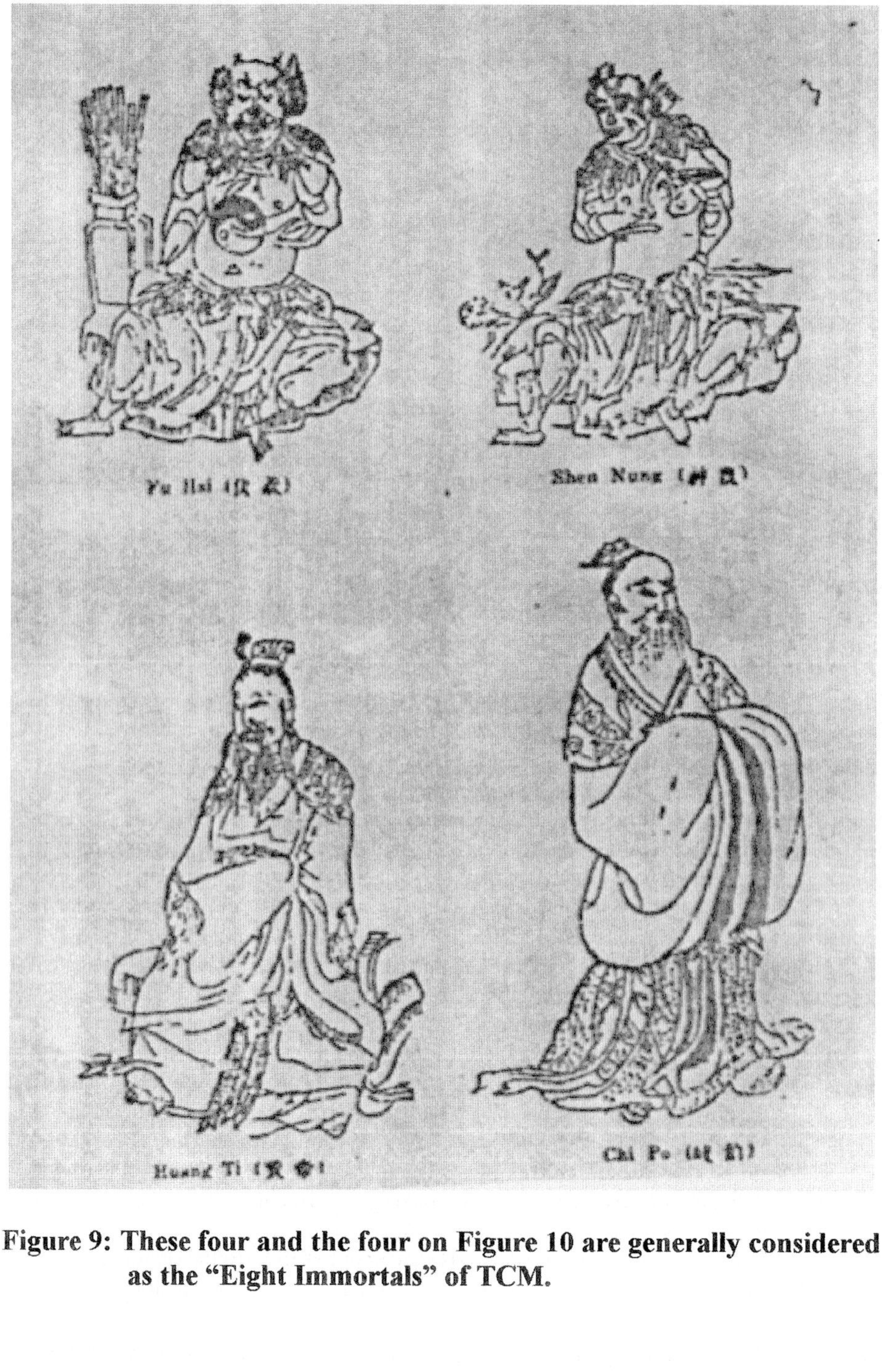

Figure 9: These four and the four on Figure 10 are generally considered as the "Eight Immortals" of TCM.

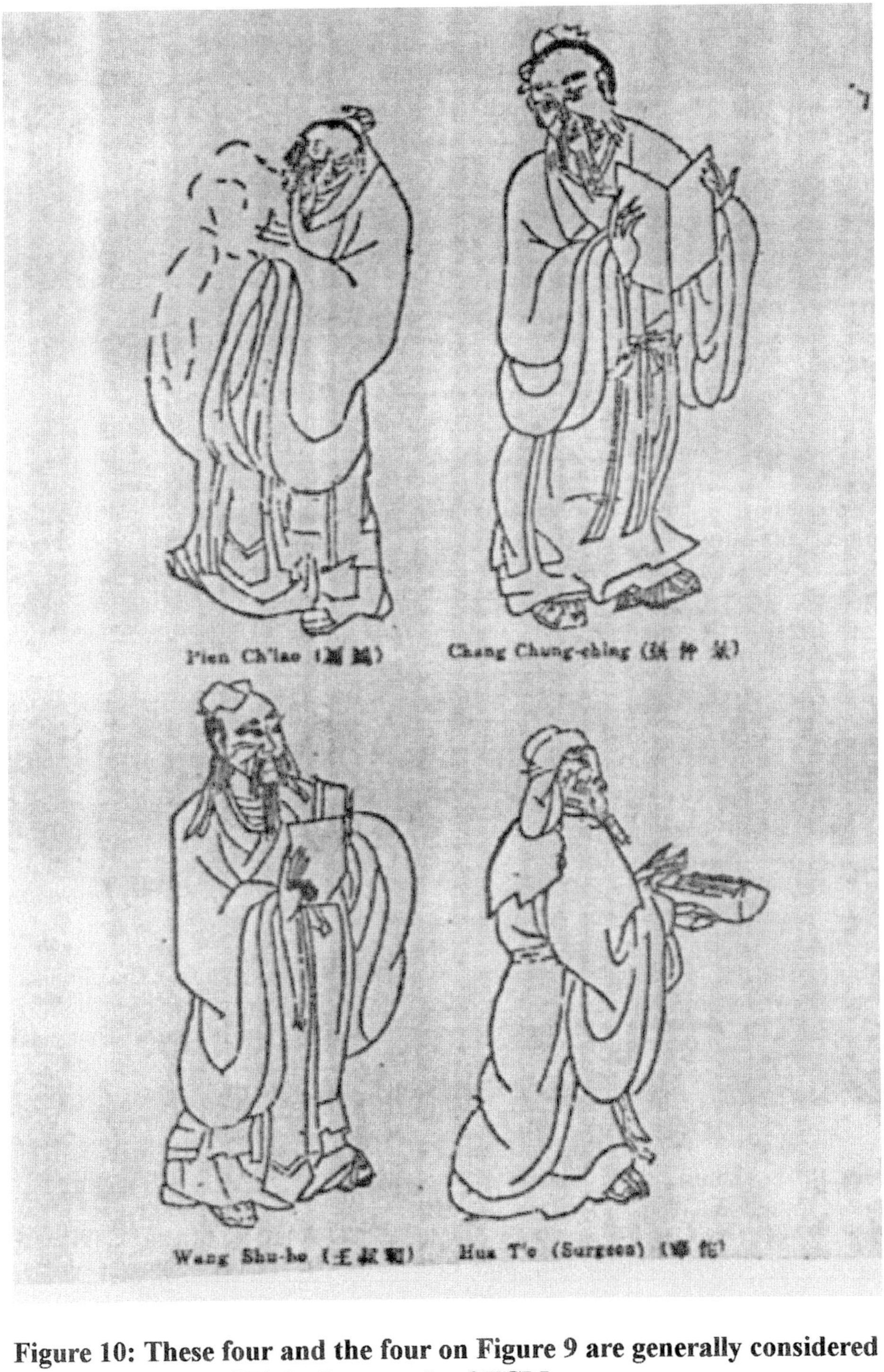

Figure 10: These four and the four on Figure 9 are generally considered as the "Eight Immortals of TCM.

time tells us the primitive people began to understand the natural phenomena through the struggle against Nature. Thousands of inscribed carapaces and bones have been unearthed in archaeological excavations, from which we know that the ancient people used simple designs and symbols to describe the world. The references to herbal medicine were appearing on oracle bones-inscriptions that are able to give us some insight into the sicknesses and diseases of that time. E.g. Massage has evolved from the instinctive action of rubbing, stroking and kneading to sooth an injured or stiff limb. The beginning of surgery dates from the moment when instruments of daily use were employed as means of healing. With such articles as thorns, fishbones, shells, flints, etc. an abscess could be opened and also blood let out. So that massage has evolved from the instinctive action of rubbing, stroking and kneading to sooth an injured and stiff limb. The commencement of surgery dates as far back as the Stone Age. With thorns, fish bones, shells, flints, etc., an abscess could be opened and also blood let out. Moxa, cupping, cautery and puncture were also practiced. "Needling" occupied a rather important position in ancient times. It developed into the art of acupuncture, which forms one of the characteristic branches of Chinese medicine.

Three of the legendary characters are regarded as the founders of the Chinese medicine. They are **[fu xi] 伏羲 Fuxi, [shen nong] 神农 Shenlong, [huang di] 黄帝 Huangdi。**

In fact. the history of Chinese begins with a myth **[huang di] 黄帝**

clearly that the ancient priest-physicians did know nothing more than all the other Assyro-Babylonian and Egyptian priest-physicians did, that is they knew a certain number of bones, the main organs (brain, heart, lungs, stomach, liver, bowels, kidneys, urinary bladder and uterus), blood vessels (but didn't make any distinction between arteries and veins); blood and urine; some very common diseases and chiefly urological ones, like strangury, dysuria, anuria and bladder stones and a lot of wounds (chiefly war wounds), among which they distinguished the mortal from the non mortal ones. It is interesting to emphasise that a wound of the urinary bladder was maintained to be mortal since that times, an idea that lived on until at least the XVII century A. D.

We must conclude that also during this period of Greek civilisation *physicians* did surely exist, but *medicine* in the sense of "*scientific medicine*" didn't at all.

Second period (from the VI century B. C.)

Philosophical and Scientific thought came into being in the VI century B. C. chiefly in Miletus (on the Middle East Aegean seaboard) and in the so-called *Magna Graecia* (South Italy) and the phenomena of the universe and of life and living animals, man included, began to be interpreted under an astronomical (that is geometrical) and anatomo-physiological point of view. But a fundamental previous statement is necessary: **ALL ANCIENT SCIENCE IS BASED ON A "QUALITATIVE" AND NOT "QUANTITATIVE" INTERPRETATION OF THE PHENOMENA**. That is to say, e. g., that

"Yellow Emperor". The legend has it that he taught men how to cultivate the five grains (i.e. millet, rye, sesame and two kinds of wheat), which has earned him the title of **[shen nong] 神农 "Divine Farmer"**. He possessed a magic whisk which was used to discover whether a plant was poisonous or not and to determine the nature of such plant. He would even taste a plant himself to examine its effects, because his transparent body allowed him to neutralise any poisonous matter. His medical practice was shown in the book **[huang di nei jing]黄帝内经 "Yellow Emperor's Classic of Internal Medicine**", which is to be discussed later.

Fu Xi [fu xi] 伏羲 also known as **[pao xi] 庖羲** lived in (2953B.C.) also-called **Fu Xishi [fu xi shi] 伏羲氏** with the dynastic appellation of **[tai gao] 太杲** Tai Gao, a legendary primitive clan society in the history of China. It is said that he has been miraculously conceived and was born after 12 years' gestation. He invented picture symbols, established rules of marriage, taught fishing and rearing of domestic animals, cooking of food, making of music instruments, etc. The legends say that he made nine kinds of needles. That was the time when the therapies of acupuncture and moxibustion were first invented. But his connection with medical history chiefly rests on his construction of **[ba gua] 八卦 "Eight Diagrams"** on which were bases the [**yi jing] 易经 "Book of Changes"**. The Ba Gua "Eight Diagrams" has been used for at least two thousand years to interpret the process of nature and is the fundamental feature in the theories which underlie philosophy, astrology, divination a stone falls not at all because of the connection between masses and distances (that are "*quantities*"), but because of the "***precipitative virtue***" which animates it and makes it to trend towards its "*natural place*", that is "*the low*", which is the its "*natural place*". So it is clear that a "quantitative" interpretation is always also an "*animist*" and therefore "*finalistic*" one. We cannot deal with mathematics, physics, cosmogony, astronomy, cosmology, zoology and botany (that all came into being as "*sciences*" in the VI century B. C.) and must confine ourselves to medicine.

Health, disease and medicine.

All the animal, vegetal, and mineral phenomena, man included, are the result of the composition of four elements: *Air*, *Water*, *Earth* and *Fire*. But this composition could not give origin to anything without the presence of a "*fifth element*" that is of heavenly origin, the famous "*quinta essentia*" (fifth essence), which is, so to say, the catalyst of the four elements, and makes it possible for each phenomenon to be born, to grow, to develop, in one word to live. When the "*fifth essence*" abandons the phenomenon, the composition of the four elements disintegrates and each element goes back to its like: Air to Air, Water to Water, etc. But one must take present that the "*fifth essence*" - as has been said - is of heavenly origin, otherwise we could not understand the joining between medicine, astrology and alchemy (that is just the research of obtaining the "*fifth essence*" by the chemical treatment of the various substances) that lasted until the XVII century. Man too, obviously, is a compound of the "*four elements*" with his

and medicine. It is also spoken of as the parent of mathematics and of written characters.

Shen Long 神农 [shen nong] (3494 B.C.) a legendary Emperor, (2838-2698 B.C.). **[san huang ben ji] 三皇本纪 "Records of the Three Emperor"** says he was the son of a princess named **[an deng] 安登** who conceived through the influence of heavenly dragon and born her child. he reigned by the influence of the agent fire, and is consequently entitled **[yan di] 炎帝 "Fire Emperor"**. He fashioned timber into ploughs and introduced agriculture to his people and to have become fascinated and intrigued by the apparent medicinal properties of various plants. According to the ancient book wrote by **[liu an] 刘安 Liu An** of the **[han] 汉 "Han Dynasty**", "Shen Long tested a hundred of herbs and came across seventy poisonous herbs each day", so the art of herbs was born .

He is usually ascribed the writing of the **[ben cao] 本草 "The Herbal"**, which is supposed to be the earliest treatise on medicine. Of the 365 drugs listed, about 240 belong to the vegetable kingdom. They are classified under three main groups, 120 being listed as "superior", 120 as "medium" and 125 as "inferior", the total corresponding to the number of days in a year.

The superior drugs are supposed to be non-poisonous, possessing rejuvenating properties and can be taken for long periods without harm. The medium drugs are said to have tonic effects, their tonicity depending on the dosage. The inferior drugs are only employed for curing diseases, being considered poisonous and should not be taken for any length of time. He is "*fifth essence*" (the soul), but he is characterised by the presence of "*four humours*": *blood*, *phlegm*, *yellow bile* and *black bile* (or *melancholy*). Moreover both elements and humours are characterised by the "*four qualities*", hot, cold, moist and dry, variously combined each other: blood is hot and moist; yellow bile is hot and dry; black bile is cold and dry; phlegm is cold and moist. Obviously these "*four qualities*" characterise also the "*four elements*": Air is hot and moist; Fire is hot and dry; Earth is cold and dry; Water is cold and moist. But the "four qualities" characterise also the four seasons: Spring is hot and moist; Summer is hot and dry; Autumn is cold and dry; Winter is cold and moist. Moreover, the life of men too is characterised by the "*four qualities*": infancy is hot and moist; youth is hot and dry; maturity is cold and dry; old age is cold and moist. So we have these four correspondences:

1 - blood - air - spring - infancy
2 - yellow bile - fire - summer - youth
3 - black bile - earth - autumn - maturity
4 - phlegm - water - winter - old age.

Man is a "*microcosm*" into the "*macrocosm*" (which we can call "*environment*", stars, planets and heavens included), each characteristic of the second has repercussion on the former, on the balance of his humours, that are generally well balanced (health), but may be unbalanced by a change of the balance of the qualities of the "macrocosm": e. g. in Winter cold and moist prevail and cause an increasing of phlegm and therefore an imbalance of the humours. This imbalance is the cause of a "*phlegmatic disease*" like cold, cough,

venerated as the "Father of medicine".

Besides **[ren shen] 人参 "Ginseng"** (Panax Ginseng), numerous other medical plants mentioned in Shen Long's book are still used today. The properties of each drug are described. Ginseng, for example, is said to invigorate the **[wu zang]五脏 " Five Organs"** and calm the mind, as well as for prolong life". And the place where each medicinal plant grows is also given. The preparation of such medicinal plants is also concisely described.

[huang di] 黄帝 "The Yellow Emperor" (2695-2598B.C.) is another important figure in Chinese healing art. With the aid of the sage physician **[qi bo] 歧伯 Qi Bo**, one of his ministers, he is said to have written the famous classic **[nei jing] 内经 "Internal Classic"**. Hence the medical profession is sometimes spoken of as the art of **[qi huang] 岐黄 "Qi and Hunag"**. But the historical researches proved that this work was not composed by him but was a later production most probably written about the end of **[zhou] 周 "Zhou Dynasty"**.

The fables had it that he visited most of the immortals and obtained knowledge of medicine from them. He got the formula of the "nine gourd powder" from the True Middle Emperor, and "nineteen gold and silver prescriptions" from the spirit of **[huang kai] 黄楷 Huangkai** and composed the chapters on diagnosis and the pulse from other goddesses. It is said that he invented the nine needle for acupuncture and wrote a treatise of 18 volumes on medicine and surgery.

Qi Bo 歧伯 the most famous assistant of **[huang di] 黄帝**. The legends had it

pleurisy, pneumonia, etc. Therefore the disease is nothing but an "*imbalance of humours*" cause by the prevalence of one (the "*materia peccans*", that is the "*sinning matter*") upon the other humours, and nature provides to eject the prevailing humour: when suffering from a cold, e. g., we eject from the nose a lot of "*phlegm*", that is a lot of mucus. This is the "*vis medicatrix naturae*", the "*the healing virtue of nature*". But we must aid this "*healing virtue*", and this is the main task of medicine: to aid nature to eject the "*materia peccans*" fighting against the disease on the basis of the therapeutical principle of "*contraria contrariis*" (contraries against contraries) and "*similia similibus*" (similars against similars), that is sometimes medicines must be contrary to the qualities of the disease: we fight against a cold and moist disease prescribing hot and dry simple medicines; sometimes they must be similar to the qualities of the disease: we fight against a hot and dry disease with hot and dry simple medicines. If the disease is a compounded one (e. g. both cold-moist and dry-hot, like pleurisy) the physician fights against it with compounded medicines. The Arabian physician Al Kindi (813 c. - 873 A. D.) made an addition to the doctrine of the "*four qualities*"and started a real algebra of the qualities, maintaining that each quality can be present in four degrees and four half-degrees so that one must take present both the degrees and the half-degrees in preparing a compound medicine. One of Al Kindi's prescriptions can make all clear: prescription against cough:

that the emperor asked Qi Bo to taste various kinds of herbs and to study medicine and pharmacy. The first and greatest medical work in China, **[nei jing] 内经 "Classic of Internal Medicine"**, was written in the style of questions and answers between Huangdi and Qi Bo on problems of medicine and pharmacy.

[huang di nei jing] 黄帝内经 (2698-2590B.C.) **"Huangdi's Internal Classic"** or **"Canon"**. The authorship is traditionally ascribed to the ancient Emperor Huangdi. Actually the work was a product of various unknown authors during the **[zhan guo] 战国 "Warring States"** period. There is also much uncertainty regarding the exact number of volumes of the book. Eighteen is the usual number given; The book consists of two parts: **[su wen] 素问 "Plain Questions"** and **[ling su] 灵枢 "Miraculous Pivot"**.

(1) "Plan Questions" consists of nine volumes including a variety of subjects, such as prevention treatment of diseases, health preservation, man and nature, the application of the theories of Yin and Yang and Five Elements to medicine and the theory of promotion of Qi.

(2) "Miraculous Pivot" consists of nine volumes with more detailed description of meridians and needling acupuncture and moxibustion. In introducing basic theories and clinical practice, the two books supplement each other. The surviving written records on stones, clay, parchment or papyrus give us some ideas of the past history.

Some ideas of this medical work

	Hot	**Cold**	**Moist**	**Dry**
Cardamom	1	½	½	1
Sugar	2	1	1	2
Indigo	½	1	½	1
Myrobalan	1	2	½	1
Total	4½	4½	2½	5

The general quality of this compounded medicine will be characterised by the degrees of the total.

Moreover sometimes nature cannot succeed in healing the affected body, and medicines cannot be efficacious, as in cases of wounds, fractures, bladder stones, etc., and therefore medicine must have recourse to surgery (traumatology, orthopaedics, incisions, etc.).

The correct cure of a disease needs a correct prognosis, that can be made only on the basis of the "critical days", that is the fourth and the seventh: the seventh can be foreseen on the basis of the fourth. If the disease is "chronic" (that means nothing but "lasting") the computation must be made on the basis of the "continuous weeks", that is: the 14th day was the last of the second week and contemporary the first of the third week, that ended at the 20th day, that was the first of the fourth week, that ended at the 26th day; from this day on the computation started again with the following day, that is the 27th, for other two weeks (27th - 33rd days and 34th - 40th days), and so on.

are as follows:

Anatomy. The internal organs are divided into two kinds-the [wu zang] 五脏 "Five Zang" – the heart, liver, spleen, lungs, and kidneys and **[liu fu]** 六腑 "Six Visca" – gall-bladder, stomach, large intestine, small intestine, bladder, and the **[san jiao]** 三焦 "Three Energizers". The function of Zang is supposed to be solid, storing up not eliminating; while Fu is hollow, eliminating not storing.

Dissection of the human body appears to have been attempted. Some measurements of the alimentary tract are giver. E.g. distance from lip to teeth 9/10 inch; width of mouth 2.5 inches; distance from teeth to epiglottis 3.5 inches; capacity of mouth and pharynx 5 Ho (ho means one-tenth of a pint); weight of tongue is 10 oz., length 7 inches, width 2.5 inches; length of stomach, stretched 2 feet 6 inches, circumference 1 foot 5 inches, capacity 3 dous and 5 shengs (ancient Chinese measures which are different from those of the present day), etc.

Physiology. The physiology described in the "Classic of Internal Medicine" was not something scientific. The functions of different organs are a kind of imagination. The heart is the prince of the body, all the blood is under the control of heart, which is considered as the seat of the vital spirit. The lungs are the ministers who regulate one's action. The gall-bladder is the center, courage dwells in it. etc.

The blood circulation was not quite understood. According to one passage, the blood stream is said to start from the foot and circulate to the kidneys, the

Anatomy and Physiology.

The ancient physicians did not ignore that some diseases affect the whole body (like fever, that was thought to be not a symptom, but a disease, chiefly because of the great spread of malaria in ancient times), while some others affect only a particular organ or a particular apparatus, like renal calculosis, diarrhoea, hepatitis, etc., and thought the human body to be formed by "*similar*" and "*dissimilar parts*": e. g. if one cuts a vein until he reaches its smallest part, this will have the same characteristics of the whole vein, and therefore is a "*similar part*" (something like our "*tissue*", though no ancient anatomist or Physiologist or physician had even the palest idea of what we mean with "*tissue*"!) while if one cuts the heart until he reaches its smallest part, he will find some parts of vein, some of artery, some of muscle, etc. and therefore this is a "*dissimilar part*" (something like what we call "*organ*", though no ancient anatomist or physiologist or physician had even the palest idea of what we mean with "*organ*" and "*apparatus*"). So to the great Alexandrine anatomists - whose knowledge has been inherited by Galen (129 *c.* - 199 A. D.) - the human body was composed by the skeleton (which is the supporting structure they knew very well), a complex net of blood vessels (only after the half of the IV century B. C. veins have been distinguished from arteries, most probably by Praxagoras of Cos) and nerves (which the ancients considered to be a third vascular system)

heart, the lungs, the liver, the spleen, and then from the spleen back to kidneys, thus making a complete circuit.

The liver has a rancid odor, a sour taste, a brown color, and is the seat of anger. The heart has an odor of toast, a bitter taste, a brownish-red color, and is the seat of happiness. The spleen has a fragrant odor, a sweet taste, a yellow color, and is the seat of thought. The lung has a fishy smell, a hot taste, a white color, and is the seat of sorrow. The kidney has a putrid smell, a salty taste, a black color, and is the seat of fear.

According to **[nei jing] 内经 "Classic of Internal Medicine"**, diseases are commonly divided into two groups, external injuries (diseases caused by external pathogenic influence such as wind, cold, dryness, moisture etc.) and internal injuries (diseases caused by internal emotions such as joy, grief, anger ,fear ,etc. "Failure to keep a sound mind may weaken resistance and invite attacks by pathogenic factors", therefore, it is imperative, for the sake of preventing diseases and promoting longevity, to keep a sound mind. Man has seven emotions and six desires (joy, anger, melancholy, anxiety, grief and terror) when excessive will cause disorder of the function of **[zang fu] 脏腑 "Zang and Fu"**, as it is stated in book **[nei jing] 内经 "Classic of Internal Medicine"**, "Anger harms the liver, joy the heart, anxiety the spleen, grief the lungs and fear the kidney".

The book also gives an early description about the physiologic phenomena of the human body. That is the female begins to have menses at the age of 14, the male at the age of 16 begins to ejaculate semen. At this period, both male and female begin to have the and by a "*parénkhyma*", that is coagulated blood whose task was for fill the empty spaces of the vascular net (and therefore is a mass without any structure and quite another thing from what we mean with "*parenchyma*", that is a structured tissue).

As for physiology, the ancient physicians - starting from Empedocles of Agrigentum and Alcmaeon of Croton (flourished during the VI/V century B. C.) - had realised that man - like all other animals - can live only if has aliments, breathing and blood. We must take present that until the XVII century no ancient anatomist or physician or physiologist did realise that blood circulates: they thought it moved from the center (liver) to periphery through the veins and from the center (heart) to periphery through the arteries, and finally it was transformed into "*spirits*" that too moved from the center (cerebellum) to periphery through the nerves. Each part (veins, arteries, nerves, stomach, heart, bowels, liver, etc.) is endowed with four "*virtues*": "*attractive virtue*", "*retentive virtue*", "*transforming virtue*" and "*ejecting virtue*". Foods, prepared into the mouth, are attracted through the oesophagus by the stomach, which retains them, transform them into gastric chyme and eject them through the "*pylorus*" (that means the "*doorkeeper*"); the bowels cooperate with the ejecting virtue of the stomach attracting the gastric chyme, that is retained, transformed into chyle end ejected through the *vena portae* (that is the "*porta hepatis*", the "*liver door*"); the liver cooperates with the ejecting virtue of the bowels attracting the chyle, which is retained, transformed into venal blood,

reproductive function called in TCM [**tian kui zhi] 天癸至 "Arrival of Tiankui"**. In his book, there are some descriptions about the male organs, e.g., **[jian] 菅 "surgical resection of penis or testes", [zong jin] 中筋 "penis", [jing chui] 筋捶 "penis and testes", [gao] 睾 "testicle" etc..** The pathogenic factors of the diseases are considered as **[liu yin] 六淫 "Six Excesses of Xie Qi":** wind, cold, summer-heat, dampness, dryness and fire (heat), etc..

Particular significance is attached to the atmospheric changes of the four seasons. The vital spirit should harmonize with the seasons, the five elements, the Yin-Yang principles and various other factors. Sickness will arise, if these forces are deranged.

In those early times all matters, both public and private, were closely related to religion. By the time of the **[yin] 殷 "Yin Dynasty"** (about 1500 B.C.), worship, sacrifice, astrology, divination, healing ,etc. were in the hands of the priests and sorcerers. The healing art at this early stage consisted chiefly of divination, incantation, sacrificial offerings, propitiations, magic, prayer and other superstitious practices. The profession was entirely under the control of **[wu yi] 巫医 "Priest-doctor"**. At the same time religion and astrology merged into healing and, as in all early civilizations, the first doctor was a priest and the first priest was a doctor.

charged it with "*natural spirit*" and ejected through the *vena cava* through whose branches it reaches all the parts of the body providing to its growth and preservation. Thanks to its "*transforming virtue*" it "*assimilates*", that is becomes similar, to the parts that need to grow or to be restored: e. g. the growth needs bones increasing; the venous blood becomes similar to bones and increase them; on the other hand, if a bit of skin has been cut by a knife, the venal blood becomes similar to the skin and repairs the wound. Finally it reaches the right heart, passes through the ventricular sept (that up to Andreas Vesalius (1514 - 1564) and Realdus Columbus (1520 - 1559) has been thought to be pervious) and reaches the left heart. Here it is retained and transformed into arterious blood, charged with "*vital spirit*" and is ejected through the aorta. The aorta attracts and distribute it to all the parts of the body, providing to movement, relation life, etc. The arterious blood is attracted by the carotids and reaches the "*rete mirabile*" (the "*wonderful network*", called also "*arbor vitae*", "*life plant*", a network of minute vessels on the under-surface of the brain, that doesn't exist in man, as Vesalius proved, but is found in the brains of many animals, especially those with hooves, and from these it has been constantly referred to man!). Here the arterious blood is attracted, retained, transformed into "*animal spirit*" and reaches all the specific places devoted to the five senses: the eyes, where it becomes "*spiritus visivus*" ("*visual spirit*"), the nose, where it becomes "*spiritus olfactivus*" ("*olfactory spirit*"), the mouth, where it becomes "*spiritus gustativus*" ("*gustatory spirit*"), the ears, where it becomes "*spiritus auditivus*"

	("*auditory spirit*") and all the surface of the body, where it becomes "*spiritus tactilis*" ("*tactile spirit*"). All these anatomo-physiological theories, all the above mentioned and described pathology ant therapy were organised by Galen in a great scientific edifice, that dominated for more than fourteen centuries and began to be demolished only at the beginning of the XVII century, when the Galilean scientific revolution inaugurated a "*quantitative*" interpretation of the whole Universe and all its phenomena: the Universe is nothing but an immense machine and all phenomena obey to mechanic laws, so that in the whole Universe and in each phenomenon there is no "virtue", no "end": the phenomena happen as they happen only because they cannot do else! A stone falls down not because of its natural "precipitating virtue" and not because of its trending to its "natural place", but only because it cannot do else than falling down because of the mechanical connection of "quantities", that is the mass of the stone, the mass of Earth, the distance between stone and Earth. As the mass of the stone is lesser than that of the Earth, the stone falls towards the Earth. Would the mass of the stone be greater than that of the Earth, the Earth would fall towards the stone and could not do else than falling. With the Galilean scientific revolution starts the modern and contemporary science, that has nothing to do with what science has been from the origin of human civilisation until the XVII century. One can say that with this century we enter a new scientific world and that a dialogue between scientists of the past and post-galilean scientists is a dialogue

between persons that speak languages that are unintelligible each other and to which both are absolutely deaf.

IX-VIII Century B.C.

[zhou] 周 "Zhou Dynasty" can be divided into **[xi zhou] 西周 "Western Zhou"** (1122 B.C to 771 B.C.) and **[dong zhou] 东周 "Eastern Zhou"**. Traditional historiography also refers the **[chun qiu] 春秋 "Spring and Autumn"** period (770-476 B.C) and **[zhan guo] 战国 "Warring States"** period (475-221 B.C).

With the advent of **[zhou] 周 "Zhou Dynasty"**, China gradually entered a feudal stage. The functions of the profession- doctors and priests were officially separated with the decline of hold of **the [wu yi] 巫医 "sorcery"**. Medical practice witnessed the beginning of the organization. According to **[zhou li] 周礼 "The Zhou Rituals"** there were four categories of physicians at court. There were e.g. **[ji yi] 疾医** "physicians for the cure of illness", who were concerned with internal medicine, and **[yang yi] 疡医** "physicians for the treatment of wounds" to treat cutaneous affections, injuries, traumatisms and fractures. There were also **[shi yi] 食医** "physicians for nutrition", who acted as dieticians and **[shou yi] 兽医** "physicians for animals". The medical practitioners based their diagnoses on the theory of **[yin yang] 阴阳 "Yin-Yang"** and **[wu xing] 五行 "Five Elements"** (to be discussed fuller later).

The antiquity of the principles on which traditional Chinese medicine depended has been confirmed by the

GREEK MEDICE

IX-VIII Century B.C

HOMER: described 141 wounds, some of which are of urological interest (bladder, testicles, etc.). 150 anatomical terms can be found in his poems *Iliad* and *Odyssey.* Moreover he speaks about prognosis, therapy (mainly surgical therapy) and physiology. But this doesn't at all mean that Homer was the founder of Medicine and so much the less of Urology!

During this period medicine was practiced mainly by the priests of Asclepios (the God of Medicine corresponding to the Roman Aesculapius) in the so-called *Asclepièia* (the temples of Asclepios). There were more than 200 and many "ex voto" (legs with varicose veins, ears, bladders and wombs, penis and scrota, etc.) and many votive tablets (with the description of the therapy) have been found during the excavations. This means that a lot of patients recovered their health and expressed their gratitude to the healer God. The priests were the *Asclepiàdai*, but it is sure that also lay physicians were present as medical experts.

The priests of the *Asclepieia* went on practising medicine for centuries, also after the dawn of Science and of scientific Medicine.

It is noteworthy that the members of the most famous and prestigious

1973 discovery in the number three tomb at **[ma wang dui] 马王堆 "Ma Wangdui".** They are as follows: **[huang di nei jing] 黄帝内经 "Huangdi's Classic of Internal Medicine"**, the oldest Chinese work on medicine (to be already discussed). **[wu shi er bing fang] 五十二病方 "Fifth-two Prescriptions against Fifty-two Ailments"**, it can claim to be one of the earliest Chinese pharmaceutical documents. The treatment is primarily dependent on internal medicine, surgery, obstetrics, pediatrics and medicine for "five organs". It also lists 242 drugs of mineral, plant and animal organs. **[shi jing] 诗经 "Classics of Odes"**, the earliest anthology of Chinese poems, compiled in the 6th century B.C., contains the names of fifty medical plants. Moreover, a growing interest in alchemy during Zhou times foreshadowed a medical chemistry. Alchemy meant the preparation of elixirs to prolong human life. A reading of **[zhou li] 周礼 "The Zhou Rituals"** (1066-221B.C.) reveals that earlier Chinese were preoccupied with nutritional and even sexual hygiene. Zhouli stresses on health preservation, "Striving for health", "Conserving health", "Cultivating temperament" to achieve the purpose of prolonging life. **[zhou] 周 "Zhou Dynasty"** gave medicine its theoretical framework and its status in the language and culture.	medical guild in Greece boasted of being lineal descendants of Asclepios, and therefore called themselves proudly "*Asclepiadai*"(sons of Asclepios).
VII Century	**VII Century B.C.**
The reliable history does not go further back than the middle of the **[zhou] 周 "Zhou Dynasty"** (722 B.C.). This is one of the most glorious periods in Chinese history. Literature, art,	

religion, philosophy flourished and reached a high degree of development. This dynasty is rightly represented as the age of philosophy for **[guan zi] 管子 Guangzi**， **[zhuang zi] 庄子 Zhuangzi, [lie zi] 列子 Liezi.** Towering above all these were **[lao zi] 老子Laozi, [kong zi] 孔子 Confucius, and [meng zi] 孟子 Mencius**. The study of medicine was dominated by the scholastic subtleties of visionary philosophers and was characterized by reverence for authority, petrified formalism and a pedantic excess of detail. Medicine was no longer an effective, practical art based on observation and knowledge, pretentious systems of healing have tended to become less and less practical. As the result of these varied speculations on the theory and causation of the diseases two doctrines evolved which formed the basis of the whole of Chinese medicine.

The first is the Doctrine of the Two principles called **[yin yang] 阴阳 "Yin and Yang"**.

In fact the origin of the concepts of Yin and Yang is lost in the mist of Chinese history. According to **[guo yu] 国语 "Discourses of the States"**, a history work dating form [chun qiu] 春秋 **"Spring and Autumn"** period (8th century B.C.). **[yin] 阴 "Yin"** was identified with the earth, the moon, darkness, everything feminine, coldness and passivity. [yang]阳 "Yang" was identified with heaven, the sun, light, everything masculine, warmth and energy. In the book of **[yi jing] 易经 "Book of Changes"**, (a work of divination compiled during **[xi zhou] 西周 "Western Zhou"**, it comprises a set of eight trig rams called **[ba gua] 八卦 Bagua**. It illustrates the most harmonious of the combination unite the two elements of Yin and Yang, which are seen as inseparable, each one dependent on the other. The idea of the coexistence of Yin and Yang within each being pervades traditional Chinese medicine. Good health depends on the equilibrium of these two elements, while an excess of one or the other provokes illness.

The second doctrine is that of the **[wu xing] 五行 "Five Elements"**, which are metal, wood, water, fire and earth. The human frame is supposed to be made up of a harmonious mixture of these primordial substances. So long as the proportions remain proper health results; but if the balance is distributed disease follows. That is everything in the world could be combined, exchanged and separated by the principle of **[yin yang] 阴阳 "Yin and Yang"**. According to **[yi jing] 易经 "Books of Changes"**, male belongs to Yang, while female belongs to Ying. The combination of Ying and Yang – the sexual intercourses of male and female produces life. Generally speaking, ancient Chinese began to get to know something about sex activities, and understand that the reproduction is no longer controlled by the power of God, but due to the combination of Yin and Yang -male and female.

VI-V Century B.C.

Yi He 医和 (about 600 B.C.) a famous physician in the Period of **[chun qiu] 春 秋 "Spring and Autumn"** (722-476 B.C.), who put forward the theory that abnormality in the six climatic conditions in nature, namely, **[yin]** 阴 "cloudy", **[yang]** 阳 "sunny", **[feng]** 风 "wind", **[yu]** 雨 "rainy", **[hui]** 晦

VI-V Century B.C.

THALES, ANAXIMANDER and ANAXIMENES founded both Philosophy and Science and created the so-called *School of Miletus* (on the Aegean seaboard). Anaximander maintained that water is the fundamental element from which everything originates and that even man is the result of a transformation of an original fish.

"gloomy", and **[ming]** 明 "bright", would lead to various kinds of diseases.

According to **Yihe**, there are six kinds of weather which give rise to the five tastes, the five colors, and the five sounds. Diseases are caused by excess. It forms the four seasons and follows the order of the five elements. If the balance is distributed dire consequences will result. Excessive cloudiness causes cold diseases, excessive clearness causes hot diseases, excessive wind causes painful limbs, excessive rain causes bowel complaints, excessive mist causes sensuality and excessive brightness causes heart troubles.

During the period of **[han chao] 汉朝 "Han Dynasty"**, the keepingi of the historical records was systemised. The first step was taken to record the pharmacopoeia and remedies of the herbal medicine.

The second major work appeared in the period of late**[dong han] 东汉 "Eastern Han Dynasty"** (206 B.C-AD). **[han niang xue shuo] 寒凉学说 "Discussion of Cold-Induced Disease"** together with **[jin kui yao lue] 金匮要略 "Synopsis of the Golden Chamber"**, summarizing the experience of Chinese practitioners in the prevention and treatment of disease, the book explained certain infectious diseases by describing the functioning of the major channels of the body, it also described the developed of a wide range of other diseases according to the theory of the internal, or **[zang fu] 脏腑 "Zang Fu"** organs. These descriptions later developed into a complete theory for the differentiation of symptom-complexes, which is the basis for diagnosis in traditional Chinese medicine, leading to the various schools

Only fragments of their works have been preserved.

PYTHAGORAS of Samos (570 *c.* - 489 B. C.) was the inventor of mathematics and geometry. He thought that number is the fundament of all the Universe and that the elements are four: *air*, *water*, *earth* and *fire*. Everything is a compound of these elements, each of which is characterised by a combination of four qualities, *heat*, *cold*, *dry* and *moist*. The four elements and their qualities give origin to the four humours of the human body: *blood* (warm and moist), *yellow bile* (warm and dry), *phlegm* (cold and moist) and *black bile* (cold and dry). Health, as well as the particular character of everyone, is the result of a perfect balance among them, wile imbalance is the cause of illness. This theory ruled over Medicine for more than 21 centuries, began to be censured in the XVII century, and was definitively demolished only by Virkhow in 1858.

Only fragments of his works have been preserved.

ALCMAEON of Croton (Calabria in South Italy) flourished around the year 500 B. C. and was the most distinguished among Pythagora's disciples. Is the first author we know to have written medical treatises and perhaps improved and perfected his Master's theory on the four humours. He also was the first who performed anatomical dissections and realised that the brain is center of the nervous system, the responsible for the functioning of all the organs of the human body, including the urogenital apparatus. Moreover the brain was for Alcmaeon the seat both of sensations and intelligence. This theory was

of medicine.

[chun qiu] 春秋 "Spring and Autumn"
period experienced the competition and conflict that anticipated the **[zhan guo] 战国 "Warring States"** period, a time when seven principal states engaged in interminable wars. The time of crisis and dramatic change threw up a number of significant personalities. So in the year of about 600 B.C., two giants of Chinese thinking emerged.

Confucius [kong zi] 孔子 (551-479 B.C.), celebrated as China's greatest sage, he established a code of rules and ethics which began with the premise that there is a right order and harmony to the universe, based upon a delicate balance of Yin and Yang forces, and the force exerted by man must be essentially moral. He strove to realise **[ren] 仁 "to love others**" and preached that Man must cultivate **[wu de] 五德** "Five Virtues" of benevolence, justice, properties, wisdom and sincerity in order to exert his own force in this external cycle of good and evil. Virtue was regarded as the secret of health.

According to him, early marriage was discountenanced. He thought thirty for the man and twenty for the girl as the most suitable age for marriage. The teaching of Confucius was echoed by another great sage of that era.

Lao Zi [lao zi] 老子 the founder of **[dao ja] 道家 "Daoism"**, the writer of **[dao de jing] 道德经 "Classic of the Way and Virtue".** Taking the Confucian doctrine of universal order, Lao Zi taught that man himself can only achieve personal harmony by bowing to its natural and inevitable fate and pursuing a course of inaction. Never strive nor

maintained also by Hippocrates, the Father of Western scientific Medicine, and by Galen (II century A. D.) but was rejected by Aristotle who maintained the center to be the heart. Aristotle's wrong theory gave origin, in the XVI century, to a tremendous quarrel between "Peripatetics" and "Galenists", and was finally demolished only in the XVIII century. Only fragments of Alcmaeon's works have been preserved.

interfere, he declared, because things would come to a successful conclusion without effort. Taoist theory dictated that while regular and even abandoned sex was good for the health, it had to be accomplished without release of semen to promote and nourish the vigor of the male. Even at the bed-pillow, the principle of "opposing forces" held sway. Men were Yang, and Women Yin and it was considered crucial that in the sexual union of the two the male must retain and conserve his vital essence and limited Yang while absorbing as much as he could of the female's unlimited supply of Yin essence.

V Century B.C.

Bian Que 扁鹊(407-310 B.C.), the earliest noted physician, he was the first medical to be mentioned by historians. He is better known as **[qin yue ren] 秦越人 Qin Yueren**. Some state that he was a native of **[zheng] 郑 "Zheng Kingdom"**, his family was **[qin] 秦 "Qin"** and his given name was **[yue ren] 越人 "Yueren"**; others think that he came from **[lu]** 鲁 "Lu Kingdom", a member of the **[bian] 扁 "Bian family"**, his name being **[que] 鹊"Que"**. Realistic **[han fei] 韩非 Hanfei** , a well-known Legalist of the 3rth B.C. gives a more historically accurate picture of Qin Yueren, who has become the Chinese equivalent of Aesculapius, the Greek and Roman gods of medicine. In **[si ma qian] 司马迁 Si Maqian**'s biography of Qin Yueren, he emphasises the reputation that Qin acquired in the fields of gynaecology, pediatrics, otorhinolaryngology and even psychiatry. Qin asserted that an imbalance of Yin and Yang was the principal cause of illness, and his

V Century B.C.

ANAXAGORAS of Clazomenae (on the Aegean seaboard) (born in 499 B. C.). He agreed with Pythagoras about the humours in the human body, but thought illnesses to be the result of an imbalance between only yellow and black bile. Only fragments of his works have been preserved.

EMPEDOCLES of Agrigentum (Sicily) (500 *c.* - 430 B. C.), founder of the so-called *Italic School* of Medicine. He reclaimed the marshes of the river Selinum and rescued the town of Selinunte from malaria. He agreed with Pythagoras' theory of the four humours, their balance and imbalance. He was the first to maintain that breathing occurs both through the lungs and the skin, and the heart is the center of the vascular system and the origin and the end of the comings and goings of the blood, and that the *pneuma* (the vital spirit) was carried to every part of the human body through the blood vessels.

methods of diagnosis and treatment relied on pulse taking and acupuncture. He used decoctions and fomentations in the cure of patients. He was supposed to be the author of **[Bian Que Nei Jing] 扁鹊内经 "The Internal Classic of Bian Que", [Bian Que Wai Jing] 扁鹊外经 "The External Classic Bian Que".** He was well up both in medicine and surgery. Traveling from one place to another, he treated people on the way as a specialist on eye, ear, women's or children's diseases. He practiced medicine and acupuncture and introduced the first gynaecological and pediatrician treatments. His fame was so great that aroused the intense jealousy of the court physician **[li shi] 李谧 Li Shi** who caused him to be assassinated. However, he is regarded as the most foremost exponent of the pulse lore, indispensable to native doctors for diagnosis.

He was the first to perform studies on embryology, and to maintain that the heart is the first part that forms and that breathing begins only after birth. He also anticipated the theory of evolution, yet it was rejected until Darwin. Only fragments of his poetical works have been preserved.

DEMOCRITUS of Abdera (in Thrace) (494 - 404 B. C.). Founder of *Atomism.* Atoms, separated by pores, form the human body. Atoms of the external objects, which strike our sense organs, cause sensation. Illness is an alteration of the balance between atoms and pores. He had a mechanical idea of the Universe and maintained that nothing is created, nothing is destroyed, and only the combinations among the atoms change, by nothing else than the mechanical laws of nature.

Only fragments of his works have been preserved.

DIOGENES of Apollonia (the Phrygian, not the Cretan Apollonia) flourished around 430 B. C. Put the premises of the so-called *Pneumatic School*, which suggested many physiological theories to Galen. Diogene's theories of generation, respiration and the blood are very important in the history of Medicine. Aristotle has preserved his account of the veins: he observed that the blood vessels run to the left ventricle of the heart and described the *vena cava* and its branches correctly.

EURIODES of Sicily is told by Ruphus of Ephesus (see below) to have performed nephrotomies in the year 430 B. C. Ruphus states also that Euriodes and Hippocrates were the only able to operate by incision on nephritis sufferers, but this sounds rather like a legend.

THREE SCHOOLS OF MEDICINE:

1 - The *School of Agrigentum* or Italic School that was considered by Galen equal to the other two, but about which we know little more than what has been preserved by the fragments of Alcmaeon and Empedocles;

2 - the *Cnidian School* (in the Aegean isle of Cnidos), which we know better. The followers of this School specialised in diagnosis and described the patients' symptoms so meticulously that often they mistake symptoms for illnesses, and ended by seeing an illness in any symptom. This extreme meticulousness caused a final confusion, which let us understand why Hippocrates did not agree with the theories of this School.

3 - The *School of Cos*, the greatest and the most lasting medical School, founded and immortalised by Hippocrates, who brought Greek Medicine to develop in the highest degree.

The theories and the ideas of the *School of Cos*, or "*Hippocratic School*", lasted until the century, and are still alive, chiefly for their marvelous and amazingly up to day ethical ideals.

HIPPOCRATES the GREAT of Cos (contemporary of Socrates, 469 - 399 B. C.) is considered "the Father of Medicine". His method was "*observatio et ratio*", that is "observation and reason". It is not so sure that he adhered to the doctrine of the "four humours", but it has been ascribed to him, because it is

	maintained by many of the works preserved under his name, which form the so-called "*Corpus hippocraticum*", a collection of 53 treatises in 72 books, none of which most probably has been written by Hippocrates himself, but at least four or five represent his genuine teaching, while some others are surely works of the *Cnidian School*. So being the things, some philologists have supposed that the collection was nothing else than the Library of the School, where also the works of the either direct or indirect disciples of Hippocrates were preserved. According to Hippocrates urine is a fundamental mean for a correct diagnosis, so that he can be considered the founder of "uroscopy". On the other hand, he did not know the difference between veins and arteries and, therefore, one cannot find in his works even the faintest hint to any doctrine of the pulse. Man is a microcosm into the macrocosm, and every change or imbalance of the qualities of the macrocosm cause a change and imbalance in the microcosm. Illness is due to an imbalance of one of the humours, that prevails over the others, as a consequence of an imbalance in the qualities of the macrocosm (seasonal changes, etc.). Therefore the therapy is always "evacuant", in order to expel the prevailing humour and to restore the balance. Medicines must be prescribed according to the two fundamental principles of "*contraria contrariis*" and "*similia similibus*", that is "contrary against contrary" and "similar against similar", that is to say that the medicine must have qualities sometimes contrary, sometimes similar to the qualities of the illness.

According to Hippocrates "*Nature is the physician of all illnesses*" and the physician has nothing else to do than aid Nature.

He also had a particular idea of generation and the combination of male and female parts, which may seem anticipate the biological laws of Mendel, though he thought the uterus to be double and that males were formed in the right part and by the sperm of the right testicle and females in and by the left ones.

He is told to have hindered the progress of Urology, because in the *Oath* (perhaps the most famous of hippocratic works, after the *Aphorisms*, that were considered "*the Bible of the physician*" until the XIX century) one can read: "*I will not use the knife , not even, verily, on sufferers from stone, but I will give place to such as are craftsmen therein*", but it is a nonsense. In fact this passage is a very late interpolation, inserted in the original text only during the II century A. D.

The precept "*Where there is love of man, there is also love of the Art*" is the highest expression of hippocratic Ethics.

V-IV century B. C.	V-IV century B. C.
	PLATO of Athens (428 - 348 B. C.). The great philosopher who founded the *Academia*, that lasted until 529 A. D. when the emperor Justinian closed it. He was not a physician, but his theories about the mutual relation between the *microcosm* (the man) and the *Macrocosm* (the Universe) joined with the ideas of Hippocrates and exerted a great influence on the Medicine until the XVII century. His pathology and Physiology derive from Hippocrates. **ARISTOTLE** of Stagira (in Chalcidice, the Macedonian peninsula between the gulf of Salonicco and the mouth of the Struma river) (384 - 322 B. C.). His father was a physician of the guild of the *Asclepiàdae* and most probably was his first master. Studied at the Academy of Plato but very soon rejected the theories of his Master, founded a School (the famous *Liceum*) and framed a doctrine all his own. Philip, the king of Macedonia, called him at his court to be the tutor and e Master of his son, Alexander the Great. Aristotle was one of the greatest philosophers and scientists of all times, and his works deal with Logic, Physics, Metaphysics, Politics, Arts, History, but the treatises on Anatomo-physiology, Embryology, and Natural History are the most important and the most striking for the extraordinary vastness of his researches and the astonishing sharpness of mind.

	We must confine ourselves to the urological, sexological and andrological observations. As for Urology, he observed that urine is present in the blood (a fact that Hippocrates had already observed), percolates into the pelvis (though no blood reaches it) where gathers to reach the bladder through the ureters and be discharged through the urethra. He observed that the human kidney appear like one only mass, but is composed by many parts like little kidneys joined together. He maintained that sperm derives from the blood and therefore from all the parts of the body, accumulates into the epididymis to be ejected through the urethra, but misunderstood the function of the testicles and maintained that they were nothing else than weights to keep the bending of the spermatic ducts. As for andrology he observed that the voice changes from childhood to puberty; that eunuchs become female, do never suffer from varicocele, but suffer from all the illnesses that are characteristic of women, like varicose veins in the legs, etc. In the field of sexology he was the first - and for more than twenty centuries the only one - who observed that an incorrect sexual education just at the beginning of puberty can cause great psychological and sexual troubles in ripe age. Moreover, Aristotle formulated clearly and nearly always correctly the fundamental problems of biology (embryology, biological heredity, nutrition, growth, adaptation, etc.) and made the first scientific classification of animals, on the basis of compared anatomo-physiology. His theories and statements

	dominated all the branches of Science (from Astronomy to Physics; from Politics to Art; from Biology to Psychology) for more than eighteen centuries and Scientists began to doubt them only starting from the XVII century. But some of the Aristotelian ideas (like the theory o "spontaneous generation") were definitively rejected only at the end of the XVIII century, and a lot of his observations are still exceptionally correct and valid.
IV - III century B. C.	**IV-III Century B.C.** **THEOPHRASTUS** of Eresos (a town in the isle of Lesbos) (370 - 285 B. C.) was called "The father of Botany". He studied under the guidance of Plato and Aristotle and led the *Liceum* after Aristotle's death.. Wrote treatises on Logic, Metaphysics, Psychology, Ethics, Politics, Rhetoric, Art, Music, Physics, Natural History, Zoology and Botany. In his "Enquiry into Plants"(a treatise in 9 books) he describes about 500 varieties of plants, and in book IX he deals with their pharmacological properties. Many of the plants he speaks about came from the Far East and were diuretic. **PRAXAGORAS** of Cos flourished in the second half of the IV century B. C. Many of his treatises were well known by Physicians until the II century A. D., but only fragments have been preserved. His anatomy was a strange mixture of correct and false notions. He recognised the connection between the spinal cord and the brain; on the other hand he maintained that the arteries come from the heart, taper away and finally turn into nerves. Moreover he

	considered the arteries as air-channels, a theory that will be developed by Erasistratus of Ceos and Herophilus of Chalcedon (III century B. C.), but Galen (II century A. D.) rejected it on the basis of marvelous experiments. The discovery of the arterial pulse was ascribed to Praxagoras, who practiced also surgery: his operation on the ileus is mentioned. **CHRYSIPPUS** of Cnidos flourished at the end of the III century B. C. and was the court physician of Ptolemy II Philadelphus, the second King of Egypt after Alexander the Great's death (323 B. C.). He paid great attention to the frequency of the pulse during the fits of fever.
III century B. C.	**III Century B.C.** **The great School of Alexandria** was founded by Ptolemy I Sotér and was increased by his son, Ptolemy II Philadelphus (309 - 246 B. C.). When Egypt became a Roman province (31 B. C.) the School of Alexandria went on studying and teaching for centuries and waned only in the VII century A. D., when the Arabs conquered Egypt and founded the great University of Cairo. **HEROPHILUS** of Chalcedon flourished in the first half of the III century B. C. and his school was still flourishing at the end of the I century B. C. The anatomical inquiries based on the dissection of the human cadaver are his greatest original contributions: particularly famous were his studies of the brain, which he considered as the

organ of the soul; of the liver, the eye and the sexual organs, in which he discovered and described the seminal vesicles, the seminal ampullae and, most probably, the prostate gland. He discovered and studied the rhythm of the pulse and formulated a mathematical law of its systole and diastole, which exercised a fundamental influence on the doctrine of pulse that developed during the following centuries, and is partially still valid.

Unfortunately all his works went lost and only fragments and indirect quotations (chiefly by Galen) have been preserved.

III-II Century B.C.

Nan Jing [nan jing] 难经 "Difficult Classic" or **"Classic on Medical Problems"**, a book appeared in the 1st or 2nd century B.C. with unknown authorship. No mention of it is found in the **[han shu] 汉书 " Anal of Art of the Han Dynasty"**, but is mentioned in the book **[shui tang yan yi] 隋唐演绎 "Changes of Sui Tang Dynasties"**. From this it may be inferred that the book was published before the period of **[san guo] 三国 "Three Kingdoms"**. It deals with fundamental medical theories and expounds the main points of **[nei jing] 内经 "Classic of Internal medicine"** in the forms of questions and answers. The points of acupuncture and moxibustion, the method of needling, the physiological and pathological

III-II Century B.C.

ERASISTRATUS of Ceos (one of the Aegean isles) lived in Alexandria together with and after Herophilus (first half of the III century B. C.). His school still flourished in the II century A. D. and his books were read as late as the IV century A. D. On the basis of his anatomical studies, he reached the clear distinction between sensory and motor nerves; he recognised the changes of the body due to diseases dissecting human bodies *post mortem*, and was interested in comparative anatomy. As for physiology, he studied the growth of the body and the process of digestion, and made researches that included even quantitative experiments. Like Herophilus he maintained that the blood flows through the veins, while the

conditions related to the meridians and collaterals, and the method of feeling the pulse are all discussed. Numerous commentaries have been later written about it.

Chinese medicine begins properly in **[han] 汉 "Han Dynasty"** and its scientific advancement centers in the figures of **[cang gong] 仓公 Canggong, [zhang zhong jing] 张中景 Zhang Zhongjing** and **[hua tuo] 华佗Huatuo**。

Canggong [cang gong] 仓公 also known as **Chunyu Yi [chun yu yi] 淳于意**(about 205-B.C.), " the Reverend master of Granary", for having been put in charge of the public granary of Qi Kingdom, a well-known physician with rich experience in treating diseases, who was said to have attached great importance to pulse-taking and he was the first person to keep complete personal clinical records. Unlike most of the medical writers, who usually made exaggerated accounts of successful cases, he was more modest for he admitted his failures with admirable frankness. For two purpose he kept his medical records : one is to estimate the percentage of successes and failure, the other is to find a guide for future predictions. From the 25 cases he has left us, we may have a peep into the medical thoughts of that time. The name of the patient, the name and nature of the illness, its cause, the treatment followed, the remedy used and the progress of the illness accompany each of his twenty-five observations. These case histories are not to be compared with those of Hippocrates for they are not great scientific value. Too much stress was laid on the pulse

arteries bring the *pneuma* (the vital spirit) to all the parts of the body. Galen, who based his criticism on marvelous experiments that he performed on living animals, finally rejected this theory.

Unfortunately all his works went lost and only fragments and indirect quotations (chiefly by Galen) have been preserved.

Many other famous physicians flourished in Alexandria during this period: Apollodorus, who wrote on poisons; Demetrius, a famous obstetrician; the renowned ophthalmologist Demosthenes Philalethes; Serapion, the founder of the *Empirical School* (see below), against which Galen fought tooth and nail; In particular

AMMONIUS, nicknamed "*the Lithotomist*" who invented a particular instrument with which he was able to break the stone in the bladder and then extract the fragments. This method of performing the operation for the extraction of the stones in the bladder was adopted for centuries, and the idea of breaking the stone is still fundamental in the present Urology.

In this century Medicine separated in two Schools which polemized against each other for centuries:

1 - the *Dogmatic* (or Rational)

2 - the *Empirical School.*

The former was the heir of Hippocratic Medicine, but brought the hippcratic idea of "*observatio et ratio*"

readings, which were so vague that not much could be made out of them. But the diseases listed were cancer of the stomach, several varieties of indigestion, retention of urine, cystitis, amenorrhea, intestinal worms, rheumatism, paralysis kidney diseases, etc. After him, the practice of taking clinical case histories died out until the **[song] 宋 "Song Dynasty"**.	to the level of a so complicated and quite abstract rationalism as for provoke the violent reaction of Philinus - one of Erasistratus' disciples - who flourished in the first half of the III century B. C., and, most of all, of Serapion of Alexandria. The *Empiricists* rejected any abstract theory, confining themselves only to the results of practical experience. These were the most important *Medical Schools* (or *Sects*, as they has been called), when Medicine settled in Rome. **ROMAN MEDICINE**
I Century B.C.	**I Century B.C.** **ASCLEPIADES** of Prusa (in Bithynia) died about 40 B. C., studied in Alexandria and practiced in Parium and Athens. He accepted the atomic theory, rejected all teleology and stressed the importance of phenomenal appearances. He explained health as the unhindered movement of the atoms and disease as their inhibited movement. Only fragments of his works have been preserved. **THEMISON** of Laodicea (second half of the I century B. C.) founded the *Methodical School* and was a precursor of Thessalus of Tralles. He introduced into medicine the theory of "*communia*", that is "*status strictus, fluens and mixtus*" referring to excretion which is either too much or too little, or too much from one part and too little from another.

	He was the first to study methodically the chronic diseases and encouraged their treatment by physicians. Only fragments and indirect quotations of his works have been preserved.
I Century AD	**I Century AD** **SCRIBONIUS LARGUS** (1-50c.AD). Studied in Rome during the reign of the Emperor Tiberius (14-37). His patron C. Julius Callistus, secretary of the Emperor Claudius (41-54), procured the Emperor's patronage for his writings. In gratitude, Scribonius dedicated to his patron his treatise *Compositiones* (Prescriptions). He is a follower of the Empirical School, like Celsius. In his treatise many drugs are listed for the cure of affections and pains of the kidneys, affections and pains of the bladder, dysuria, stranguria and anuria, incontinence of urine, stones in the kidney, stone in the bladder and haematuria. His work was the main source of Marcellus Empiricus. **THESSALUS** of Tralles (died before 79 A. D.). He developed Themison's ideas and brought the *Methodical School* to its maximum. Thessalus' school was the only new sect seriously to compete with the older Hellenistic schools (the *Dogmatic* and the *Empirical*) and Galen's violent and slanderous attacks are the clear expression of a reactionary archaist who did understand nothing of the modernist attitude of the Roman culture in Nero's times.

AULUS CORNELIUS CELSUS flourished under the Emperor Tiberius (14 - 37 A. D.) and wrote an Encyclopaedia comprising Agriculture, Medicine, Military science, Rhetoric, Philosophy and Jurisprudence. Only the eight medical books are preserved. Of the other sections we have nothing more than fragments. His work is the main source for the reconstruction of Hellenistic Medicine. The introduction is a brief but admirable outline of the history of Medicine up to the author's time.

The VII book deals with surgery and describes with particular exactness and exceptional wealth of details many operations so that it is difficult to accept the opinion that he was a layman, writing only for his own instruction and that of other laymen, as maintained by many scholars.

The most important operation described by Celsus is the so-called "*sectio celsiana*" or "little apparatus", that is the perineal incision for the extraction of the stones in the bladder. This technique was more or less amply described and constantly adopted by all the surgeons of the following centuries, up to 1522, when Marianus Sanctus (see below) wrote and published his treatise "*Libellus aureus de lapide a vesica per incisionem extrahendo*" (Golden booklet on the extraction of the bladder stone by incision), in which the "great apparatus" is described.

As for urological anatomy, it is noteworthy that he describes the calyces of the kidneys and the male and female genital apparatus quite correctly.

	ATHENAEUS of Attaleia practiced medicine under the emperor Claudius (41 - 54 A. D.) and was the founder of the *Pneumatic School*. He devised most elaborate dietetic rules, in which he included pedagogical as well as medical precepts, differentiated according to the different stages of life and chiefly to the puberty age. His ideas were highly esteemed by Galen. **PEDANIUS DIOSCORIDES** of Anazarbus (in Cylicia, Near East) (44 - 90 A. D.). He was an army physician and wrote "*Materia medica*", in six books, and "*De simplicibus medicamentis*" (On simple medicaments) in two books in Greek language. Almost 600 plants and nearly 1.000 drugs composed of vegetal, animal and mineral substances are studied and described, many of which are said to be efficacious against urological, andrological and lexicological diseases. He gives also many prescriptions for anaesthetic medicines to be used in performing surgical operations. All the subsequent surgeons inherited them until at least the XIX century, when modern means of anaesthesia were discovered. Dioscoride's books superseded all earlier pharmacological literature and became the standard work of later centuries both in the East and the West. All chemist's had to have by law Dioscoride's books in their library until the end of the XIX century. **AGATHINUS Claudius** (50 c. - 100 c. A. D.) was one of the pupils of the Stoic L. Anneus Cornutus' pupils and of the physician Athenaeus of Attaleia (quoted above). He was the teacher of

Archigenes (quoted below) and adopted some of the tenets both of the Empirical and the Methodical Schools, founding the Eclectic School.

ARCHIGENES of Apamea (in Syria) flourished in Rome at the time of the emperor Trajan (98 - 117 A. D.). Being one of Agathinus' (quoted above) disciples, he belonged to the *Eclectic School*, but was chiefly influenced by the doctrines of the *Pneumatic School.* Galen inherited his theory of the pulse, though he reacted against other points of Archigenes' medical theories.

I-II Century AD

Zhang Ji 张机 (150?-219?AD), also-called **Zhang Zhongjing张中景** was born in Nanyang district, Henan Province. He is often spoken of as the Chinese Hippocrates and is highly regarded as the Sage of Medicine. Very little is known about his life, what we only know is that he received his medical education from **[zhang bo zu] 张伯祖 Zhang Bozu.** In 168 AD, he graduated as a doctor of literature and about 196 AD held office as mayor of **[chang sha] 长沙 "Changsha"**. He quickly superseded his teacher in medical skills and became famous of being a capable doctor. As one of the most influential physician in the history of Chinese medicine, he is the first to advocate the methods of analysing and differentiating pathological conditions in accordance with the Six Meridians and Eight principal Syndromes and the principle of treating diseases. His medical works are **[shang han za bing**

I-II Century AD

RUFUS of Ephesus studied in Alexandria and practiced Medicine in Ephesus under the emperor Trajan (98 - 117 A. D.). In his treatise "*On the names of the parts of the human body*" he describes very clearly and carefully, besides many other parts, the ureters, the seminal ducts, the prostate gland, the uterus and its tubes. Moreover, he realised that the pulse is the result of the systole and not of the diastole, as always maintained by all the former authors. The work "*On the diseases of the kidneys and bladder*" was particularly appreciated by the following authors. In it Rufus describes quite correctly the inflammation and suppuration of the kidneys, the renal calculi, the haematuria, the disease that he calls "*diarrhoea of the urines*" and perhaps is diabetes; the cystitis, the stones and tumors in the bladder. In his treatise "*On satyriasis and gonorrhoea*" he describes perfectly the spermatic arteries and

lun] 伤寒杂病论 "Treatise on Febrile and Miscellaneous Diseases" which was published in 217 AD The original having been lost, the one handed down to the present was compiled by **[wang shu he] 王叔和 Wang Shuhe** in the third century AD The work does not, as the name implies, deal with typhoid fever alone, but with other diseases as well. The work is divided into six parts, each one corresponding to the six pairs of **[jing mai] 经脉 "meridians or channels"**, e.g. Taiyang, Yangming, Shaoyang, Taiyin, Shaoyin ang Jueyin. The section dealing with illness of Taiyin is the most elaborate.

Concerning treatment, Zhang recommended two of his favorite drugs. One is a decoction of **[gui zhi] 桂枝 "Cinnamomum cassia"**. Another is **[chai hu] 柴胡 "Bupleurum Falcatum"**. When the patient shivers with fever, breathes heavily and feels nauseous, a decoction of Cinnamomum cassia is used. To sweat or not to sweat was considered very important to his point, thus many indications for or against inducing sweating being given. Zhang was perhaps the first to employ enemas for evacuate the bowels. The directions for preparing the enema are given thus: Secure a large pig's gall; mix the bile with a little vinegar. Take a bamboo tube 3 or 4 inches long, insert half of it into the rectum and pour in the mixture.

Another book is **[jin kui yao lue fang lun] 金匮要略论 "Synopsis of prescriptions of the Golden Chamber"**. It deals with miscellaneous diseases. In his books, he described with detail about the defective ejaculation, cold semen, thin seminal fluid or deficiency of sperm due to hypo function of the kidney, which leads to sterility, veins, the epididymis, the seminal ducts and maintains quite correctly that the sperm is elaborated by the testicles and start from them, and not from the epididymis, which is not at all directly connected with the spermatic veins and arteries. This most important observation was ignored by all the anatomo-physiologists of the following centuries until Andreas Vesalius made it again and finally in 1543.

SORANUS of Ephesus 98 - 138 A. D.) was the greatest among ancient gynaecologists. His treatise "*On the diseases of women*" was the standard work of the later fifteen centuries. It is particularly noteworthy his description of the uterus that in the woman is "*like the cupping-glass of the physicians*" and, therefore, not at all double or "*two-horned*" as it is in the other animals and as it was believed to be until the XVI century. He speaks astonishingly near the truth about menstruation, fertility, the symptoms of pregnancy, the pre-natal cares, the care of the baby, the dysmenorrhea and the hemorrhages of the uterus. He maintains that uninterrupted virginity is not bad for women, because "*they become more strong and resistant against the diseases*", and describes many diseases of the external genital apparatus, like condylomas and gonorrhoea.

GALENUS CLAUDIUS (119 c. - 199). He was the greatest physician after Hippocrates and his anatomo-physiological, pathological and therapeutic system dominated on all the Western Medicine for more than 15 centuries. He gave a final assessment to the Hippocratic theories on the four

nocturnal emission and dysuria, etc..

Generally speaking, before the Han dynasty, treatment was chiefly confined to acupuncture, moxa, massage and medical draughts. Medical writing was entirely philosophical. With the advent of Zhang Zhongjing a new era was inaugurated. Diseases were studied more from a clinical standpoint, emphasis being laid on the physical signs, symptoms and course of an illness, the methods of treatment and the action of drugs rather than on the theories of the diseases. According to **[tao hong jing] 陶弘景 Tao Hongjing**, an authority on materia medica, states that "Zhang Zhongjing's book is the first treatise on treatment". The celebrated surgeon **[hua tuo**] **华佗 Huatuo** described it as a "real life-saving book".

Zhang Zhongjing had an unusual opportunity for studying of fevers, especially typhoid. At that time, people in his native village suffered from typhoid, as a result, seventy percent died. He was deeply impressed by this terrible epidemic that he devoted his time and energy to this particularly malady. Years of hard working produced him the immortal work. **[shang han lun] 伤寒论 "Essay on Typhoid"**. He lamented the ignorance and credulity of the general public concerning medical matters. He not only showed his keen power of observation but also gave the medical profession a high conception of its dignity and its noble mission in life. After his death, there appeared a big gap nearly one thousand years in medical filed due to the scientific medicine degeneration into dogmatic formalism.

Hua Tuo 华佗 (?-203 AD), the most famous surgeon, who is often

humours (blood, phlegm, yellow and black bile), the four qualities (hot, cold, dry and moist) and tried to explain every biological and physiological phenomenon as due to four fundamental "virtues" (attractive, retentive, transformative and expulsive) of each part of the body. So, for instance, the nutriments elaborated by the stomach, were attracted by the bowels, where they were kept and transformed into chyle and finally expelled towards the liver, which, in turn, attracted the chyle, kept and transformed it into venous blood, to expel it finally through the veins, etc. Moreover, he formulated the theory of the "three spirits" (natural, in the liver; vital, in the heart; animal, in the brain), but didn't have even the palest idea of the circulation of blood (as nobody else, until Harvey discovered it in the XVII century). Nevertheless Galen was the greatest anatomist before Andreas Vesalius.

As for urology, andrology (and sexology) Galen made the mistake (which Aristotle did before him) of maintaining the right kidney to be higher than the left (a mistake that was corrected only in the XVI century by Juan Valverde and Realdo Colombo), but discovered (perhaps on the way paved by Herophilus and Erasistratus) the prostate gland, the seminal vesicles and the seminal ampullae and described perfectly (as Aristotle had already done about five centuries before him) the epididymis and the seminal ducts. He thought that the female uterus was two-horned, that the woman too produce and secrete a sort of sperm, which partly contributes to the formation of the embryo; as females are cold and moist, as every left part in the body, while

worshipped as "the God of Surgery". According to **[hou han shu] 后汉书 "History of the Later Han"**, written in the fifth century AD, Hua Tuo was born somewhere about 190 AD, in the romantic period of **[san guo] 三国 "Three Kingdoms"** and had his education in **[xu zhou] 徐州 Xuzhou , [jiang su] 江苏 Jiangsu province**. He turned down offers from various eminent persons to take up an official career, choosing medicine instead Legend has it that he was fond of traveling, roaming over mountains and hills. During the course of his travels he cured the people along the way and gained medical knowledge. Numerous anecdotes concerning him still circulate today. It is said that he used very few drugs in his prescriptions and was so accurate in dispensing that he never took the trouble to weigh the ingredients. In acupuncture, he only punctured a few spots. He was also very accurate in diagnosis and could give a precise predication about the result of the diseases. Hua Tuo's fame rests chiefly on his discovery of the use of analgesics and his marvelous skill as a surgeon. He is said to have performed many operations including abdominal section with herbal anesthesia. Hou Hanshu recounts that Hua Tuo perfected an anaesthetic known as **[ma fei san] 麻沸散** (san means powder of opium), which the patient took dissolved in a fermented beverage. He used this anaesthetic in carrying out incisions of the abdomen, the first known case of laparatomy in the history of Chinese surgery. Hua Tuo is considered the first to use the blossom of a solanaceous plant **[man tuo luo] 蔓陀罗** as an analgesic (the narcotic effects of certain plants were known some time before males are hot and dry, as every right part of the body, he agreed with both Hippocrates and Aristotle that males form into the right horn of the uterus and from the sperm starting from the right testicle, and females into the left horn and from the sperm starting from the left testicle. He wrote more than 400 treatises, about 120 of which have been preserved. The most important are: *De usu partium* (On the utility of the parts), in 17 books; *Anatomicae administrationes* (On anatomical procedures), in 15 books (half of which preserved in the original Greek text and half in an Arabian translation by Hunayn and Hubaysh); *De naturalibus facultatibus* (On the natural faculties), in 3 books.

ARETAEUS of Cappadocia (150 *c.* - 200 *c.* A. D.) was the most important representative of the *Pneumatic School* and built his doctrines on the solid foundation of Archigenes (quoted above). His treatises "*On surgery*" and "*On female's diseases*" were appreciated for a long time and his descriptions of many diseases (diphtheria, tetanus, pneumonia, pleurisy, epilepsy, etc.) have become classic and remain insuperable. He was surely the first to describe clearly and perfectly the diabetes.

HELIODORUS, probably from Egypt, a very skilful and famous surgeon belonging to the *Pneumatic School*. He was the first to describe the uretral stenosis (or prostate hypertrophy) as "carunculae" (caruncles) and to remove them by an astonishing modern surgical operation. He also described and performed the dilatation of the urethra

Huatuo). It is used today in traditional Chinese medicine to soothe tracheitis, stomach-pain, toothache and arthralgia. He was the first to recommend therapeutic gymnastic called **[wu qin xi] 五禽戏 Wu Qin Xi "Frolics of Five Animals"**. It consisted of adopting the position of a tiger about to leap, of turning the head like a deer, standing erect like a bear, jumping on tiptoe like a monkey, and stretching the arms like a bird flying. It removes diseases, strengthens the legs and ensures health. The book **[zhong zang jing] 中藏经 "Treasures Classic"** is ascribed to him but it is in fact compiled by an unknown author during **[liu dai] 六代 "Six Dynasties"**. The book includes 49 articles on diagnosis and treatment, pulse, internal organs, deficiency and excessiveness syndromes, cold and heat syndromes, etc., as well as a list of prescriptions, which are particularly in the treatment of imbalance between Yin and Yang, menopathy, sterility in both male and female, impotence, dermatitis of scrotum, etc. A long list of his marvelous cures of strange diseases is recorded in the historical works dealing with that period. This including all sorts of operations, which range from venesection and acupuncture to laparotomy, excision of spleen, intestines and liver. But it is a great pity that in spite of his great discovery of the use of anaesthetics, Chinese surgery has never had a chance to develop, on account of the Confucian dogma, which holds the body to be sacred and not to be mutilated in any way. With such concepts and traditions it could hardly be expected that any progress could be made in anatomy and physiology. Without such fundamental	by copper, tin and lead sounds, but chiefly by a particular sound made of papyrus.

knowledge, no operation even the simplest one could be performed with real success. Since Hua Tuo, there is no record of further use of effective powder or other substances to cause anaesthesia, nor mention any surgeon who dared attempt major operations. **220-589 AD the Chinese "Middle Ages"** From the fall of **[han]** 汉 **"Han Dynasty"** to the succession of **[sui] 隋 "Sui Dynasty"**, China underwent 400 years. Then China was under the control of **[san guo] 三国 "Three Kingdoms"**, which was **[wei shuhan wu] 魏 蜀汉 吴** (200-280AD) At this time some dominant persons emerged, such as **[cao cao] 曹操 Caocao**, who is the founder of **[wei] 魏 "Wei Kingdom"**. Then followed by **[xijin] 西晋 Xijing** (265 – 317 AD) and **[dong jin] 东晋 Dongjing** (317-420 AD), one of the five Dynasties that ruled over the Southern China until 589 AD while North China was under the control of Northern Wei Dynasty. It is called **[nan bei cao] 南北朝 "Southern and Northern Dynasties"** in Chinese history. During this period, China was warlike, no elitist, and almost illiterate. There existed another impact on medical culture, Daoism and Buddhism. There are three great religions in China: Daoism, Confucianism and Buddhism, the last one was transplanted from India. Healing and religion are always related so that they can react on each	

other in many ways. From the end of Han to the Northern and Southern Dynasties, Taoists persevered with their quest for longevity. Their founder is **[zhang dao ling] 张道凌 also-called [tian shi] 天师 "Heavenly Teacher",** popularly known to foreigners as the Taoist pope, composed a book of charms for the curing of diseases and expelling of demons.

The legends have it that Zhang refused the offer of the emperors into the service of the state, he retired to seclusion in the great mountains, and there he devoted himself to the study of alchemy. His search for the elixir of life was successful, at the age of 123, after compounding and swallowing the grand elixir, he ascended to the heaven to enjoy the bliss of immortality.

Similar to the conditions existed in Europe in the 15th and 16th centuries, the search for the elixir of life reached its height during the **[tang] 唐 "Tang Dynasty"**. Daoism, medicine and alchemy are influenced each other. Magicians, doctors and alchemists everywhere tried to carry out experiments with herbs and minerals in an attempt to discover a substance, which could give everlasting life and beauty after people drink it. **[lian dan shu] 炼丹术 "Art or technique of purifying cinnabar"** was highly developed, and promoted the development of pharmaceutical science.

Among the host of herbs supposed to possess the remarkable power of conferring immortality , the cypress and the pine hold the first place. The seeds and resin are highly valued. The minerals such as cinnabar, gold, silver, jade, talc, were considered to be able to prolong life.

Another product of Daoism that influences medicinal development is the art of deep breathing.
Qi is the foundation of life: "long, deep breathing" and "physical and breathing exercises and massage" could regulate Qi; "Normalizing breathing with mind at the still state and attention concentrated with eyes closed" could maintain Qi., etc. With gradual practice, one could keep fit and health.

The second great influence exerted on medicine was the introduction of Buddhism from India about 67 AD It influenced great branches of learning, art, science, mathematics, astronomy and medicine. According to Buddhism, "Humanity suffers from two kinds of afflictions: physical and mental. For physical ailments the drugs of Ben Cao will be effective but for the mental affections noting but Buddhist remedies is required". Once Buddha told one of the physicians: "You go and heal his body first , I will come later to treat his mental sufferings". It is said that faith-healing, hypnotism, autosuggestion and other psychotherapeutic measures mostly originated from Buddhism. The art of **[zuo shan] 坐禅 "Meditation"** was also practiced. It is a system of mental exercises, which can lead the mind to be relaxed. It is considered the gateway of health, the highroad to immortality.

Another contribution by Buddhism is the system of physical exercises commonly known as **[quan] 拳 "Boxing". Bodhidarma or [da mo] 达摩** was an ardent advocate of the principle of “A sound mind in a sound body. He is said to have sat for nine years with his face to wall, wrapped in meditation. **[shi ba luo han quan] 十八罗汉拳** which is practiced by the monks at Shao Lin monastery, was attributed to him. Even the Taoist writing were frequently viewed and studied by Buddhist, which is clearly evident in the case of **[tao hong jing] 陶弘景 Tao Hongjing**. One of his medical works evoked the Buddhist concept of the 101 ailments.

The Doctrine of the Pulse

Traditional Chinese medicine has always attached to examination of the pulse, but the art of pulse feeling is a most mysterious and misunderstood subject. Chinese physicians assert that the entire superstructure of medical practice is built upon the theory of the pulse-the nature, location, course and treatment of every disease depends on this. The exact date when feeling of the pulse to locate diseases originated in China is unknown. It is said that [bian que] 扁鹊 Bianque was the first exponent of this idea. **Wang Shuhe 王叔和(265-317 AD),** a court physician is generally acknowledged as the greatest authority. Drawing from the experience of his predecessors, Wang Shuhe compiled **[mai jing] 脉经 "Pulse Classic"**, which brought together all the knowledge accumulated in this area since the compilation of "Huangdi Neijing". 24 kinds of pulse were described and differentiated, among which we have e.g. **[fu]** 浮 "floating", **[hua]** 滑 "Smooth", **[jin]** 紧 "tense", **[shen]** 深 "deep", **[wei]** 微"faint", **[se]** 涩"uneven", **[xi]** 细"fine", **[ruo]** 弱"weak", **[huan]** 缓 "moderate" etc. Maijing also refers to the three radial positions for examining the pulse: the anterior pulse **[cun]** 寸"inch", the middle pulse **[guan]** 关 "bar", and the posterior pulse **[chi]** 尺 "cubit". As Chinese doctors lay great stress on the pulse, Maijing is regarded as one of the outstanding works on medicine.

Huangfu Mi 皇甫谧(215-282 AD) , a literary man, suffering from rheumatism, turned to study medicine and became a famous acupuncturist and compiled the book **[Zhen Jiu Jia Yi Jing] (about 259 AD) 针灸甲乙经 "A Classic of Acupuncture and Moxibustion" or "Systematic Classic of Acu-moxi-therapy**", the book consists of 12 volumes and is divided into 123 chapters. It is a special treatise on acupuncture and moxa, in which the names and number of points of each meridian and their exact locations are defined. The work outlines the theory and nature of the meridians (the twelve regular channels and the eight extraordinary channels) with the traditional concepts of anatomy and physiology. The technique of manipulating the needles is mentioned as the clinical application of acupuncture and moxibustion and the art of acupuncture are explained minutely.

III Century AD

Ge Hong 葛洪(283-343 AD), more popularly known as [**ge zhi chuang**] **葛稚川 Ge Zhichuang**, a famous physician. He was a native in [jiang su] 江苏 Jiangsu Province. When he was young, his father died. He began to study Confucian in his early age and at the age of twenty he was introduce to alchemy by a disciple of his great-uncle. As an alchemist and Taoist Adept in search of drugs to prolong life, his experiment paved the way for the development of chemical pharmacy. With the desire to prolong human life and the idea of

III Century AD

A little number of very modest followers of Galen lived and wrote during this century, among whom one is only worthy to be remembered:

QUINTUS SERENUS Most probably he must be identified with the poet **Quintus Serenus Sammonicus**, one of the friends of the emperor Gordianus I (born in 159 AD c.). He was the master of the Emperor Gordianus II (192c.-235c.). chapter XXIV of his *Liber Medicinalis* (Medical Book) deals with lumbago and pains of the kidneys, while

nourishing the vital principle, he made many experiments. He not only worked with cinnabar, the principal substance for Chinese alchemists, but also with many other minerals such as realgar, sulphur, steatite, saltpeter, alum, lodestone, mica, iron, and tin. He is the author of **[bao pu zi] 抱朴子**, also his pseudonym, "A treatise on Alchemy, Dietetics and Some Magical practices", in which details of his experiments were described, including many valuable descriptions records about diseases as well as their treatments. Besides mineral drugs, some medicinal plants he mentioned are still used today: the resin of the conifer, the rhizome of the rhemannia glutinosa, rhizomes of the Coptis chinesis etc. Being an ardent Taoist Ge Hong devoted much of his time to experimenting with the elixir of life. In his book **[zhou hou bei ji fang] 肘后备急方 "A Handbook of Prescription for Emergencies"**, he intended to try every possible means to give a quick and cheap cure. He also recommended therapeutic measures such as acupuncture and moxibustion, including massage and cure by fumigation. The lists of the diseases mentioned in his books are typhoid, dysentery, malaria, erysipelas, smallpox, leprosy and cholera. Sometimes the symptoms are arbitrarily described. Preventive measures were another of his concerns, he used prophylactic drugs and the quarantine of the patients to deal with contagious diseases. **Gong Qingxuan** 龚庆宣, a surgeon and expert in **[nan bei chao] 南北朝 "Northern and Southern Dynasties"** (317-617AD) who compiled the book **[liu juan zi gui yi fang] 刘涓子鬼遗方**	Chapter XXXI with therapy of the bladder and of bladder stones. Serenus suggests only pharmacological therapy and doesn't make even the palest hint to surgical operations.

"Remedies Left Over by Ghosts", the earliest extant medical book on surgery which recorded the procedures carried out by a certain Liu Juanzi. The book provides a lot of information on the experience gained up to the fifth century, e.g. the treatment of wounds caused by metal instruments, ailments affecting the skin, boils, anthrax and abscesses. Mercurial ointment was used in the cure of skin diseases.	
IV –V Century AD	**IV-V Century AD**
Tao Hongjing 陶弘景 (456-536AD), a native a Jiangsu, he had numerous interests which led him to study medicine, astronomy and geography. He is especially renowned as the author of **[Ben Cao Jing Ji Zhu] 本草经集注 "Commentary on Sheng Nong's Herbal"**, which revised and annotated, increasing the number of herbal drugs and compiling one of the most valuable books on materia medica in China, describing 730 varieties of medical substances including vegetable, animal and mineral drugs. From the Taoist point of view , he discussed a great deal on the principles of health preservation and their concrete implementation, and put forward the various taboos in preserving health in his book **[Yang Xing Yan Ming Lu] 养性延命录 "Recordings of the Art of Health and life Preservation"**, including many forms of [qi gong] 气功 "Qi Gong" exercises e.g. physical and breathing exercises, expiration and inspiration and massage etc. Chinese Dao school pays great attention to the close relationship between mental activities and health: "Integrating spirit with body" is its	**MARCELLUS EMPIRICUS** was born probably in Bordeaux. In 388 was appointed Archiater and minister of Theodosius the Great (395 AD). He wrote a treatise entitled *De Medicamentis* (On Drugs), having chiefly Scribonius Larus as source. Like by Scribonius, many drugs are listed by Marcellus for the cure of affections and pains of the kidneys, affections and pains of the bladder, dysuria, stranguria and anuria, incontiunence of urine, stones in the kidney, stones in the bladder and haematuria. He made also some additions of his own, but he draws inspiration from magic and spells, and therefore tells nothing but nonsense. **ORIBASIUS** (325 - 403 a. d.). He was a famous but not at all original physician, who wrote - among many other works - the *Collectiones medicae* (Collections of Medicine) (in 50 books). This very ample anthology of passages chiefly from Galen but also from a lot of other Authors whose works have been lost, is the main source whence we can get some information about Physicians and Anatomists who would be ignored otherwise. He never quotes any surgical

established theory, which puts stress on the guiding position of regulation of the spirit in health care. **[jing] 精** "Essence" **[qi] 气** "Vital energy", **[shen] 神** "Spirit" are regarded as three treasures of one's life, granting longevity as well as resistance to diseases if they are conserved and cultivated.	operation for the extraction of the bladder stones that means that this operation was no longer performed by physicians at his times, but was a matter only for craftsmen.
VI century AD	**VI Century AD**
In [sui] 隋 "Sui Dynasty" (589-681), the government began to organize the cultivation of the drugs. E.g. three hundred **[mu]** 亩 (Chinese acre or one-sixth English acre) of fertile land were located at the capital for the purpose of cultivating drugs. Young people from sixteen to twenty years of age were assigned to study as apprentices. After they finished their study, they were promoted as keepers of the farm with the restored kinal plants, gather them in the right season, and as **[yao yuan shi] 药园师 "Keeper of the Drug Farms"**. Their duties were to cultivate them in the proper places. **Xu Zhicai 徐之才** (505-572AD), a well-known physician in the Northern and Southern Dynasties, who was especially proficient in preparation of drugs and made a great contribution to pharmacology with his new classification of the action of drugs. In his book **[Yao Dui] 药对 "Pharmacy and Compatibility"** on the basis of **[lei gong yao dui] 雷公药对 "Lei's Pharmacy and Compatibility"**, he divides them in ten categories: **[xuan] 宣** "Carminatives", **[tong] 通** "Diuretics", **[bu]** 补 "Tonics", **[xie] 泄** "Purgatives",	**AETIUS of AMIDA**, is the only great author of this century. He lived in the first half of the century. His great treatise *De medicina libri undecim* (Eleven books on Medicine) is a syncretistic compilation mainly inspired by Galen and Archigenes. He can be considered as the founder of systematic "uroscopy", which many pages of his work deal with. Aetius is not at all so original, but his work is important because it was considered - together with the work by Paulus of Egina - as a sort of "Bible of Medicine and Surgery" by the Arabs. **ALEXANDER OF TRALLES**. Was a contemporary of the Emperor Justinianus (527 - 565). His father was the Physician Stephanus and his brother was Antemius, the architect of St. Sophia's in Constantinople. Alexander practiced medicine in Rome. During the last years he wrote the great treatise *Therapeytiká* (The cures) in 12 books, in which he deals with a series of diseases under both the therapeutic and surgical aspect. He is chiefly an intelligent and very original practician and is as brave as to censure even Galen's doctrines. As for the urological diseases, he has an

[se] 涩 "Astringents", **[hua]** 滑 "Laxatives", **[zao]** 燥 "Diaphoretics", **[shi]** 湿 "Demulcents", **[qing]** 轻 "Alternatives" and **[zhong]** 重 "Sedatives". Later he added the other two, stimulants and antipyretics, forming the total 12. **[sui tang] 隋唐 Empires (589-907 AD)** **[sui] 隋 "Sui Dynasty"** came into power in 581 AD, titled **[sui wen di] 隋文帝 Sui Wendi**. Then peasant revolts led by **[li yuan] 李原 Liyuan** and his son **[li shi min]李世民 Li Shimin** overthrew **Sui** and founded **[tang] 唐 "Tang Dynasty"** under the name of **[tang gao zu] 唐高祖 Tang Gaozu** (618-626) and **[tang tai zhong] 唐太中 Tang Taizhong** respectively. The end of the 7th and the beginning of the 8th were under the control of **[wu ze tain] 五则 天** "conforming with heaven", she was described as China's "female Calamities". The 8th century belonged to the Emperor **[xuan zong] 旋宗 Xuanzong** (712-756 AD), called **[kai yuan] 开元 "Kaiyuan Period"** (713-741AD, one of the prosperity times during the history of China. In 755, the rebellion of **[an lu shan] 安庐山 An Lushan** brought this "golden age" to an end. During this period, medicine and pharmacy, underwent a rapid progress enriched by new experience. The Tang era has been described as China's "Second Classical Period". Chinese civilisation at this time attained one of its high peaks. It was a time when there was an extraordinary outburst of poetic talent and when Buddhist influence in China reached its zenith. Medicine and pharmacy, enriched by	absolute preference for the pharmacological cure against surgical operations.

new experience, witnessed a rapid growth during the Tang. Medical and pharmaceutical works during this period revealed the high level of development. Etiology and semiology were important achievement, which can be seen in **[chao yuan fang] 巢元方 Chao Yuanfang's [zhu bing yuan hou lun] 诸病源侯论 "Treatise on the Causes and Symptoms of Illness"**. The work discussed the risk of infection from wound as well as the causes for parasitic diseases such as tapeworm. At the same time, various preventive measures were adopted. Hospitals for lepers were established. The ways were sought to guard against rabies, smallpox and typhoid. On the pharmaceutical field, the Tang Dynasty was a rich period for **[ben cao] 本草 "treatises on herbal medicine"**. Here we have **[xin xiu ben cao] 新修本草 "Newly-revised Herbal Medicine"**, also known as [**tang ben cao] 唐本草 "Herbal Medicine of the Tang"**. With the flourishing of Tang, China also opened to foreign influence. So far as the exchanges with medicine and pharmacy is concerned, China's relationship with Japan, Korea, Vietnam, India and Persia brought about greater progress. China can be described as the medical center of Asia.	
VII Century AD	**VII Century AD**
Chao Yuanfang 巢元方 (550-630 AD), imperial physician of Emperor **Yangdi [yangdi] (炀帝)**. He is the most significant medical figure during Sui Dynasty, who took charge of the compilation of the well-known book **[Zhu Bing Yuan Hou Zoing Lun] 诸病源候总论 "General Treatise on the Etiology and Symptomatology of**	**PAUL OF AEGINA** (625c.-690c.) Studied in Alexandria and traveled through Greece and about all the Mediterranean Countries. The VII book of his treatise *Compendium medicinae* (Outline of Medicine), in 7 books, deals with surgery and gives a good description of the surgical operation on sufferers from stone in the

Diseases", writing about etiology and semiology. The book is in 50 volumes and is divided into 67 headings with 1720 chapters., which exerted a profound influence on the further development of Chinese medicine. The book deals with internal medicine, surgery, gynaecology, pediatrics, otorhinolaryngology, ophthalmology and dermatology. The book also gives details on infectious and contagious disease such as smallpox, measles, scarlet fever, tuberculosis and parasitic afflictions.

The formation of calculi in the body was also discussed. He spoke **[shui]** 水 "liquid" being transformed into **[shi]** 石 "stone"- what is known today as the formation of stony concretions in the bladder and urinary tract. In the book mentioned above, he classified abnormalities of micturition into **[lin zheng]** 淋症 "Lin Symptom Complex", which is mainly manifested by frequency of urination, urgency of urination, painful micturition or incontinence of urination. Such as **[shi lin]** 石淋 "stranguria due to urolithiasis"; **[qi lin]** 气淋 "stranguria due to disturbance of Qi"; **[lao lin]** 劳淋 "stranguria caused by overstrain"; **[gao lin]** 膏淋"stranguria with chyluria"; **[xue lin]** 血淋 "stranguria with haematuria" ; **[re lin]** 热淋"stranguria due to heat".

Sun Simiao 孙思邈(581-682 AD) a native of **[shan xi]** **山西** **Shanxi Province**, a prominent physician of [tang] 唐 "Tang Dynasty" and author of **[Qian Jin Yao Fang]** **千金药方** **"Prescriptions Worth a Thousand Gold"** (652 AD) and **[Qian Jin Yi Fang]** **千金翼方** **"Supplement to prescriptions Worth a Thousand**

bladder, but it is shorter and not at all different from the perfect description made by Celsus about five centuries before. The descriptions of the surgical operations on carcinoma, abscess of the liver, inguinal hernia and of the catheterism of the bladder are particularly interesting.

Notwithstanding that Paulus - like Aetius of Amida - was not at all original, but he is most important because he and Aetius were the first and the greatest intermediaries between the Graeco-Roman and the Arabian Medicine and Surgery.

THEOPHILUS PROTOSPATHARIUS: his name means "colonel of the Imperial Guard". Lived in Constantinople and was court Physician of the Emperor Heraclius (575-641). He wrote a valuable treatise on Anatomo-physiology, but his most famous works were the two treatises *De urinis* (On ruins), in which he organised finally the rules of "uroscopy" and expounded minutely the meanings of the various aspects of urine in the "matula", and *De pulsibus* (On pulses), that is nothing else than a summary of Galen's treatises on the argument. The *De urinis* was one of the foremost texts every medical student had to read and expound before his doctorate. He correctly maintained that the kidneys transformed the residue of the blood into urine and therefore have not only a "filtering", but also and chiefly a "transforming" function, that is to say that the kidneys are not at all simply passive, but are active organs as for diuresis.

Gold" (682 AD), which has been considered as an agglomeration of the medical achievements before the 7th century. In this work, more than 700 drugs were classified according to the origin: minerals, plants, animals, insects, fish, fruits, vegetables and cereals. His knowledge of medical substances, earned him the reputation "the king of medical herbs". Influenced by Confucianism, Daoism and Buddhism, he reflected his "humanistic" notions in his writing. He thought every good physician should study the Confucian Five Classis, including "Book of Changes" and the "Classic of Odes". If not, he will not follow the way of **[ren yi] 仁义** the virtues of benevolence and righteousness advocated by Confucius.

Sexuality, in fact, was one of the preoccupations of Chinese physicians at this period. Thus an entire section of the Qianjin Yaofang is devoted to sexual questions or "the art of the bedroom". According to Sun Simiao, people should follow regualr sexual life, and he writes taboos for sexual life: sexual intercourse with no tipsiness; sexual intercourse with no anger, terror and tiredness; sexual intercourse in usual weather (no thunderstorm, lightning or extreme coldness or hotness). In his book "Qianjin Yaofang", sexual activities and the "art of bed" were discussed: "A man must not engage in sexual intercourse merely to satisfy his lust. He must strive to control his sexual desire so as for be able to nurture his vital essence. He mustn't force his body to sexual extravagance in order to enjoy carnal pleasure giving rein to his passion".

In his books, he describes different kinds of diseases, such as **[shan qi] 疝气** "a collective term for diseases of the

external genitalia, testicles and scrotum"; abscess of scrotum; shrinkage of scrotum; the emission of seminal fluid during sleep and premature ejaculation; enuresis and difficulty of urination etc.. He thought a suitable treatment was the harmonious combination of acupuncture and drugs. **Su Jing** 苏敬 (500-674 AD), also known as Su Gong, a court official in the Tang Dynasty, who submitted a written statement to the Emperor Gaozong about the necessity of systematization of the herbals and was ordered by the Emperor to review traditional herbals with several others scholars and physicians. As a result of their hard work, in 659AD, **[Xin Xiu Ben Cao] 新修本草 "Newly Compiled Materia medica"** also-called **[tang ben cao] 唐本草 "The Tang Materia Medica"** was published as the first Official pharmacopoeia in China. It was the first Chinese official pharmacopoeia, preceding by eight or nine centuries the first pharmacopoeia in the west, such as the "Nuovo Receptario", which was published in Florence in 1498. The work describes the therapeutic qualities of about 850 drugs., and classifies them in nine categories according to the origins; minerals, herbaceous plants, trees, quadrupeds, birds, insects and fish, fruits, vegetables and cereals. Chinese pharmacy during the Tang Dynasty was further enriched with another text **[ben cao shi yi]** 本草拾遗 **"A Supplement to the Herbal"**, written in 10 volumes by **[chen cang qi] 陈藏器 Chen Cangqi,** who lived during the eighth century in the Tang Dynasty. The book further alluded to the omissions	

and even the errors in the works of Tao Hongjing and Su Jing.

VIII-IX Century AD

Wang Tao 王涛 (about 670-755AD), a distinguished physician of the Tang Dynasty. He compiled a book of his own, entitled **[Wai Tai Mi Yao] 外台秘要 "Medical Secrets of an Official"** (752 AD), in 40 volumes in which a comprehensive and exhaustive study of medicine is made with 1,104 issues of medical problems discussed and over 6,000 prescriptions recorded. There are over 30 prescriptions particularly in treating of stranguria. This magisterial work is a summary of all the fields explored by Chinese medicine from the origin to the eighth century: internal medicine, surgery, gynaecology, obstetrics, pediatrics, dermatology, orthopedics, otorhino-laryngology and ophthalmology. Wang Tao was particularly skillful in dealing with deficiency-induced illness; he recommended, for example, treating beriberi with plants rich in vitamin B1, such as plantain (Plantago asiatica). To cure goitre, he advised the use of algae such as sargasso, or gulf-weed (Sargassum pallidum; Sargassum fusiforme, and laminaria (Laminaria japonica), which is still used today.

Following in the footsteps of Sun Simiao, Wang Tao advocated the adoption of measure to ensure maternal and infant care, insisting that special attention has for be paid to the health of a pregnant women, particularly at the time of giving birth. Wai Tai Mi Yao

VIII-IX Century AD
The Arab medicine

During these centuries both Hippocratic and Galenic theories and doctrines migrate form the Western to the Middle-East countries where they met an exceptional favor. The works of the *Corpus hippocraticum* and Galen's main treatises were translated firstly directly form Greek into Syriac and Hebrew, then from Syriac and Hebrew into Arabic and only starting form the IX century directly from Greek into Arabic. These translations were very important, because the first translations into Latin of Hippocrates' and Galen's works were not at all made from the original Greek, but form the Arab text. So one can say that Graeco-Roman Medicine was inherited by Arabs, who brought it back to Western Europe, mainly through the great schools of Cordoba, Seville and Granada.

IOANNITIUS (Hunain Ibn Ishaq) (809-873/77). Translated directly form Greek into Arabic and expounded with very ample knowledge a lot of medical and philosophical works, most of all the main treatises of Galen. His son Ishaq and his nephew Hubaish continued his work.

Medical School of SALERNO:
The foundations of this most famous school were laid in these two centuries.

and Qian Jin Yao Fang both occupy an important place in the history of gynaecology and obstetrics in China. **JianZhen鉴真** (688-763AD) Jian Zhen was born at **[yang zhou] 扬州 Yangzhou**, he entered the monastic life when he was young and later traveled to **[changan] 长安 Chang An** and **[luoyang] 洛阳 Louyang,** the capital of old China, to study Buddhist doctrines, architecture, fine arts and medicine. His reputation became known by the Japanese Buddhist missionaries in Chang An, who invited him to Japan. Jianzhen had a great influence in Japan, especially in the field of medicine. When he became blind, he could recognise a medicinal plant by its odor, touch and taste. His medical knowledge, especially in the realm of phytotherapy, earned him reputation in Japan. The prosperity of Tang Dynasty brought China open to the foreign influences. The exchange of medicine and pharmacy with Japan, Korea, Vietnam, India and Persia enhanced great progress. The influence of Buddhism made people seek for the knowledge of India. And Arab medicine was able to borrow from China not only alchemy but also pulsology. From Persia , the relation between China and the Byzantine empire developed. **Zan Yin 昝殷**(about 797-860 AD), a specialist in women's diseases and author of **[Jing Xiao Chan Bao] 经效产宝 "Tested Treasures in Obstetrics"**, one of the earliest books on obstetrics existing today, which was written during 852-856 AD In the book diseases during pregnancy, at the time of parturition and	

after delivery are diagnosed and treated.	
XIV - XV century A. D. **The Ming Dynasty (1364-1644)** With the avent of the four famous doctors of **[jin yuan si da jia] 金元四大家** Jin and Yuan Dynasties, several innovations were introduced into ancient theory and medical art became divided into many schools, they were generally grouped under five main headings: 1. **[yang yin pai] 养阴派 "The Yin-nourishing school"**. The members were chiefly the followers of **[zhu dan xi] 朱丹溪 Zhu Danxi** who is well known for using the methods of nourishing Yin and relieving fire heat. They thought Yin was always insufficient and should be nourished by tonics. They were **[dai yuan li] 戴原礼 Dai Yuanli**, **[xu yong cheng] 徐用诚 Xu Yongcheng** and **[liu chun] 刘纯 Liu Chun** etc. 2. **[wen bu pai] 温补派 "The Warming and Invigorating School"**. They thought Yang Essence was the most important to life. It was easy to lose but difficult to get. So the doctors should always nourish the Yang Essence instead of killing it by cooling medicine. 3. **[gong xia pai] 攻下派 "The Purging School"**. They thought the pathogenic evil factors should be expelled and fevers should be reduced by appropriate measures by purging. **[wu you ke] 吴又可 Wu Youke**, one of the best exponents of	**XIV – XV century A. D** **PIETRO DELL'ARGELLATA** († 1423). He graduated in 1391 in Bologna where became professor of Anatomy. He was the greatest surgeon of his time and wrote *Chirurgiae libri VI* (Seven books on Surgery). Described ulcers and cystis of the bladder, ulcers of the penis, and pustules of venereal origin. He advised washing the penis with water in summer and with urine - to which he attributed great therapeutical properties - in winter. **GUARNERIO ANTONIO**. He flourished between the second half of the XIV and the first half of the XV century and graduated in Padua, where was appointed Professor to the University in 1412. Wrote a commentary on the IX book of the *Liber Almansoris* of Rhazes and a treatise *De mulierum affectionbus* (On the diseases of women). He tried to relieve the dramatic problem of urine retention due to bladder stones by turning his patients upside down and shaking them, but suggested also to have recourse to "*candelam subtilem ceraceam vel virgulam stanneam aut argenteam*"(either a subtle wax bougie, or a thin either tin, or silver bar) for the cure of urethrostenosis. **MARCELLUS OF CUMA** (XV century). He was one of the later disciples of Pietro dell'Argellata and described several and multiple ulcers of the penis, most probably due to syphilis.

the "purging school" adopted saltpetre and other drastic measures in his book **[wen bing] 瘟病** "On Plague", and **[zhang zi he] 张子和 Zhang Zihe**, who is well known for using purgative, diaphoretics and emetics.

4. **[xing gu pai] 信古派 "The Conservative School**".

Many Ming doctors thought the ancient medical literature had been lost and distorted by compilers and commentators. So their aim was for restore it as far as possible. **[miu xi yong] 缪希雍 Miu Xiyong**, **[fang you zhi] 方有执 Fang Youzhi** were among them.

5. **[zhe zhong pai] 折衷派 "The Moderate School"**. The members of this school had no particular ideas of their own, they simply selected all the good points from the previous writers. The two prominent moderates were **[ni wei de] 倪维德 Ni Weide** and [**wang ken tang] 王肯堂 Wang Kentang.**

A medical Encyclopaedia

[yong le da dian] 永乐大典 "Great Dictionary of the Yobgle Regin" was published in 1408, including 22,877 entries originally, only 795 survive today, seventy-two of which are of particular interest for medicine and pharmacy. It provides a clear idea about certain illness. E.g. the section on 'children's nosebleeds' contains a list of bibliographical references, citing the **[zhu bing yuan hou lun] 诸病原候论 "Treatise on the Causes and Symptoms of Illness"** by Cao Yuangfang and **[qian jin yao fang] 千金药方 "Prescriptions of the Thousand Ounces of Gold**" by Sun Simiao etc., and a description of a

NICOLAUS OF CUSA (or CUSANUS) (1400/1401 - 1464). He wrote books on Mathematics, Theology and Philosophy. In 1476 was published his treatise *De staticis experimentis* (Experiments with steelyard) in which he suggests to weigh water, blood and urine, in order to compare their weights in state of health and disease. With this treatise he paved the way to Santorio Santorio (1561 - 1636) and his treatise *De statica medicina* (On medicine with the steelyard).

number of remedies culled from various sources with extracts from various materia medica. It also brings together medical texts such as **[shang han lun] 伤寒论 "Treatise on Febrile Diseases"**, which has been richly annotated with commentaries by experts in Song Dynasty. **Hua Shou 滑寿** (1304-1386AD), author of a very useful treatise on acupuncture **[shi si jing fa hui] 十四经发挥 "Exposition of the fourteen meridians"**(1341 AD) and **[Nan Jing Ben Yi] 难经本义 "The genuine meaning of the difficult classic"** (1361 AD). **Lou Ying 楼英** (1332-1402AD), author of **[Yi Xue Gang Mu] 医学纲目"Compendium of medicine"**, in which diseases are classified into various types and categories according to Yin-Yang **Dai Sigong 戴思恭** (1324-1405 AD), a physician of the Ming Dynasty, court physician and president of the Imperial College of Physicians, he was the faithful follower and creative successor of Zhu Danxi. He wrote **[zheng zhi yao jue] 证治要诀 " Principles of Diagnosis and Treatment", [zheng zhi yao jue lei fang] 证治要诀类方 "Classified Prescriptions according to the Principle of Diagnosis and Treatment" and [tui qiu shi yi] 推求师意 " An Inquiry into the Master's Doctrine"**. With the description of aetiology, symptomatology and therapeutic measures to treat fifty illness, Zhu's theory of nourishing Yin was expounded. The first three sections of the book, entitled "Various Illness", described the afflictions during the fourteenth century:	

malaria, diabetes, abnormal elimination of urine, sore throat, cough, urticaria, tuberculosis, haemoptysis, palsy, gonorrhoea, dysuria, diarrhoea, dysphagia and arthralgia.

Another interesting example concerned ejaculation of semen during sleep. It described the case of a twenty-year-old insomnia. And various methods of treatment were recommended to treat the involuntary emission of sperm. There is a section dealing with gynaecology and obstetrics, including an account of the foetus, gradual formation of its shape, and a method to determine the sex of foetus.

Xiong Zongli 熊宗立, a physician of the Ming Dynasty, author of **[ming fang lei yi shu da quan] 名方类证医书大全 " A complete medical work of proved recipes"**, also-called **[yi shu da quan] 医书大全 " A complete work of medical books"**(1446 AD

XV - XVI century AD

Han Mao 韩懋 a physician of the Ming Dynasty, author of **[han shi yi tong] 韩氏医通 "Han's Book on Medicine"** (1522 AD), in which the importance of the four methods of diagnosis in the treatment of diseases is stressed and improvement in case history is made.

Syphilis is motioned in several medical works of the time, but **Wang Ji 汪机** (1463-1539 AD) was one of the bests to deal with syphilis. According to his view of no external treatment without internal treatment, he combined the use of decoctions and ointments and prescribed a decoction of the four rulers

XV - XVI century AD

JOHANNES ARCULANUS (1419 - 1484). He was born in Verona and was appointed Professor to the University of Bologna, where taught Logic, Moral Philosophy and Medicine. From Bologna he moved to Padua and then to Ferrara, where taught Medicine and died. The *Expositio noni libri Almansoris* (An exposition of the 9th book of Almansur, by Rhazes), published in 1480, is the most famous of his works. In 1483 a new treatise was published, *Practica medica* (Medical practice), that contained another commentary to the IX book of Rhazes, with the description of syringes and flexible catheters He discovered that lesions in the *cervix*

(Panax ginseng, Atractylodes macrocephela, Poria cocos and Glycyrrhiza uralensis) to increase vital energy. He also applied an ointment from the golden and silver flower on the patient's ulcers. His decoction of the eight precious ingredients is still used today in TCM as a tonic for energy and for the blood. He is the author of several medical books such as **[zhen jiu wen da] 针灸问答 " Catechism of Acupuncture and Moxibustion " (1530 AD)**, which is clear, simple and kept to essentials, and is very useful for beginners, **[wai ke li li] 外科理例 "Surgery with Illustrations" (1531AD) and [Yi Xue Yuan Li] 医学原理 " Principles of Medicine"**, etc. Wang Ji was not only engaged in fighting against syphilis, he was also skilled in acupuncture and surgical practice. He thought surgical instrument should not be used excessively, on the other hand one should not hesitate to operate if it was absolutely necessary.

Xue Ji 薛己 (about 1487-1559 AD), a famous physician, one of the forerunners of the "Warming and Invigorating School". Xue Ji began his medical career as a specialist in skin diseases, then through various medical practice he became a physician with high reputation and was able to deal with all kinds of diseases in internal medicine, surgery, gynaecology, paediatrics etc.

He compiled many medical works such as **[Nu Ke Cuo Yao] 女科撮要 "Essentials of Obstetrics and Gynecology"** (1548AD). His and his father's works were edited by [**wu guan**] **吴官 Wu Guan** and entitled **[xue shi yi an] 靴氏医案 "Xue's medical Records"**, which consists of 24 books such as **[wai ke shu yao] 外科枢要 "Essential of** *vesicae* caused retention of urine.

NORCINES and PRECIANS. A long series of surgical craftsmen who practiced between the XV and the XVII century, and performed surgical operations on sufferers from bladder stones, cataract, hernia and toothache. They came from Norcia and the burg of Preci and practiced almost regularly epicystotomy, preceding Pierre Franco (who was given the credit for inaugurating such an operation) by more than a century.

LEONARDO DA VINCI (1452 - 1519). He made a lot of anatomical drawings from autopsies, which he had to perform in great secret, to avoid the dangers and the punishments he would have incurred. He is said to have been the renewer of Anatomy and the founder of modern Anatomo-physiology, but in fact he did nothing else than illustrate - albeit with masterly skill - the descriptions of Galen, or rather of Mondino de' Liuzzi , whose mistakes he repeats, though clearly in contrast with the results of his autopsies. So he puts erroneously the right kidney higher than the left, according with both Galen (whose works he surely had not read!) and Mondino; he draws the cornea as a continuation of the dura mater, repeating the mistake made by Galen and Mondino; he draws the "*rete mirabile*" (wonderful net), or "*arbor vitae*" (life's tree) that Galen and Mondino describe above the cerebellum, and which doesn't exist at all. Although he made some discoveries, they had no meaning for the progress of Anatomy: since he didn't ever publish any of the results of his anatomical studies, he

Surgery" (1571 AD), etc.

Xue Ji's therapy was based essentially on the principle of invigorating spleen and kidneys with remedies. E.g. he recommended many herbal drugs belong acting upon the spleen meridian; **[gui pi tang] 归脾汤 "decoction of drugs acting on the spleen"** was one of them. There was also a decoction to treat inappetence and fatigue, a decoction to regularise the Middle Jiao and increase energy. He also used the decoction of the hare's ear (a species of bupleurum) to treat the case of man who felt pain in his penis and who complained of urinary problems accompanied sometimes by itching.

Zhao Xianke 赵献可, a physician of Ming Dynasty. He was considered as the supreme master of the **[wen bu]** 温补 "Warming up and Invigorating" school. Xue Ji mentioned above was its founder. Zhao Xianke expanded on the teachings of Xue Ji to formulate the theory of the **[ming men]** 命门 "Gate of Life". According to Zhao, it was not the heart that governed the body but the "Gate of Life". The intensity or the weakness of "fire" corresponded with the expansion or diminution of energy. Insisting on the dual relationship between water and fire, Yin and Yang, he maintained that in order to strengthen the body, the physician had only to nourish the Yin and Yang - water and fire. His famous **[ba zhen dan] 八珍单 "The Pill of Eight ingredients" and[liu zhen dan] 六珍单 "The Pill of Six Ingrediants"** were used to reinvigorate fire and reinvigorate water respectively.

Wang Luan 王銮 a pediatrician in the 16th century, author of **[you ke lei**

caused no advance whatsoever. His famous *Quaderni Anatomici* (Notes on Anatomy) were only finally discovered at the end of the XIX century, and published at the beginning of our century.

BENIVIENI ANTONIO (1440 *c.* - 1502). His treatise *De abditis nonnullis ac mirandis morborum et sanationum causis* (On some hidden and wonderful causes of disease and recovery) was published by his brother Girolamo in 1507. This is the first treatise on pathological anatomy ever published. In it Benivieni describes the muscle fibres and the sphincter of the bladder (which Galen had already discovered), and observes (as Galen had done) that the oblique entry of the ureters into the bladder have been provided by Nature in order to prevent the reflux of urine.

DA VIGO GIOVANNI (1450 c. - 1525) was born in Rapallo and was the son of the famous lithotomist Battista da Rapallo. Practiced in Saluzzo and Savona and was appointed personal surgeon of the Cardinal Giuliano della Rovere, the future Pope Giulio II. From then on he lived in Rome, where published his famous *Practica in arte chirurgica copiosa continens novem libros* (Ample practice of surgery in nine books). He described the wounds from firearms for the first time and suggested the use of mercurial ointments in the cure of syphilis. Though he doesn't add anything to what his predecessors in the field of urological surgery, had already said, he is important because was one of the masters of Mariano Santo (1488 - 1565 *c.*).

cui] 幼科类萃 "Collection of Pediatric Cases " (1534AD), a comprehensive work summarizing the current knowledge on the subject, in which each ailment was dealt with according to pulse diagnosis, method of treatment, acupuncture and prescriptions.

Lu He 卢和 a distinguished herbalist in the 16th century, author of **[shi wu ben cao] 食物本草 "Dietary Materia Medica"**, in which Lu gave explanations on the laxative value of vegetables and their good effect on the health of man. He advocated vegetable diet and advised that meat should be eaten sparingly.

Sun Yikui 孙一奎 (1520-1600 AD), author of **[chi shui xuan zhu] 赤水玄珠 " Black Pearl of the Red River", [Yi Zhi Xu Yu] 医旨绪余 "Supplement to Principles of Medicine" and [Yi An] 医案 "Medical Records"**, in which he advocated the combination of various schools and maintained that a doctor should be conversant with all the theories in order to master the whole art of healing, and his chief aim should be the conquest of all diseases.

Xu Chunfu 徐春甫 lived in the 16th century and was the author of **[gu jin yi tong da quan] 古今医同大全 "A Complete Work of Ancient and Modern Medicine"** (1556 AD), in which rich and valuable materials in various fields of medicine were accumulated. Xu warned that healthy people should avoid company of patients with consumptive diseases, mainly pulmonary tuberculosis.

Li Yan 李延 a physician of the

BERENGARIUS OF CARPI (1470 - 1530) was one of the greatest anatomists of his time and, together with Bartholomaeus Eustachi, Gabriele Falloppio and Ieronymus Fabrici (or Fabricius) of Acquapendente, was the real renewer of the anatomical studies and the founder of modern Anatomy. He wrote *Carpi commentaria cum amplissimis additionibus super Anatomia Mundini una cum textu eiusdem in pristinum et verum nitorem redacto* (Commentaries of Carpi on Mundinus' Anatomia, with very ample additions and the text of the work brought back to its former and true correctness), printed in Bologna in 1521. Injecting water through the vena emulgens, Berengarius discovered that the liquid - which, obviously, followed the same route of urine - did not flow directly into the pelvis, but accumulated into the substance of the kidney. By dissecting the kidney (surely the kidney of a pig) from the convex side, he discovered the papillae through which the water percolated into the pelvis. He also described the seminal vesicles, already discovered by Herophilus, clearly described by Galen but forgotten for centuries and defined by Berengarius "*sperm receptacles*".

SANTO MARIANO (1488 - 1565) was born in Barletta (Puglia region) and studied Surgery in Rome at the *S. Maria della Consolazione* Hospital under the guidance of Giovanni da Vigo (or di Vico), Giovanni de Romanis and Giovanni Antracino. Worked in Rome, Milan, Ragusa, Hungary and Venice. Was appointed Teacher of Surgery in Rome and Venice and was military

16th century who summarized the prescriptions used in that period in medical practice and divided them into 18 different kinds. He was the author of **[yi xue ru men] 医学入门 "Elementary Medicine" (1575AD) and [xi yi gui ke] 习医规格 "Rules for Medical Study"** (1575AD)

Li Lian 李濂 (1489-1569?AD, a literary man in the Ming Dynasty. He wrote **[yi shi] 医史 "History of medicine"** (1513 AD). It is said that the earliest work on medical history was **[li dai ning yi shi ming] 历代名医姓名 "Names of Famous Physicians"** by **[gan bo zong] 甘伯宗 Gan Bozong** (923-936 AD), but this book existed only in name. Li Lian's book consisted of 10 volumes and contained the names of 65 persons, recording the lives of distinguished physicians. Li was the earliest biographer of ancient medical professionals.

Li Shizhen 李时珍 (1518-1593AD), also-called **[li dong bi] 李东壁 Li Dongbi** or **[li bin hu] 李濒湖 Li Binhu**, a great physician and naturalist. He was a native of Qi Zhou, **[hu bei] 湖北 Hubei province**. His father **[li yan wen] 李延文 Li Yanwen** was an accomplished medical practitioner. Carrying on his father's profession, Li concentrated his mind on medical studies and his medical skill gained a wide acknowledgment by his contemporaries. At the age of thirty he began his researches on medicine and for forty years he devoted all his time to these studies. With a wide knowledge he felt dissatisfied with the **[ben chao] 本草 "Materia Medica"** of his time, particularly because of the confusion of nomenclature. He undertook a close and

Surgeon during the war of the emperor Charles V against the Turks. He improved and popularised the technique of lithotomy later known as "*great apparatus*" or "*Sectio Mariana*", that was invented by his teacher Giovanni de Romanis, and perfected by Mariano. He wrote the *Compendium in chirurgia utilissimum volentibus eam exercere* (Summary of Surgery very useful to those who want practice it) (Rome, 1516), but his fame is due to the *Libellus aureus de lapide a vesica per incisionem extrtahendo* (Golden booklet on the extraction of the bladder stone by incision) (Rome, 1522), with which he divulged the new technique, that was widely applied for more than two centuries with more or less important additions and changes.

DEVILLE OCTAVIANUS († 1556) He practiced surgery in Rome where became friends with Mariano Santo, who taught him the extraction of the stones from the bladder with the "treat apparatus". When Mariano moved from Rome to Venice, Deville was left alone and began to be called everywhere, but chiefly in France. During his trips he was fond of crossing the town of Trensel, near Troyes, in Champagne, where he became friends with Laurent Collot, who learnt from him the new technique. When Octavianus went back to Rome and died, Laurent Collot was the only surgeon in Europe who was able to perform the perineal incision with the "*great apparatus*". The new technique was kept secret by the Collot, who handed it down from father to son until 1727, when François Collot divulged it in a posthumous work, the *Traité de la lithotomie* (Treatise on lithotomy),

methodical reading of **[zheng lei ben cao] 症类本草 "Classified Materia Medica"** of Tang Shenwei, one of the most important herbalists during the Song Dynasty. **He began to work on [Ben Cao gang Mu] 本草纲目 "Compendium of Materia medica"**1552 AD and finished in 1578 AD This monumental work consists of 52 volumes, in addition to the preface, introduction, 2 volumes of index of diseases, and 3 volumes of illustrations. Out of 1.892 drugs that the book lists, 1.518 were already known to Chinese herbalists. Li introduced a total of 374 new drugs in his materia medica, drawing on a variety of sources. There are 11.091 from ancient and modern recipes, selected from previous writings. Of the drugs listed 1.074 are derived from plants, 443 from animals, and 354 from minerals and other substances. Under each drug the proper name is first given, then its popular names are collected, corrected, and explained as for their origin and meaning. Generally speaking, he pharmaceutical work of this book can be summarized under four parts: expanding the content of the materia medica, revising the classification of drugs, correcting errors in the work of his predecessors, and establishing guidelines for preparation as well as the usage of drugs.

The classifications of the drugs in Bencao Gangmu are different from the others. The Shen'nong Bencaojing divided drugs by virtue of their 'toxicity'. In the eleventh century, Tang Shenwei arranged drugs in his Zhenglei Bencao under the headings of jade and stone, plant, tree, products of human origin, quadruped, bird, insect, reptile, fish, fruit, grain, cereal and vegetable. Li Shizhen, in his Bencao Gangmu, used the together with the heap of experiences that 8 generations of lithotomists had accumulated.

FRANCO PIERRE (1500 *c.* - 1580 *c.*). We know very little about his life. He was born in Turriers, in Provence, practiced surgery in Lausanne, where he seems to have studied anatomy. He perfected the technique of the "*great apparatus*" and performed a lot of successful operations with his personal method, which he exposed in the treatise *De la cure de la pierre avec gros ferrements* (On the cure of the stone with the great apparatus). In his *Petit Traité de chirugie* (published in 1561), which contains the descriptions only of operations for hernia and bladder stones, he reports the first case of a suprapubic incision he performed on a ten years old boy who had a bladder stone the size of an egg. This incision, which Franco himself judge "*a great folly*", was abandoned until the XVIII century. Franco partly modified the "alphonsinum" invented by Alfonso Ferri, and transformed it into a lithotrite that paved the way to Civiale's instruments. Moreover he used a double-edged razor (the so-called "*razor of Franco*") and was the first to preconize the incision in two stages when the stone was too big to be extracted at the first stage. His *Grand Traité* (Great treatise), published in 1571, is a complete treatise on surgery, obstetrics and oculistics. Ambroise Paré leaned very much from Franco, although he doesn't ever quote him.

FERRI ALFONSO (1500 *c.* - 1595 *c.*) He was archiater and court surgeon of the Popes Paul III, Paul IV

headings of water, fire, earth, metals and stone, plant, cereal, vegetable, fruit, tree, products derived from 'garments and tools' insect, creatures with scales (reptiles, fish), creatures with shells, bird, quadruped and products of human origin. Bencao Gangmu is undoubtedly the best work on Chinese materia medica. It is the most varied and comprehensive known. Not only does it mention all sorts of most extraordinary substances, ranging from tiger bones to bat's dung, but also a host of articles, which are officinal in modern pharmacopoeias, are also included. Besides, it contains not a few valuable products as Kaolin, Eumenol, Chaulmoogra oil and ephedrine, which have only recently come to be known to western scientists.

Li Shizhen condemned the false advice of charlatans who prescribed drugs to 'prolong life'. According to him, to believe, for example, that a certain mushroom such as **[ling zhi] 灵芝** (Ganoderma lucidum) could enable a person to avoid death was foolish. But his Bencao Gangmu includes many (more than 500) remedies to "strengthen the body" and "prolong life". More than fifty of these remedies were devised in the course of Li's own medical experiments.

Li's was not only a herbalist with high reputation but also a famous physician. The other works written by Li include **[bin hu mai xue] 濒湖脉学 "The Pulse Studies on Binhu" and [qi jing ba mai kao] 奇经八脉考 "A Study on the Eight Extra meridians"**, etc.

Pharmacognosist, pharmacologist and physician, but also a botanist, zoologist and mineralogist, Li Shizhen contributed a lot to the medical world and his popularity has survived to the present.

and Julius III. Wrote a treatise entitled *De sclopetorum sive archibusorum vulneribus libri tres* (Three books on wounds from gun and harquebuses) in which described and illustrated a particular instrument for the extraction of the bullets from the wounds, that he proudly called "*alphonsinum*" He also studied and perfected the use of wax bougies and sounds to cure urethral stenosis, and eliminated the so-called "*caruncula*e" (most probably either urethral stenosis or prostate hypertrophy) with the aid of cutting sounds, like those used by Heliodorus in the I century A. D., and performing a true and proper internal urethrotomy. As for the extraction of the bladder stones by perineal incision, he adapted to this operation his "*alphonsinum*", that was a three-pronged pincer, very similar to a pencil lead holder, but much bigger. The three long divergent prongs were characterised by a crescent- shaped section with internal tooth, a short and solid handle, and a movable ring, and could be closed as a sort of sound, when the ring was moved towards the tip of the prongs. Once the sound had been introduced, the ring was lowered again and the prongs diverged again, surrounded the stone (or the bullet), were closed again by moving the ring up and gripped firmly the stone allowing its easy extraction.

ROUSSET FRANCOIS (XVI century). We don't know the place and the date either of his birth, or of his death. We know only that he was court physician of the Duke of Savoia, and was one of Ambroise Pare's friends. His fame is due to the caesarian section, of which he was a staunch supporter and to which he dedicated all his works: *Traité*

Chen Shigong 陈实功 (1555-1636), one of the outstanding in surgery .He wrote the book **[wai ke zhen zhong] 外科正中 "Orthodox Manuel of Surgery"**, which was published for the first time in 1617. In the book he described a way of stitching the gash resulting from suicide attempt to cut the throat and mentioned the cancer of lip and the cancer of breast. He also suggested several causes for such a serious affliction; in addition to psychological factors such as profound distress, Chen spoke of localised inflammation due to the eating of fried, spicy or burnt food and advocated that external and internal treatment had to be harmoniously combined.

Zhang Jiebin 张介宾(about 1563-1640 AD), also-called **[zhang jing yue] 张景岳 Zhang Jingyue**, author of several books on specified subjects, such as pulse, gynecology, pediatrics and surgery. Being especially versed in **[nei jing]** 内经 "Internal Classic", Zhang was the author of **[lei jing]** 类经 "Systematic Compilation of the Internal Classic" being the result of forty years of labor. His complete works **[jing yue quan shu] 景岳全书 "Jingyue's Complete Works"** appeared in 1624 AD The book includes studies of theories, pulse, febrile diseases, internal medicine, gynecology, pediatrics, surgery, materia medica, modern prescriptions, ancient prescriptions, etc. The author extracted the essence of various schools and made a systematical analysis of the diagnosis and treatment of diseases based on differentiation of their symptoms and signs. Advocating the theory "Yang is ever in excess and Yin never sufficient", he recommended using warm, tonifying drugs and wrote 2 whole

nouveau de l' hysterotokotomie ou enfantement césarien, qui est extraction de l'enfant par incision latérale du ventre et matrice de la femme grosse, ne pouvant autrement accoucher; et ce, sans préjudicier à la vie de l'un ni de l'autre, ni empêcher la fécondité maternelle par après (Paris, 1581); *Roussettii assertio historica et dialogus apologeticus pro partu caesaro* (Rousset's historical assertion and apologetic dialogue pro the caesarian section) (Paris, 1590) and *Brevis apologia pro partu caesareo in dicacis cujusdam chirurguli theatralem invectivam* (Short apology pro the caesarian section against a treacherous and poor surgeon's theatrical diatribe) (Paris, 1598). In 1581 he demonstrated with the section of a cadaver that when the bladder is full and the body lies on its back, it can be incised without any fear of injuring either the peritoneum or the bowels. Therefore he suggested this technique of operation for the extraction of bladder stones.

MASSA NICOLA (1504 c. - 1569). He studied at the University of Padua and published an *Anatomiae liber introductorius* (Introductory book of anatomy). He is not at all an original anatomist, but maintains clearly that no *filtering membrane* is present into the kidney, dividing the pelvis into two parts, and that the only visible membrane is the panniculus formed by the branches of the vessels, covered by their membranes (as had been already maintained by Galen, whose words had been misunderstood by the following anatomists).

PARÉ AMBROISE (1509 *c.* - 1590). Almost fanatical admirer of Vesalius, he was court surgeon of the

volumes of new prescriptions. In his book there are also some part about the sexology, including the selection of the spouse, eugenics, the proper time and places for sexual activities, the treatment of sterility, etc.

He served in the army when he was young. This military trait could be seen throughout his writing. He created the eight forms of therapeutics called **[ba zhen] 八阵** "battle array" and grouped his prescription under these headings: 1. **[bu zhen]** 补阵 "stimulant plan", 2. **[he zhen] 和阵** "truce plan", 3. **[gong zhen]** 攻阵 "attack plan", 4. **[san zhen] 散阵** "dispersal plan", 5. **[han zhen] 寒阵** "cold plan", 6. **[re zhen]** 热阵 "hot plan", 7. **[gu zhen] 固阵** "consolidation plan", 8. **[yin zhen] 因阵** "reasoning plan".

He was particularly skillful in using the herbal medicine **[shu di huang] 熟地黄** 'Rehmannia glutinosa' considered by him highly as a tonic and useful in weakened conditions of the body. On this account he was often called Zhang Shidi. He belonged to the **[wen bu]** 温补 "Warming up and invigorating" school and exerted considerable influences on the medical practice of the Ming and Qing Dynasties.

The word **[wen yi] 瘟疫** is a kind of fatal epidemic disease caused by rats. In this field **Wu Youxing 吴有性** also-called **[wu you ke] 吴又可 Wu Youke** claimed to have a leadership. He focused on this disease in his book **[wen yi lun] 瘟疫论 "On Pestilence"**. This little treatise consisted of only two thin volumes and was published in 1642. Throughout the centuries all fevers were regarded as typhoid. Wu pointed out this fallacy and made a distinction between these diseases. He proposed the theory of

Kings Henry II, Francis II, Charles IX and, finally, First Surgeon of King Henry III. He can be considered the founder of modern Surgery. His *Cinq livres de chirurgie* (Five books on Surgery), printed in 1572, had the same influence on the development of modern Surgery that Vesalius' *Fabrica* had for modern Anatomy. In the second edition of *Les Oeuvres de M. Ambroise Paré, conseiller et premier chirurgien du Roy, avec les figures et portraicts tant de l'anatomie que des instruments de chirurgie et de plusieurs monstres* (Works of Ambroise Paré, councilor and first surgeon of the King, with the tables and the figures both of anatomy and surgical instruments and of several monsters), printed in Paris in 1575 for the first time, he added three important booklets: *Des chaudes-pisses* (On the clap); *Des pierres* (On the stones) and *Des rentions d'urine* (On urine retentions). He was chiefly a military Surgeon, but was very able also in the field of urological surgery: he performed easily catheterisations also in military camps; his operation for urethral stenosis is the same performed and described by Heliodorus in the I century A. D. but surely reinvented by Paré, because he did know neither Greek, nor Latin; he observed clearly the retention of the testicle and suggested transillumination for the diagnosis of hydrocele. As for the clap, he too - like many other of his time and of the following centuries, up to Philippe Ricord (1799 - 1889) - muddled syphilis and blennorrhoea.

COLLOT LAURENT (XVI century). He was disciple of Octavianus Deville, and one of Paré's friends. Surely owing to the great influence of Paré, he was called to Paris where a

[li qi] 戾气 "excessive influences", pathogenic agents, responsible for the spread of pestilence which penetrated the body through the "mouth and nose"

Culture Aspects of the medical practice.

The medical practice has been divided into a number of branches since the very early time. **[zhou]周 Zhou Dynasty** distinguished four branches, **[tang] 唐 Tang Dynasty**, seven, and since **[song] 宋 Song Dynasty**, thirteen are classified according to **[song shi] 宋史 "Song History"**

1. Wind diseases, 2. Typhoid fever, 3. Diseases of adults, 4. Women's diseases, 5. Obstetrics, 6. Acupuncture and moxa, 7. Throat, 8. Mouth and teeth, 9. Ulcers, 10. Bone-setting, 11. Wounds, 12. Conservation of life, 13. Praying cures.

Medicine in **[yuan] 元 Yuan dynasty** was similarly split up but here the list is given as: 1. Diseases of adults, 2. Miscellaneous diseases, 3. Diseases of children, 4. Wind diseases, 5. Obstetrics, 6. Women's diseases, 7. Eye diseases, 8. Mouth and teeth, 9. Throat, 10. Bone-setting and wounds, 11. Acupuncture and moxa, 12. Charms and incantations, 13. Chin k'e or forbidden subject.

[ming] 明Ming dynasty followed the Yuan but with a slightly different version. The divisions were: 1. Diseases of adults, 2. Diseases of children, 3. Women's diseases, 4. Ulcers and inflammations, 5. Acupuncture and moxa, 6. Eye diseases, 7. Mouth and teeth, 8. Bone-setting, 9. Typhoid fever, 10. Throat troubles, 11. Wounds, 12. Massage, 13. Charms and incantations. The list from the Institutes of Ming

special appointment of lithotomist was created for him at the Hôtel Dieu. In 1556 Laurent was appointed *Chirurgien pour la taille*" (surgeon for the perineal incision) of the King Henry II. The Parliament of Paris charged him with an evaluation (by a post mortem incision) to the suprapubic incision proposed and performed (but only on a cadaver) by Rousset and he wrote in his report that he could not think to such an operation without shuddering!

EUSTACHI BARTOLOMEO (1510 c. - 1574) Was born in Sanseverino (Marche region) and died while traveling from Rome to Fossombrone. Was appointed Archiater to the Pope and professor of anatomy to the Sapienza. He had planned a great treatise on Anatomy, for which 54 "Tabulae" (plates) (7 of which were lost; the remaining 47 were discovered and published by Giovanni Maria Lancisi only in 1714 in Rome) had been prepared by the painter De Musis, but death frustrated his plan. Nevertheless Eustachi published a *Libellus de renibus* (Booklet on the kidneys) (reprinted together with a series of other booklets in *Opuscula anatomica*, Venice, 1564), thanks to which he can be considered the Columbus of the new kidney". He realised (as Realdo Colombo did) that the right kidney is lower than the left; discovered the adrenal capsules. Eustachi (like Berengarius of Carpi and Gabriele Falloppio) distinguished the unipapillary kidney of the dog from the pluripapillary human kidney; through vascular injections, insufflation to the point of laceration of the fibrous tunic and scarification was able to describe the vascular tree of the kidney and its terminal arches, the uriniferous tubules in

Dynasty proposes to enumerate thirteen but concludes by only naming eleven as follows: 1. Disease of adults, 2. Typhoid fever, 3. Diseases of children, 4. Women's complaints, 5. Mouth and teeth, 6. Throat troubles, 7. Surgery, 8. Bone-setting, 9. Smallpox and measles, 10. Diseases of the eye, 11. Acupuncture and moxa.

The most important event in the mediaeval period was the founding of **[tai yi yuan] 太医院** "College of Imperial Physicians". In former times the medical establishment in China was called **[yu yao ju] 御药局** "Imperial Drug Bureau". The College of Imperial Physicians was the first independent medical institution, properly organized with definite administrative power. The main functions were to direct all medical matters, to dispense medicines for the Imperial Household and to supervise the work of the medical officers. The government regarded the profession very highly and put the officials in charge of the institutions as high as the 2nd grade, which used to be only 7th to 9th grade. The personnel of the college consisted of one director of 2nd grade rank, two co-directors of 3rd grade, two senior assistants 3rd grade, two junior assistants 4th grade, two junior assistant 4th grade, two associates 5th grade, two chief secretaries and two assistant secretaries, all 7th grade, four clerks 8th grade and a number of writers, translators, interpreters, keeper of seals, etc.

In course of time the College declined until under the **[qing] 清 "Qing Dynasty**". In fact, a decline of Chinese appeared from the Ming Dynasty reaching its lowest ebb in the Qing period. Under the Tang and Song Dynasties, medical schools flourished the

the medulla (which, however, he interpreted as furrows incised in the renal substance"), the papillae (already described by Berengario of Carpi) and their urinary pores, and the funnel-shaped opening of the ureter and was the first to suppose that urine originated from arterial and not venous blood.

VESALIUS ANDREAS (1514 - 1564). He is considered the restorer of Anatomy", but, although he was so bold that rebelled against Galen's authority with his most famous *De humani corporis fabrica libri septem* (Seven books on the fabric of the human body) (Basel, Oporinus, 1543), on the one hand he repeated many of Galen's mistakes (e. g. he described and illustrated erroneously the right kidney in a higher position than the left), on the other agreed without reserve to Galen's physiology, based on the four qualities, the four humours and the particular *virtues*" of each part of the body. Moreover: he had not even the palest idea of blood circulation; he dissected the unipapillary kidney of dogs and extrapolated his observations to humans, without having checked his accuracy on human cadavers; he didn't see the seminal vesicles in describing the male urogenital apparatus; though he observed correctly that there is no direct anastomosis between the plexus pampiniformis and the epididymis, and that the testicles present an internal vascularization, he maintained (like Galen) the sperm to originate from the blood transformed by the testicles as the chyle is transformed into blood by the liver. In his controversy against Gabriele Falloppio (*Andreae Vesalii anatomicarum Gabrielis Falloppii*

empire, there existed now only one Imperial College of Physician in Beijing. Its only service was for train physicians for the Imperial Family. The ordinary practitioners had no chance to prepare themselves to be qualified physicians. Anyone can set up as a doctor. An ordinary laborer who inherits a few prescriptions from his ancestors, or a woman who has some experience from rearing her children, will put up a signboard and start practice. In a higher grades of medical practice, a
person who wants to have the knowledge of medicine can serve as an apprenticeship either under an old doctor, or in a druggist shop. People have great confidence in those who spring from medical families. The inspiration of creating something new was inhabited.

Another reason for the decline of the native practice was the numerous divisions and sects of medical profession, which blocked the development of medicine. Some advocated the orthodox teachings of Han. Others spoke of the Tang, the Song, the Qing and Yuan or the Ming respectively. New cults were formed and different schools branched out. They can be generally divided into two main schools – ancient and modern. Some urged to return to the classics of Huang di, the others favored the teaching of the modern masters. In addition to these two schools, there were so many outstanding figures, each having a group of followers, that they eventually fell into smaller cliques, which enabled Chinese medicine to remain in a setback until the early part of the nineteenth century when the occidental art broke its way into China.

observationum examen, Andrea Vesalus'examination of Gabriele Falloppio's anatomical observations) he shows to have understood none of Falloppio's descriptions of the pluripapillary human kidney and to have mistaken the calyces discovered by Falloppio for the offshoots of the membranous corpus he had observed in the unipapillary kidney of the dogs.

COLOMBO REALDO (1516 *c.* - 1559). He was born in Cremona, studied at the University of Padua and succeeded Vesalius in the chair of Anatomy in 1542. In 1546 was appointed professor of Anatomy in Pisa and in 1549 the Pope Paul III called him to Rome, where he stayed until his death. He published his *De re anatomica libri XV* (XV books on Anatomy) in Venice in 1559. He discovered - perhaps after having read the *Christianismi restitutio* (Restoration of Christianity) of Miguel Servet (Servetus) (1509 - 1553) - and described clearly and demonstrated the lesser circulation. As for Urology, he bravely writes (*De re anatomica libri XV*, book XI, chapter IX): *it is amusing indeed to observe what a great to do was made by Galen so anxiously attempting to discover why Nature placed the right kidney higher than the left. But no doubt our poor simple-minded Galen...made a useless inquiry...because what he maintains appears clearly and immediately to be false, if only one observes human anatomy*".

FALLOPPIO (or FALLOPPIA) GABRIELE (1523 - 1562). He was born in Modena and died in Padua. Antonio Musa Brasavola (or Brassavola) (1500 - 1555) was his master. He graduated in

Different Medical Schools in the History of Traditional Chinese Medicine

[jin yuan si da jia] 金元四大家 "Four Schools of Medical Practice in Jin and Yuan Dynasties" (1279-1368 AD)
It refers to **[liu wuan su]** Liu Wuansu 刘完素
[zhang zi he] Zhang Zihe 张子和 **[li dong yuan]** Li Dongyuan 李东垣 and **[zhu dangx i]** Zhu Dangxi 朱丹溪 four famous medical experts and their schools in Jin and Yuan Dynasties.

[han liang pai] 寒凉派 "The Cold and Cool School "
The school of medical practice, represented by the famous medical expert, **[liu wuan su]** Liu Wuansu 刘完素 of **[jin yuan]** 金元 "Jin and Yuan Dynasties" (1279-1368 AD), who is well known for his excellence of using the drugs with cold and cool properties.

[gong xia pai] 攻下派 "The Purging School"
The school of medical practice represented by the famous medical expert, **[zang zi he]** Zhang Zihe 张子和 of **[jin yuan]** 金元 "Jin and Yuan Dynasties" (1279-1368 AD), who is well known for using the purgatives, diaphoretics and emetics.

[bu tu pai] 补土派 "The Earth-Nourishing School"
The school of medical practice represented by the famous medical expert, **[li dong yuan]** Li Dongyuan 李东垣 of **[jin yuan]** 金元 Jin and Yuan Dynasties (1279-1368 AD), who is well known for using the methods of

1547, in his *Observationes anatomicae* (Anatomical observations) (Venice, 1561). In spite of his deference and admiration for Vesalius, whom he always calls "divinus Vesalius" (Divine Vesalius), he maintains that his Master" (though Falloppio never attended any of Vesalius' lectures) had made some great mistakes, chiefly as regards the structure of the kidney. By dissecting (from the concave part, like Berengarius of Carpi, and not from the convex one) human and not canine kidneys, he describes perfectly the calyces and the papillae. Thanks to this technique, Falloppio could realise that the pelvis *is endowed with many ducts...like perforated fingers; on each duct there is a fleshy operculum...formed by the same substance of the kidney, which reaches that duct...in order to let urine flow downwards*" and observe the complete vascularization of the kidney for the first time.

ACQUAPENDENTE GIROLAMO FABRIZIO of (1533 - 1619) He was one of the greatest anatomists and surgeons of his times. He was one of Gabriele Falloppio's disciples and in 1565 was appointed professor of Surgery and Anatomy. In 1609 the chair was divided and Fabrizio was lecturer only of Anatomy. He wrote a lot of treatises not only on Surgery and Anatomy, but also and chiefly on Comparative Anatomy and Embryology, two sciences of which he can be considered one of the founders. Notwithstanding that, he gives very little contributions to urological surgery in his *Opera chirurgica in duas partes divisa* (Works on Surgery in two parts) (Padua, 1617), the first part of which he had already published in 1592 with the title

nourishing the spleen and stomach.

[zi yin pai] 滋阴派 "The Yin-Nourishing School"
The school of medical practice represented by the famous medical expert, Zhu Dangxi 朱丹溪 of **[jin yuan]** 金元 "Jin and Yuan Dynasties" (1279-1368 AD), who is well-known for using the methods of nourishing Yin and relieving fire (heat).

[shi fang pai] 时方派 "The Contempore School"
The school of medical practice that is well-known for using the formularies employed after **[han]** 汉 "Han Dynasty" (206 B.C.-220 AD)

[shang han pai] 伤寒派 "The Shang Han School"
The group of practitioners using Shanghan Theory as the basis of their medical practice. Shanghan theory refers to external pathogenic factors as causes of febrile diseases advocated by the famous medical expert, **[zhang zhong jing]** Zhang Zhongjing 张中景 of **[han]** 汉 "Han Dynasty" (206 B.C.-220 AD) **[shang han za bing lun]** 伤寒杂病论 "Treatise on Febrile and Miscellaneous Diseases".

[jing fang pai] 经方派 "The Classic-Formula School"
(1) The school known for using the empiric formularies before the Song Dynasty. (2) The school of medicine practice that was known for using the formularies in the two classical works of traditional Chinese medicine, **[shang han lun]** 伤寒论 " Treatise on Febrile Diseases" and **[jin gui yao lue**

Pentateuchos chirurgicum (Five books on Surgery). The only interesting passages are those where he describes catheters made of silver, copper, brass and horn (already suggested by Avicenna), maintains that "*the Ancients made only a single orifice at the end of the catheter, while the Moderns make holes also at side*" (a shape adopted also by Mariano Santo) and describes catheters made of textile, impregnated with wax and moulded on a silver sound (a technique already adopted by Heliodorus in the passage on the operation of the "*carunculae*" quoted by Oribasius).

HELMONT JOHANNES BAPTISTA VAN (1577 - 1644). He took a degree in Philosophy at the University of Leuven in 1594 and in 1599 he graduated in Medicine. He spent several years traveling through France, Spain, and England. Then he moved to Bruxelles where practiced until his death. He was the founder (on the way paved by Paracelsus) of the *Iiatrochemical School* or simply *Iatrochemistry, which* will carry on a long and relentless controversy against the *Iatromechanical School*, or simply *Iatromechanics* during the XVII and XVIII centuries. From his *Hortus medicinae*, which contains both printed and unprinted works and was published by his son Franciscus Mercurius in Amsterdam in 1648, he appears to have been the first to measure the specific gravity of urine. As for the stones in the bladder he maintains that the adrenal glands have the task of secrete a particular humour that prevents the stones from forming. As for catheterisation, he applied the same principle of Fabrici of Acquapendente, but instead of textile he

fang] 金匮要略方' Synopsis of prescriptions of the Golden Chamber". **[wen bing pai] 温病派 "The Wenbing School"** The group of practitioners using Wenbing Theory as the basis of their medical practice. Wenbing Theory refers to acute febrile diseases due to external affection, of which the aetiology, diagnosis and therapeutic principle of the acute infectious diseases were first elucidated by the famous medical expert, **[wu you xing]** Wu Youke 吴有性 in his **work [wen yi lun]** 温疫论 " Treatise on Acute Epidemic Febrile Diseases" and that is created by famous medical experts **[yie tian shi]** Yue Tianshi 叶天士, **[xue shen bai]** Xue Shenbai 薛生白, [wu ju tong] Wu Jutong 吴菊通 and **[wang meng ying]** Wang Mengying 王孟英 in **[ming qing]** 明清 "Ming Qing Dynasties" through their long term clinical practice. **[shi san ke] 十三科 "The Thirteen Medical Specialties"** In Yuan and Ming dynasties medicine was divided into thirteen specialities. In the **[yuan]** Yuan Dynasty (1206-1368), they were internal medicine, miscellaneous medicine, "wind" speciality, pediatrics, obstetrics, ophthalmology, stomatology and dentistry, laryngology, orthopedics, traumatology, acupuncture and moxibustion, supplication, and non-recorded diseases. The thirteen specialties of the Imperial medical Institute in Ming Dynasty (1368-1644) were: internal medicine, pediatrics, gynecology, carbuncle and ulcers, acupuncture and moxibution, ophthalmology, stomatology and dentistry, laryngology, febrile diseases, orthopedics, sword and archery	used chamois skin, treated outside with white lead and linseed oil. He introduced his catheter with the help of a stylet made of whalebone. This allowed him to catheterise the same patient even forty times a day.

wounds, massage, and supplication. **[tang dai si ke] 唐代四科' The Four medical Specialties of Tang Dynasty"** In [tang] Tang Dynasty (618.907 AD) traditional Chinese medicine was divided into four specialties: medicine, acupuncture, massage and supplication. **[song jiu ke] 宋代九科' The Nine Medical Specialities of Song Dynasty"** In [song] Song Dynasty (960-1279 AD) traditional Chinese medicine was divided into nine specialties, namely, internal medicine, pediatrics, ulcerations and abscesses with traumatology, ophthalmology, obstetrics, "wind" speciality, stomato-laryngology and dentistry, acupuncture and moxibustion, and sword and archery wound with non-recording diseases. **[qing dai jiu ke] 清代九科 "The Nine Specialities of Qing Dynasty"** In **[qing]** Qing Dynasty (1644-1911) traditional Chinese medicine was divided into nine specialities. They were internal medicine, febrile diseases, gynecology, pediatrics, ulcers and abscesses, ophthalmology, disease of mouth-tooth-throat, acupuncture and moxibustion, orthopedics.	

Chapter Two

Brief Introduction to T. C. M. in Urology An Entry for a Medical Dictionary

Traditional Chinese Medicine, as a part of medicine in the world, is a great treasure-house, which in fact is a discipline dealing with human physiology and pathology, diagnosis, treatment and prevention of diseases. It has a specific, integrated system of theory with a history of several thousands of years rich in clinical experience. TCM has summed up the experience of the Chinese people in their long struggle against diseases, thus developing into a peculiar system of medical theory through long-term clinical practice under the influence and direction of ancient simple empiricism and ideas. As a result, it has contributed much to the promotion of health of Chinese nation and further development of medical sciences all over the world. In recent years, through the cultural exchanges between the East and the West, many people in the Western countries have recognized the importance of Chinese system of medicine. Some of its component parts, such as acupuncture, moxibustion and Shiatsu therapy have become known as "wonder-making art of healing" and the Chinese herbal medicine has aroused an increasing interest among Westerns, because of its confirmed therapeutic effects and less toxic and less side effects. A great zeal is shown by a rapidly growing number of people from all parts of the world for knowledge about traditional Chinese medicine as well as an increasing demand for books on the subject. To facilitate the process of introducing traditional Chinese medicine to the Western world and to meet the ever-increasing demand of medical professionals, Chinese and foreign, for a systematic concise reference book, we, the compilers of the dictionary and the references, take it our duty to offer something useful and beneficial for the medical workers all over the world.

The dictionary involves in the comparative study of the medical history. The "comparative medicine" is to carry out the comparative researches and investigation on the medical system in different times, different races, different places and different cultural backgrounds, to study the similarities and the differences of its basic theoretic systems, the causes and conditions of its existence, the properties and the features, the study methods and philosophical thinking. The study of comparative medicine is the basis for the unity of the medical world. In our dictionary, we are going to focus on the discussion of pharmacological treatment of urological diseases.

Traditional Chinese medicine and Pharmacology (TCMP) has a unique, comprehensive scientific system including both theories and clinical practice. In order to understand the urological diseases and the therapeutic methods of TCMP, first of all, we should have a general idea of the urological system of TCM. The following is a brief introduction of TCM theory.

1. [zhong yi de ji ben te dian] 中医的基本特点 "The Characteristics of TCM"

The theoretic system of TCM consists of the doctrines on [Yin] 阴 [Yang] 阳 and the five elements phase of [Zang Fu] 脏腑 organs (viscera), meridians [jing luo] 经络, pathogenesis syndrome, techniques of diagnosis, therapeutic principles, health preserving, five elements' motion and six natural factors. TCM has the unique concept of wholism, which refers to a general view of the proper human body as an integral whole, closely interconnected by Zang Fu organs, channels and collaterals and maintaining close link with the outer world. In the recognition of diseases, TCM has four diagnostic techniques correlated with the principles of diseases, eight principles as its guideline of treatment. Generally speaking, the characteristic of TCM can be summarised in two outstanding features: (1) the concept of wholism, and (2) the application of treatment according to the differentiation of symptom-complexes.

The functional physiological activities of the Zang-fu organs are different, but they work in coordination. Pathologically, a dysfunction of the Zang-fu organs may be reflected on the body, and the diseases of body surface may also affect their related Zang-fu organs. The affected Zang-fu organs may also influence each other through internal connections. So regulating the functions of Zang-fu organs is one of the traditional Chinese treatments in dealing with the pathological changes. The human body is not only viewed as an organic whole, but it is also a unified entity within nature, so changes in the natural environment may directly or indirectly affect it. According to TCM, the principles of treatment are expected to accord with the different seasons and environments, which are the factors to be considered when diagnosis and treatment are carried out.

Application of treatment according to the differentiation of syndromes is another characteristic of traditional Chinese medicine, the purpose of which is to analyze the disease condition in order to know its essentials, to identify the causative factors, the location and nature, and to obtain conclusions about the confrontation between pathogenic and antipathogenic factors. Treatment in traditional Chinese medicine stresses the differences of syndromes, but not the differences of diseases. Therefore there are different treatments for the same disease and different diseases can also be treated by the same method.

2. [yin yang wu xing] 阴阳五行 "Yin-Yang and the Five Elements" (see Figure 11).

The ancient Chinese regarded the material world, which was constantly evolving due to the dynamic movement and as the result of the antagonistic movement of two opposing forces: Yin and Yang. They applied these two theories in the medical field to explain the physiological activities and pathological changes of the human body, and to serve as a guide to the clinical

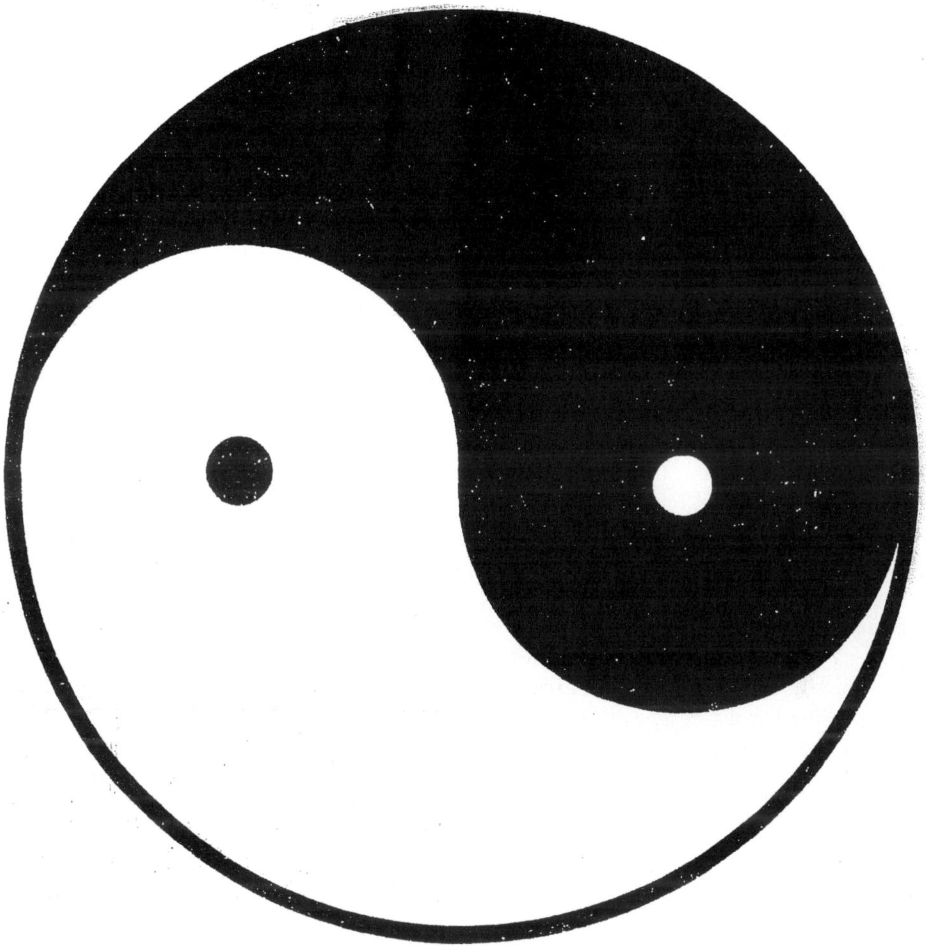

Figure 11: The “Celestial Wheel” of the “Two Modalities”, Yin (black) and Yang (white). Both are represented like two big commas, the head of one of which corresponds to the tail of the other. The two big points (white in Yin and black in Yang) mean that each modality contains the germ of its opposite.

Figure 11.1 [illegible] Yin (black) and Yang (white) [illegible]

treatment on the basis of differential diagnosis. Originally, their connotations were quite simple, meaning "turning away from" or "facing the sunlight" respectively. Afterwards, Yin and Yang were extended to describe weather (cold or warm), position (downward or upward, right or left, internal or external), moving condition (mobile or static), etc.. Each phenomenon has two aspects: negative and positive. That is to say Yin and Yang exist in everything in nature, not only in inanimate objects, but also in living things. In all situations, they are interdependent. Yin does not exist without Yang, nor does Yang exist without Yin, thus forming the concept of the unity of opposites. Generally speaking, matters and phenomena, which are hot, dynamic, vigorous, external, upward, ascending, brilliant, progressive, hyperactive, or pertaining to functional activities, belong to Yang. Those, which are cold, static, weak, internal, downward, descending, dull, retrogressive, hypoactive, or pertaining to materials, belong to Yin. The following is a system that encompasses five basic ideas of Yin and Yang.

- All phenomena can be classified as either Yin or Yang.
- Yin and Yang are relative concepts.
- Yin and Yang are interdependent.
- The relationship between Yin and Yang is constantly changing.
- Under certain conditions Yin may transform into Yang, and Yang into Yin.

2.1. [yin yang de dui li tong yi] 阴阳的对立统一 "The Unity of Yin and Yang as Two opposites"

"Excessive Yin will transform into Yang and excessive Yang into Yin. Excessive cold leads to heat and extreme heat to cold" in **[su wen]** 素问 "Plain Questions". Yin and Yang manifest themselves mainly in their mutual restraint and struggle and form the basis for understanding the "unity of opposites" in the Yin – Yang theory. **[Lei Jing Fu Yi-Yi Yi Yi]** 类经附翼医易义 "Illustrated Supplementary to the Classified Canon" (1624 B.C.), says "Violent motion should be suppressed by tranquility, and hyperactivity of Yang restrained by Yin", which means that there is a relation of mutual restraint and mutual struggle between motion and tranquility-Yin and Yang. The theory of Yin and Yang, when applied to medicine, describes the human body as an organic whole, unified but with opposing aspects. So when the human body is in a normal physiological condition, Yin and Yang, the two opposite, do not exist in a single steady entity, they are opposed to and always struggle with each other. Through the process of opposing and struggling against each other, the dynamic equilibrium is established. And all things develop and change with constant restraint and struggle of Yin and Yang.

2.2. [yin yang de xiang dui gai niang] 阴阳的相对概念 "Relative Concepts of Yin and Yang"

Every object can be divided into two aspects, Yin and Yang. Yin can be subdivided into Yin and Yang; so can Yang. The part of Yang may be re-divided into two parts, one of which is the component part of Yang within Yang, while the other is the component part of Yin within Yang and Yin in the viscera. The example is day and night. Day is Yang; night is Yin. But both can be subdivided. The morning of the day represents the Yang part of the day. It is said to be the Yang within Yang. The afternoon is the Yin part of the day-the Yin within the Yin. They are so-called **[yang zhong zhi yang yang zhong zhi yin]** 阳 中 之 阳 阳 中 之 阴 " The Yang part within Yang and the Yang part within Yin". In the interrelationships among the Viscera, the stomach belongs to the category of Yang and itself may be subdivided into the stomach-Yang and stomach –Yin. On the other hand **[yin zhong zhi yin, yin zhong zhi yang]** 阴 中 之 阴 ， 阴 中 阳 "The Yin part within Yin and the Yin part within Yang". E.g., in the interrelationship among the Viscera, the kidney belongs to the category of Yin and itself may, in turn, be subdivided into the Kidney-Yin and the Kidney-Yang.

2.3. [yin yang hu gen] 阴阳互根 "Independence between Yin and Yang"

The existence of Yin must depend on the prior existence of Yang, on the contrary, the existence of Yang must depend on the prior existence of Yin. Yin and Yang are opposed to each other, and they are also interdependent of each other. Neither can exist in isolation. **[Yin Yang Ying Xiang Da Lun]** 阴阳应象大论 "Great Treatise on Yin-Yang Classification of Natural Phenomena) of **[su wen]** 素问 "Plain Questions" (2698-2589 B.C.) says: "Yin is installed in the interior as the substantial basis of Yang, while Yang remains on the exterior as the manifestation of the function of Yin". The existence of the one being the prerequisite of the existence of the other. If one of the two opposites ceases to be the condition for the other's existence, neither of them can exist and flourish independently. At the same time, Yin or Yang may transform itself into the opposite under certain circumstances. The mutual transformation of Yin and Yang is a process of qualitative change. Such transformation would be impossible without this interdependence, which is often seen in the development of certain diseases. In TCM, this theory is used to explain human physiology and pathology, as well as the effect of climatic variations on the body.

2.4. [yin yang xiao zhang] 阴阳消长 "Wane and Wax of Yin and Yang"

The opposition, mutual restraint, interdependence and interaction between Yin and Yang are not in a static or unchangeable condition. Rather they are constantly moving and changing. The fundamental pattern of this motion is described as the interconsuming and intersupporting of Yin and Yang. That is to say within certain limits and during a certain period of time the alternation of "Wane of Yin followed by wax of Yang" and " Wane of Yang followed by wax of Yin" exists in order to maintain a relative balance between Yin and Yang. The process of transition from cold to heat through spring warmth from winter to summer represents the waning (or consumption) of Yin and the waxing (or increasing) of Yang, while the transition from the heat of summer to the cold of winter represents the waning of Yang and waxing of Yin. Take the physiological function of the human body as an example. In daytime, Yang is overabundant, so the physiological function of the human body is characterized mainly by excitement, while at night

Yin prevails and this is marked by inhibition. After middle night, Yang begins to grow, at noon, Yang-Qi (Yang Vital Force) will be excessive and the body's function turns gradually from being inhibited into exciting. Under normal conditions the mutual consuming and increasing of Yin and Yang maintains a relative balance. Under abnormal conditions there is an excess or insufficiency of either Yin or Yang, which leads to the occurrence of diseases. Therefore, the wane and wax of Yin and Yang help to maintain a dynamic equilibrium of the human body.

2.5. [yin yang zhuan hua] 阴阳转化 "Transformation of Yin and Yang"

Yin and Yang are interchangeable each other under certain conditions. That is to say when the consuming relationship between Yin and Yang reaches a certain stage of development, Yin may transform into Yang and vice versa. The rise and fall of temperature within a season may be viewed as stages of quantitative change while the intertransformation of Yin and Yang in the change of seasons represents a qualitative change. The Yin and Yang of the human body, like that of the universe, are constantly changing in their relationship to each other. Physiologically speaking, in the course of life activities of the body, the process of changing between substance and function represents the process of transformation between Yin and Yang. For example, nourishing substances (Yin) is constantly transformed into functional activity (Yang), and vice versa. But the transformation between Yin and Yang is to occur under certain conditions, and is not likely to appear without these given conditions.

2.6. [yin ping yang mi] 阴平阳秘 "Equilibrium of Yin and Yang"

In a healthy body, as in the universe, the relationship between Yin and Yang is constantly changing. Yin and Yang continuously support and consume each other, which is known as "mutual restraint" of Yin and Yang; it produces a dynamic equilibrium-a balance-in the body. So the normal life activities of the body result from harmonious relationship of the unity of the two opposites, Yin and Yang. The dynamic equilibrium between Yin and Yang is indicative of good health of the human body. If the pattern of mutual restraint fails, the balance of Yin and Yang is lost. Then the body is transformed from its healthy state into a morbid condition. So TCM stresses the physiological relation of equilibrium between Yin and Yang in the human body.

2.7. [yin sheng ze yang bing] 阴胜则阳病 "An Excess of Yin Leads to Deficiency of Yang"

A morbid condition with overabundance of Yin-cold leads to the hypo function of Yang-energy. It is meant that Yin in state of absolute excessiveness is a factor contributing to illness. Yin is associated with cold, excessive Yin will cause cold syndrome. An example is chronic nephritis with symptoms of intolerance to cold, cold limbs, and edema. In this case, the vital function of the spleen and kidney is too weak to perform the functions of transporting and transforming nutrients and body fluids. As a result, an accumulation of fluids, dampness, and cold would occur, thus suggesting deficiency of Yang and excessiveness of Yin.

2.8. [yang sheng ze yin bing] 阳胜则阴病 "An Excess of Yang leads to Deficiency of Yin"

A morbid condition with hyperactivity of Yang-heat leads to consumption of the Yin-heat. This means that Yang, when in a state of absolute excessiveness, serves as a factor contributing to illness because an excess of Yang produces heat syndrome. Such conditions are typical of acute infectious diseases; they are always accompanied by a flushed face and high temperature. The endogenous heat (a Yang factor) would injure vital essence and body fluid (Yin). Yang in excess may be manifested as fever, thirst, a scant amount of urine and constipation.

2.9. [yin yang pian shuai] 阴阳偏衰 "Insufficiency of Yin and Yang"

Insufficiency of Yin or Yang is a pathological change in which either Yin or Yang is below normal level. In [su wen] 素问 "Plain Questions" (2698-2589 B.C), it is stated that "deficiency of Yang is to lead superficial cold syndrome, while that of Yin to interior heat syndrome". According to the principle of dynamic equilibrium between Yin and Yang, the deficiency of either will necessarily lead to hyperactivity of the other. This pattern in the development of disease will be "no Yin can be formed without Yang" and "Yang fails to appear without Yin". That's to say, the impairment of Yang would impede generation of Yin. When in a morbid state, the Yang-Qi (Yang's vital energy) in the body is often failed to promote the production of Yin fluid, this results in insufficiency of Yin. On the other hand, when Yin is deficient, it will lead to relative hyperactivity of Yang and asthenic heat-syndrome. Therefore the impairment of Yin would also impede the production of Yang-Qi in the body, thus leading to insufficiency of Yang. In general, a deficiency of both Yin and Yang is most common in cases of chronic disease.

2.10. [tiao zheng yin yang] 调整阴阳 "Regulation of Yin and Yang"

[su wen] 素问 "Plain Questions" say: "Observe the relationship between Yin and Yang carefully, and make adjustments to bring about "equilibrium" and "Treat the Yin aspect for a disease of Yang nature. Treat the Yang aspect for the disease of Yin nature". According to TCM, the root cause of development of disease is the excessiveness or deficiency of Yin and Yang. So the basic principle therapy is regulating Yin and Yang in order to reduce the superfluous, making up the insufficiency, and restoring relative equilibrium of Yin and Yang, keepingi the body in balance and healthy state.

3. [wu xing] 五行 "The Five Elements"

The ancient Chinese used the five basic materials in everyday life to symbolize the behavior of all objects and phenomena in nature. These five elements are metal, wood, water, fire, and earth, which are in constant movement and change.

Everything on earth is dominated by one of these elements. They are indispensable and most fundamental elements in constituting the Universe. There exist enhancing, inhibiting and restraining relationships among them. It is a way of describing the process of all changes and activities in nature.

3.1. [wu xing xue shuo] 五行学说 "Five- Elements Theory"

The Five Elements theory is an ancient philosophical concept, which is used in TCM to expound the unity of the human body and the natural world, the physiological and pathological relationship between the internal organs. It holds that nothing is in an isolated or static state, and everything is in a state of harmonious balance during the process of the constant motion of inter-generation and inter-restriction. The early Chinese philosophers summarized nature in terms of the five elements. In the book **[shi shu]** 史书 "History Book" they are described as "Water moistens and flows downward. Fire flares upward. Wood is flexible. Metal may be transformed through casting. And earth serves for the sowing and growing of crops". Each of the five elements may be used to characterize phenomena in nature and in TCM is chiefly used to explain the properties of viscera of the human body, their mutual relations and pathological changes.

Moreover, the five elements again interact on each other, having five generators and five subjugators thus:

Wood	generates	Fire	Wood	subjugates	Earth
Fire	,,	Earth	Earth	,,	Water
Earth	,,	Metal	Water	,,	Fire
Metal	,,	Water	Fire	,,	Metal
Water	,,	Wood	Metal	,,	Wood

3.2. [wu xing xiang sheng] 五行相生 "Interpromoting Relation of the Five Elements"

The theory refers to promoting and accelerating aspects of the mutual generation of matters according to the Theory of the Five Elements. The Ancient thinkers found in actual practice that one thing is often closely followed by another or one thing is positively influenced by another, the promoting relationship is also known as the **[mu zi guan xi]** 母子关系 "mother-son relationship". The mother element gives birth to the son element. The son cannot promote the mother directly. Thus, the mother-son relationship defines a cycle of change that occurs in a specific direction and order. The regular order of generation would be in the following sequence: wood, fire, earth, metal and water, in which each has a generative and a subjugative influence on the other. The evolutive cycle proceeds as follows: wood burns to generate fire; fire produces ashes, which generates earth; earth generates metal; which can be mined from the ground; when heated, metal becomes molten, like water; and water promotes growth of plants, thereby generating wood.

3.3. [wu xing xiang ke] 五行相克 "Counteracting (Restricting) Relation of the Five Elements"

According to **[su wen]** 素问 "Plain questions" [yang sheng pian] 养生篇 "Treatise on How to Keep Healthy", "With metal, wood is felled. With water, fire is extinguished. With wood, earth is rooted and loosened. With fire, metal is melted. And with earth, water is obstructed". So another major relationship among the five elements is the restraining and expelling function among matters. Besides the principle of generation, the ancient thinkers also realized an opposite universal phenomenon in nature, that is that one thing can be often inhibited or restricted by another. The regular order for the restriction of the five Elements is wood restricts earth, earth checks water, water checks fire, fire checks metal, metal in turn restricts wood. Nature and life processes are full of vitality and also free from exceeding one another because of this inhibitive and restrictive action.

3.4. [wu xing xiang cheng] 五行相乘 "Encroachment in the Five Elements"

It means that one excessively inhibits another beyond the normal extent. It shows the overacting and counteracting relationship among the five elements. Overacting is a type of excessive control, which shows that the subjugation of one of the five elements to another surpasses the normal level. For example, in the cases of deficiency, wood can overact on earth if the latter is deficient. Or in the cases of excess, if wood is too exuberant to be restrained by mental , it will form an aggressive invasion against earth. The latter element is made weak and insufficient.

3.5. [wu xing xiang wu] 五行相侮 "Violation in the Five Elements"

It implies that one element reversibly restricts the other, which should restrict the former. This is known as "reverse restriction" or "counteraction". For instance, wood should be restricted by metal, however when wood is excessively strong, it is not restricted by metal, on the contrary, it restricts metal, which is known as "wood violates metal". In fact, it is a morbid condition in which one element fails to restrict the other in the normal, regular order, but in reverse order.

4. [zang xiang xue] 脏象学 "The Theory of Viscera" (see Figure 12).

In TCM, there is a theory of **[Zang Xiang]** 脏象学 "Zang" viscera. It refers to internal organs of the body; "Xiang" phase refers mainly to the outward physiological and pathological manifestations. The five-element theory is used to explain the physiology of the body as well as its relationship to the environment. The heart, lungs, spleen, liver and kidneys are together called as the Five-Zang organs. The gallbladder, stomach, small intestine, large intestine, urinary bladder and **[tri-jiao]** 三焦 "triple energizer" are collectively known as the six Fu-organs. And the extraordinary Fu-organs **[qi heng]** 奇恒 comprise six organs, namely, the brain, marrow, bone, vessels, gall-bladder and uterus. The Zang organs of Yang nature are the heart and the liver and the Zang organs of Yin nature refer to the spleen, the

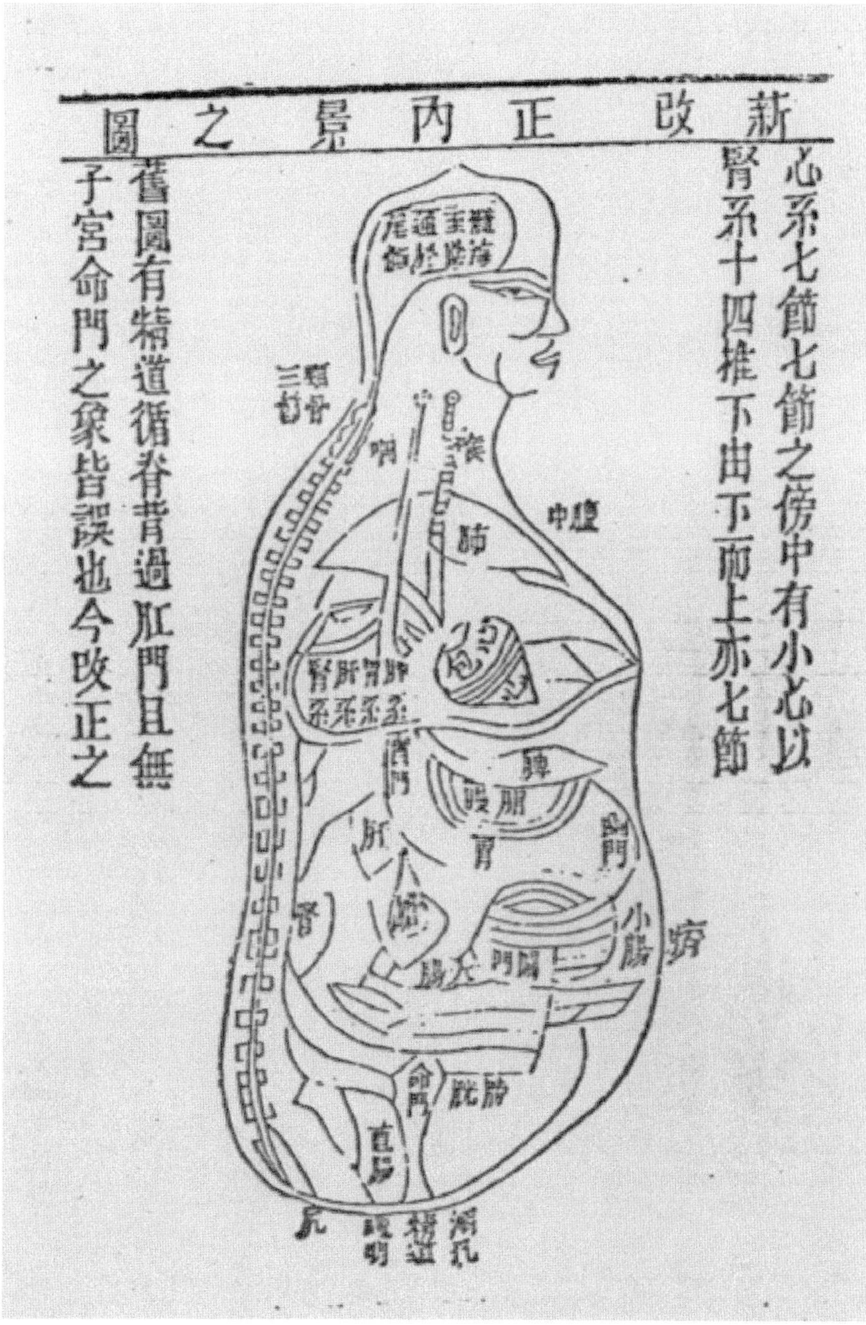

Figure 12: The internal organs.

lungs and the kidney. And the liver, heart, spleen, lungs and kidneys correspond to wood, fire, earth, metal and water respectively, they are metaphysical concepts used to explain the qualities of the body parts. The Five Zang organs are solid, installing but not discharging (essence, energy, blood or body fluid). The main functions of "the six Fu organs" are supposed to receive and digest food, supply the Fu organs with food essence but not to keep it for themselves, and discharge the waste from the body. So there are the following relationships:

***Table of Organs and Their Relationships**

	Heart	Liver	Spleen	Lungs	Kidneys
1 Element	Fire	Wood	Earth	Metal	Water
2 Color	Red	Green	Yellow	White	Black
3 Taste	Bitter	Sour	Sweet	Pungent	Salt
4 Climate	Hot	Windy	Moist	Dry	Cool
5 Odor	Scorched	Rancid	Frangrant	Goatish	Putrid
6 Emotion	Joy	Anger	Desire	Worry	Fear
7 Number	Seven	Eight	Five	Nine	Six
8 Fruit	Apricot	Plum	D Date	Pear	Chestnut

4.1. [wu zang suo zhu] 五脏所主 " Those Controlled by the Five Zang Organs"

The heart controls the blood, the lungs control the skin, the liver controls tendons, the spleen controls the muscles and the kidneys are said to control the bones respectively.

4.2. [wu zang suo wu] 五脏所恶 "Intolerance of the Five Zang organs"

The heart is said to be intolerant of heat, lung to be intolerant of cold, the liver to be intolerant of wind, spleen and kidney are said to be intolerant of dampness respectively.

4.3. [wu zang suo cang] 五脏所藏 "Storage of the Five Zang Organs"

Mind is stored in the heart, the soul in the lungs, the spirit in the liver, the desire in the spleen and the will in the kidney.

4.4.1. [mu xi tiao da] 木喜条达 "Wood has the property of growing freely and unfolding"

The liver belongs to wood. That is a metaphor to explain the physiological properties of the liver. The main function of the liver is to soothe flow of Qi (Vital Energy) and blood. This function should be carried on smoothly and should not be suppressed. If it is depressed, symptoms of stagnancy would occur. Depression of the liver gives rise to the fire syndrome, marked by headache, dizziness, flushed face, haematemesis, haemophthysis, or even mania. Fire of the liver injures the lung (the lung belongs to metal) by impairing the latter's essence and fluid and brings about dry cough, chest pain and even haemophthysis.

4.4.2. [mu yu hua huo] 木郁化火 "Hyperactivity of Wood generating Fire"

This is a fire-syndrome caused by the stagnation of liver-energy because wood is used to represent the liver. It is manifested as headache, dizziness, flushed face, redness of eyes, haematophthysis, haematemesis, anger, red tongue, wiry pulse and even mania, etc.

4.4.3. [mu yu hua feng] 木郁化风 "Hyperactivity of Wood generating Wind"

This is a wind-syndrome caused by the stagnation of liver-energy (wood represents the liver). Wind in TCM refers to certain unsteady, abrupt, wandering, and uncertain symptoms and signs. In such case, some wind symptoms, such as tremor, numbness of the extremities and of the tongue, dizziness or vertigo, and seizures may appear.

4.4.4. [mu huo xing jin] 木火刑金 "Wood-fire impairs Metal"

This is a morbid condition with consumption of Lung-Yin (the lungs belong to metal) resulting from the hyperactivity of liver-fire, manifested as dry cough, pain over the chest and hypochondria, bitter taste in the mouth, restlessness, haematophthysis, etc.

4.5. [huo xing shang yan] 火性上炎 "Fire has the property of Warming and Flaring up"

The heart belongs to the fire, fire tends to flare upwards. This is a figuration which states the fact that the symptoms caused by fire tend to appear in the upper part of the body, especially in the head, such as headache, sore throat, blood-shot eye, gum bleeding, and epistaxis.

4.5.1. [huo bu sheng tu] 火不生土 "Fire fails to generate Earth"

Fire is used to represent the Kidney-Yang (the vital fire). Earth represents the spleen. When the Kidney-Yang is deficient and weak, and the vital fire is not vigorous, the spleen and the stomach cannot receive the warmth of the Yang. The processes of digestion, absorption, and the transportation of nutriment and water will be impaired. In fact, this is a morbid condition of deficiency of Spleen-Yang and Kidney-Yang due to hypo function of the spleen resulting from the insufficiency of

Kidney-Yang, which will be manifested as backache, chilliness of knees, intolerance to cold, anorexia, dyspepsia, dysuria, puffiness or edema, diarrhea before dawn, etc.

4.5.2. [huo sheng xing jin] 火盛刑金 "Blazing Fire damaging Metal"

(1) When the liver fire becomes excessive, the lungs may be damaged. (2) When the heart fire becomes excessive, the Lung-Yin may be damaged. Metal represents the lungs.

4.6. [tu sheng wan wu] 土生万物 "Everything in Nature grows out of the Earth"

The Earth represents the spleen and can produce everything, which is the source of nutrition for building up the body. So this is a physiological characteristic of the spleen and stomach (earth), which provides the material foundation for the whole organism by digesting food and supplying nutriments.

4.6.1. [tu xi wen zao] 土喜温燥 "Earth is fit for Warmth and Dryness"

Earth represents the spleen, and one of the functional characteristics of the spleen is to drive out water or wetness. Warmth and dryness are in favour of this function, otherwise retention of water or wetness would appear because warmth and dryness enhance the capability of transporting moisture by the spleen, while coldness and dampness impair the Spleen-Yang, and this would reduce the capability of transporting moisture by the spleen, thus causing morbid conditions.

4.6.2. [tu bu zhi shui] 土不制水 "Earth fails to control Water"

Earth represents the spleen, but the spleen is too weak to transport water, so that moisture becomes stagnant and overflowing in the body. A morbid condition manifested as thin whitish sputum, semi liquid stools, edema, frequent loose stool etc. would occur.

4.7. [jin qi xiao jiang] 金气肃降 "Metal has the property of Purifying, Descending and Astringing"

Metal represents the lungs. This is one of the physiological characteristic of the lung necessary for the maintenance of its normal functional activities. That is to say that the lung should keep its Qi clear and descendant, otherwise cough, dyspnea, expectoration of sputum and stuffiness in the chest will occur.

4.7.1. [jin han shui leng] 金寒水冷 "Chilly Metal and Cold Water"

Metal represents the lungs, and water represents kidney. This is a morbid condition resulting from the damage of both the lung and the kidney during a chronic disease; classified as two types, i.e., Yin-deficiency and energy-deficiency of both the lung and the kidney.

4.8. [shui xing liu xia] 水性流下 "Water is flowing Downward"

The kidney belongs to the water, water tends to run downward: a metaphor to explain the downward tendency in pathological change due to dampness such as diarrhea, heaviness and edema of the lower extremities.

4.8.1. [shui bu han mu] 水不涵木 "Water fails to nourish Wood"

Water represents the Kidney-Yin; wood, the liver. When Kidney-Yin is deficient, the liver cannot be nourished, and Liver-Yin will become deficient. Thus this is a morbid condition of the deficiency of Liver-Yin with the hyperactivity of the asthenic wind resulting from the inability of Kidney-Yin to nourish the liver, manifested as dizziness, tinnitus, nocturnal emission, thirst, even convulsion.

4.8.2. [shui huo xiang ji] 水火相济 "Water and Fire coordinate each other"

Water refers to Kidney-Yin, while fire to heart fire. The coordination between Kidney-Yin and Heart-Fire is a physiological function necessary for the maintenance of normal activities of the organs.

4.8.3. [shui huo bu ji] 水火不济 "Water and Fire Fail to Coordinate Each Other"

Water refers to Kidney-Yin, while fire to heart fire. When the Kidney-Yin is deficient or the heart fire blazes, there is a loss of control by either of them. Disturbance of the equilibrium of the physiologic dynamics of both would result. So this is a morbid condition caused by the incoordination between Kidney-Yin and heart-fire, manifested as restlessness, insomnia, nocturnal emission, etc.

5. [jing qi xue jin ye] 精 气 血与津液 " Essence, Qi, Blood and Body Fluid"

Essence, Qi, Blood and Body Fluids are the four fundamental substances of the human body, which sustain the normal physiological functions of the Zang-fu organs and tissues.

5.1. [jing] 精 "Essence"

Essence is the fundamental material-the source-of living organism. It is of two types: the congenital (or innate) essence inherited from the parents, and "acquired essence", which originates from foodstuff and fresh air inhaled from the external atmosphere by means of the combined actions of the lungs, spleen, stomach, kidneys and other Zang-fu organs. The two types are interdependent and promote each other. Congenital essence, which is present before birth, provides the fundamental materials for the latter development of acquired essence, while acquired essence after birth continues to nourish congenital essence, rplenishing and invigorating it, through the transporting-transforming function of the spleen and stomach. Essence can be transformed into Qi- that is, into energy or movement-thus helping to maintain life activity because everyone has for depend on the spleen and stomach for absorption of nourishment from foodstuff, meanwhile, the congenital essence-Qi also relies on essential substance from foodstuff for replenishment.

5.2. [qi] 气 " Qi (Vital Energy)"

In TCM, Qi refers to the essence, which constitutes the human body and maintains its life activities. **[zhang jing yue]** 张景岳 "Zhang Jing Yue" said in **[jing yue quan shu]** 景岳全书 "Jing Yue's Complete Works" (1624 AD) "The life of a human being relies totally upon Qi". Qi has many respects in TCM. The predominant one is a kind of substance that is constantly in motion. As Qi has the properties of powerful vigor and constant movement and processes, it is regarded as the basic element or energy, which supports the life activities, and because it is also a substance, Qi is considered as one of the fundamental materials for building up the human body.

5.2.1. [qi de fen lei] 气的分类 "The Classification of Qi"

The classifications of Qi in the human body vary with its distribution, origin, and function, which are described as follows.

5.2.1.1. [yuan qi] 原气 "Primary Qi"

Primary Qi is known as genuine Qi. It is the most important and fundamental Qi originating form the congenital essence. It is nourished and replenished by the fundamental substance of food after birth. It exists everywhere in the human body by the **[san jiao]** 三焦 "Triple energizer" functions. It also arouses and promotes the activities of the Zang-fu organs and tissues, activating them as the primary motive force for life activity.

5.2.1.2. [zong qi] 宗气 "Pectoral Qi"

Pectoral Qi is a combination of the air inhaled and the digested food essence that has been transformed by the stomach and the spleen and stored in the chest, and has the function of nourishing the lung and the heart, and promoting the movements of blood, serving as the dynamic forces of proper respiration and voice.

5.2.1.3. [ying qi] 营气 "Nutrient Qi"

Nutrient Qi is a substance originating from the food collected and transformed by the spleen and the stomach. It flows through the blood vessels and becomes a component of blood, moving through the body and supplying it with nutrients.

5.2.1.4. [wei qi] 卫气 "Defensive Qi"

Wei Qi defends the surface layer of the body to guard against any invasion by external pathogenic factors. Defensive Qi is mainly derived from the essential substances of food and water, which form a part of the human body's Yang Qi, also called "defensive Yang". It moves outside the vessels, travels through the skin and flesh. Its physiological functions are 1) defending the body surface against the invasion of exogenous pathogenic factors; 2) warming and nourishing the parts and organs, and 3) controlling the opening and closing of pores.

5.2.2. [qi de gong neng zuo yong] 气的功能作用 "The Functions of Qi"

Qi, as a vigorous essence, plays a promoting and activating role in the growth and development of the body, the physiological activities of various Zang-Fu organs, channels and collaterals, the production and movements of blood, the formation, distribution and excretion of body fluid, etc. The four basic patterns of movement of Qi is ascending, descending, exiting, and entering. The channels are the passageways for the Qi to carry out the movements. In addition to activating the body, Qi performs several other functions. They are stated as follows:

5.2.2.1. [qi you wen xu zuo yong] 气有温煦作用 "Warming Function of Qi"

[nan jing er shi er nan] 难经 二十二难 "Classic on Medical Problems. Problem 22" says: "Qi is responsible for warming the body". That is to say, it is the source of the body heat. Only through the warming action of Qi the body's temperature can be kept constant, can all Zang-Fu organs, channels and collaterals and other structures perform their respective physiological functions and can such liquid substances as blood and body fluids carry on regular movements. As the saying goes: "blood flows in warm circumstances but coagulates in cold".

5.2.2.2. [qi you fang yu zuo yong] 气 有防御作用 "Defending Function of Qi"

The defense mechanism of the body against disease is very complicated and involves the coordinated action of Qi, blood, body fluids and Zang-Fu organs, channels, collaterals and other structures. Nevertheless, Qi plays a role of considerable importance here. The defensive function of Qi is reflected mainly in protecting the body surface against external pathogens.

5.2.2. 3. [qi you gu she zuo yong] 气有固摄作用 "Controlling Function of Qi"

This function refers chiefly to the action of Qi in reserving liquid substances, such as blood and body fluids, i.e., keepingi the blood flowing within the vessels in order to prevent its extravasation, controlling the amount of the secretion and excretion of sweat, urine, saliva, stomach-fluid, intestine-fluid, semen, etc, to prevent their wasteful consumption.

5.2.2.4. [qi you qi hua zuo yong] 气有气化作用 "Transforming Function of Qi"

Transforming function implies various forms of conversions due to the movement of Qi, namely, transformation of the essence (Qi), blood or body fluids and their mutual transformations respectively. For instance, the essence derived from the food and drink is transformed into Qi, blood and body fluids, the body fluids after being transformed are converted into sweat and urine, and the residues of food after digestion and absorption are turned into feces, etc. All these processes are concrete manifestations of the transforming action of Qi.

5.3. xue] 血"Blood"

Blood is the red fluid flowing through the blood vessels and nourishing the body parts. Blood is a product of nourishing Qi, transformed from food essence and the nutriments taken in the spleen and vital essence stored in the kidney. **[nan jing]** 难经"Classic on Medical Problems - problem 22" says: "The blood is in charge of nourishing the body". The internal movements of the blood bring the nourishing and moisturizing effects on all the organs and parts of the body, e.g. to the Zang-Fu organs, and to the skin, muscles, tendons and bones externally allowing them to perform their individual functions.

"Blood and Qi are the spirits of man" says [su wen] 素问 "Plain Questions". Blood is also considered as the material basis for mental activities. Pathological changes of blood cause symptoms of palpitation, insomnia, unconsciousness, delirium, etc. Qi and blood are inseparable and have equal importance. Qi is essential for blood to perform its functions. If Qi is affected, whether by emotions or environmental factors, blood will also be affected. When Qi is impeded, so is blood. Stasis of blood is therefore often treated by promoting the flowing of Qi, and persistent bleeding by enhancing Qi to bring about haemostasis.

5.4. [jing ye] 津液 "Body Fluids"

"Body fluids" is a general term for all the normal liquid components of the body, including the inner fluids existing in various organs and their normal secretions, such as saliva, stomach fluids, synovial fluids, and tissue fluids. They also refer to such secretions as tears, nasal mucous, sweat, and urine that have not been discharged. Like Qi and blood, the body fluid is also a kind of essence constituting the human body and contributing to the maintenance of its life activities.

5.3.2. [jin ye de gong neng] 津液的功能"Functions of the Body Fluids"

The body fluids perform two functions: moistening and nourishing. For instance, when distributed in the body surface, they moisten the muscles and skin with hairs, when permeating through the body orifices, they moisten and protect eyes, nose, mouth and other openings; when infiltrating into the vessels, they nourish and smooth the vessels as the basic component of blood; when pouring into the internal organs, they nourish and moisten them and when seeping into the joint cavities, marrow cavities and the skull, they lubricate the joints, nourish and moisten the bone marrow, spinal cord and brain. Furthermore, the body fluids also perform the function of the proper elimination of wastes: the maintenance of a normal body temperature, and the regulation of the balance of Yin and Yang in the body all depend on body fluids.

5.4.1. [qi wei xue zhi shuai] 气为血之帅"Qi as the Commander of Blood"

As commander of blood, Qi performs three main functions:1) the production of blood; 2) the propelling of blood, and 3) the control of the blood movements. For example, Qi can produce blood, activating it and governing its flowing. That is to say Qi serves as the dynamic force of blood flow, keeps the blood moving through the vessels, and promotes blood regeneration, and hence stagnancy of Qi will make blood stop flowing, thereby producing morbid products as blood stasis, and deficiency of Qi is bound to affect the generation, transportation and distribution of blood and body fluid, thereby giving rise to many pathological changes of blood and body fluid. And blood serves as the carrier of Qi, supplying Qi with adequate nutrients as the old saying in Chinese "Blood is the mother of Qi". Deficiency of blood may lead to weak syndromes of deficiency type-insufficient Qi (vital energy) with the following clinical symptoms: male complexion, pale lips, dizziness, palpitation, lassitude, listlessness, emaciation, etc. and massive loss of blood my cause prostration of Qi manifested as collapse.

According to the theory of TCM, body Fluid and Blood are derived from water and food essence, hence they are said to have "a common source", and so they are closely related physiologically and pathologically. So blood and body fluid usually influence each other under certain pathological conditions. In clinical practice, blood loss and fluid loss are often mentioned together. So preservation of fluids is as essentially important as preservation of blood.

6. [zang fu] 脏腑 "Five-fu Organs" (see Figure 13).

Chinese medicine recognizes two classes of organs: the [zang] 脏 Zang and **[fu]** 腑 Fu. There are five Zang organs: the heart, liver, spleen, lung and kidneys (see Figure 14).The task of the Zang organs is to maintain a full and vital supply of Qi. If they fail to perform their functions, that are to say if Qi becomes stagnant, illness occurs.

The Fu organs are six: gallbladder, stomach, small and large intestines, urinary bladder (see Figure 15), and triple energizers. They digest, absorb and excrete. Their function is to take in and digest food, then discharging the waste products.

Zang and Fu are all internal organs, the function of Zang is to store and preserve the vital forces and Qi whereas the Fu organs propel and digest food. They are opposing but related to each other, they work in pairs. Each Zang organ is bound in a relationship with each Fu organ both exteriorly and interiorly

6.1. [xin] 心 "The Heart"

The heart is one of the five solid organs and the most important one of the body. Its main function is to maintain the normal blood movements. In TCM the heart belongs to the element of fire, it is the ruling member of the Zang-fu organs. It governs the life and activities of the entire body and controls the life process of the human body. It is considered as closely related to the functional activities of the higher nervous system, mental and emotional activities, and the secretion of sweat glands and even the changes of tongue, and has an **[biao]** 表 "exterior" and [li] 里 "interior" relationship with the small intestine.

6.1.1. [xin zhu xue mai] 心主血脉 "Heart controls Blood Movements"

In **[su wen]** 素问 "Plain Questions", it is said "the heart is in charge of blood vessels". Blood flows through the vessels under the power of heart Qi because

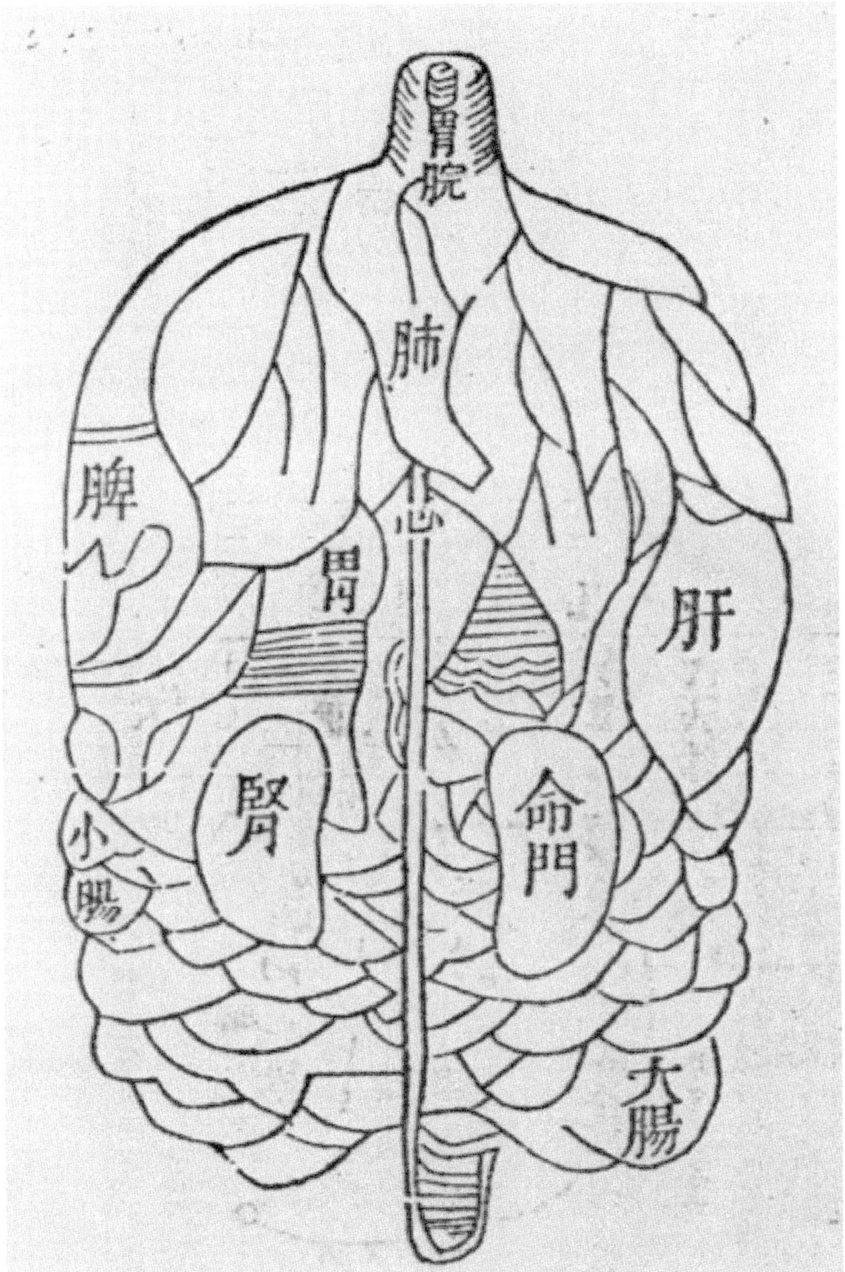

Figure 13: The position of the "five viscera", the stomach, the large and the small intestine. The kidneys are indicated as the seat of the imaginary called "The gate of life".

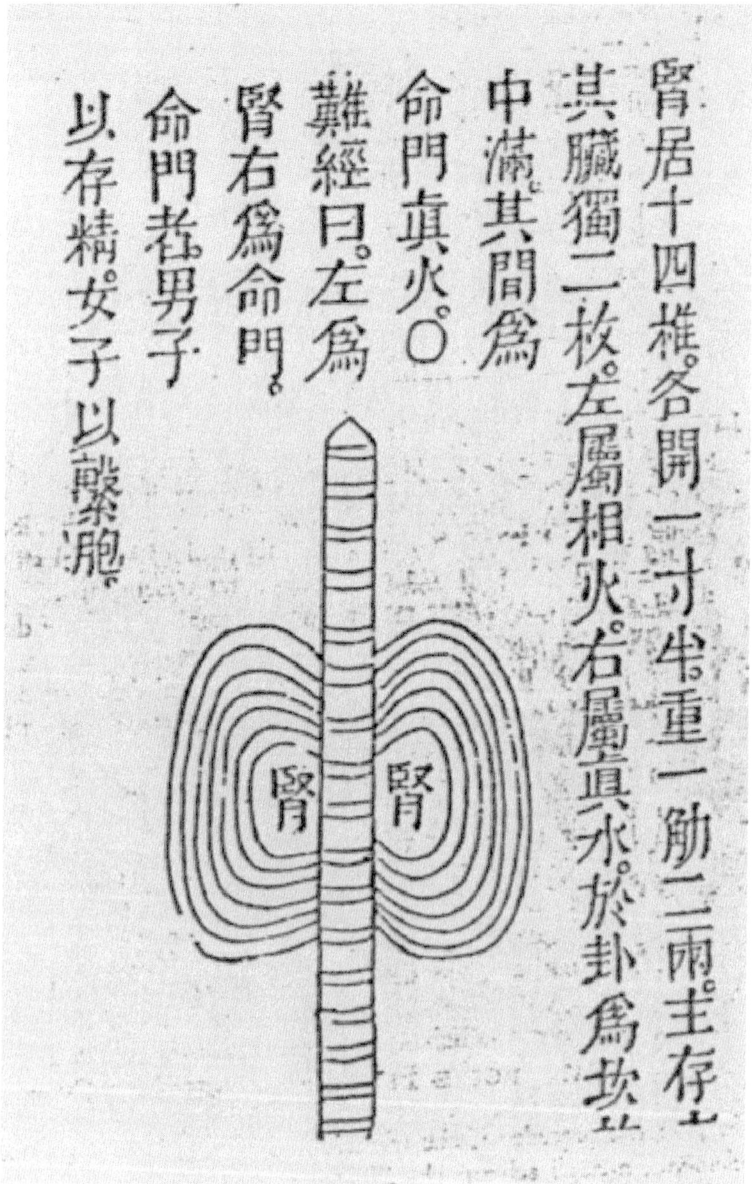

Figure 14: The kidneys.

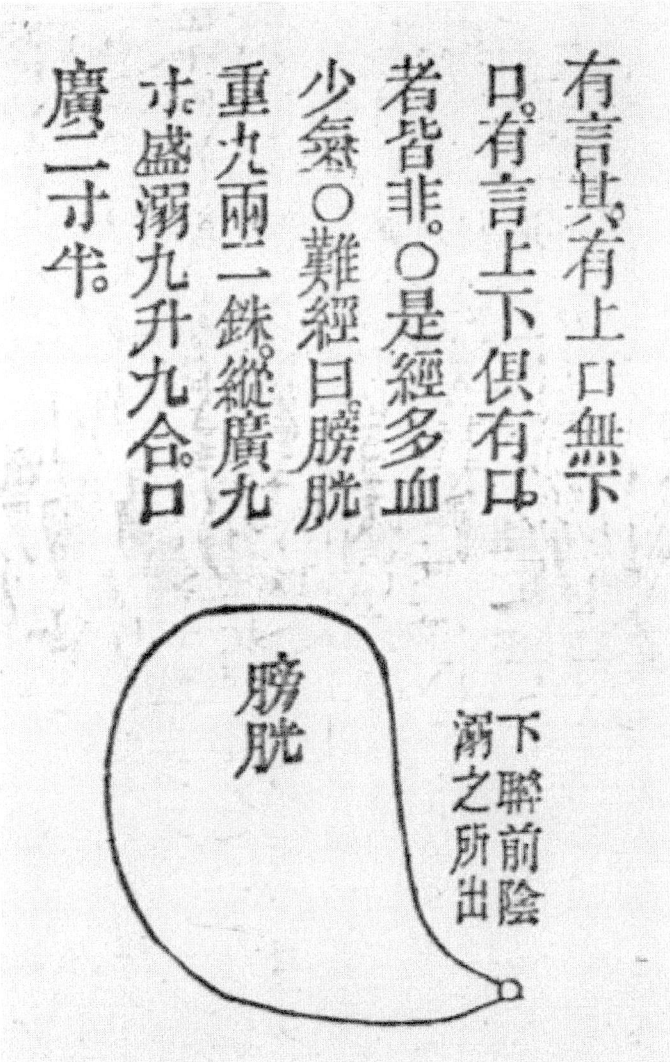

Figure 15: The urinary bladder.

the heart is the motive power of blood movements. When heart Qi is abundant and the blood vessels are full, the pulse beats normally and forcefully and facial complexion is rosy with luster. If the heart is insufficient, the vessels will be empty, the pulse feeble and weak or irregular and the facial complexion pale. Insufficiency of heart Qi may lead to blood stagnation, resulting in diseases. So the heart is the root of life.

6.1.2. [xin zhu shen ming] 心主神明 "Heart controls Mental and Emotional Activities"

According to TCM, mental activity is a general term for the life process and the heart accomplishes the process of thinking. Western medicine holds that mental activities are controlled by the brain while TCM says that it is the heart that governs these activities as was maintained both by Aristole (IV Century B. C.) and his master Plato (V-IV century B. C.) in ancient Greek culture. Mental disorders arise when the heart is injured in some way. And if the heart is weakened, disturbed by emotions, or invaded by external evils, the person may suffer from fearfulness, anxiety, insomnia, forgetfulness, mental confusion and so on.

6.2. [gan] 肝 "The Liver"

One of the five solid organs, its main function is to store and regulate blood, control the movements of the joints and tendons and adjust the digestive function of the spleen and stomach. It is also closely connected with mental activities.

6.2.1. [gan zang xue] 肝藏血 " The Liver stores Blood"

The liver stores blood and regulates the volume of the blood that is in moment and needed by various organs. The demand for blood is increased when the body is active. The blood is released from the liver to meet the need of this demand by increasing the volume of flowing blood. If the liver's blood storage function is abnormal, there will be an affect on normal body activities causing haemorrhagic diseases.

6.2.2. [gan zhu shu xie] 肝主疏泄 "The Liver regulates the Flow of Qi"

TCM says that the liver "favours a smooth flowing of Qi and has an aversion to stagnancy". That is to say it is responsible for the ascending, descending, and harmony of body Qi. If the Qi in the body is harmonious and its ascending and descending are normal then the internal organs will continue their normal physiological activities. The smooth flow of Qi has two functions. First it regulates emotional activities; TCM considers that the normal or abnormal function of free releasing of Qi is directly related to emotional activities, and that the mental state is not only dominated by the heart but also by the liver. When liver Qi does not flow smoothly or is obstructed, abnormal emotional activities such as depression or moodiness may occur. Second, liver Qi regulates ascending function of the spleen and descending function of the stomach. It can also control the secretion of bile. If liver Qi loses its harmonious flowing activities, it will affect the digestive function of the spleen and stomach and the secretion and elimination of bile may become abnormal, leading to the pathological symptoms of jaundice or dyspepsia. In addition to maintaining normal emotional and digestive activity, the smooth flow of Qi ensures the normal functioning of the triple energizers. When liver Qi is impeded owing to liver troubles, the channels may be obstructed by blood stasis, and the accumulated fluid may result in ascites.

6.2.3. [gan zhu jin] 肝主筋 "The Liver controls the activity of the Tendons"

One of the functions of the liver is related to the activities of the ligaments, tendons, muscles and joints. The normal function of the tendons relies on the nourishment of liver blood. The movements of limbs and joints are not only the result of tendon flexing but are also related to the strength or weakness of liver blood. If the liver blood is insufficient and fails to nourish the tendons, the patient might experience symptoms such as tremors of the hands or feet, numbness of the limbs, or even difficulty in flexing and extending the limbs, thus resulting in spasm and atrophy.

The conditions of the liver can be also seen in the conditions of the nails. The dryness or moisture of the nails can reflect the sufficiency or insufficiency of liver blood. When liver blood is plentiful, strong nails develop. When liver blood is insufficient and incapable of nourishing the tendons, the nails become thin and flexible, or even deformed. In **[su wen]** 素问 "Plain Questions", it is said: "The liver communicates with the tendons. The health of the liver is reflected in the luster of the nails". Thus, the condition of the liver can be determined by observing the condition of the nails.

6.3. [pi] 脾 "The Spleen"

The spleen is located in the **[zhong jiao]** 中焦 "the Energizer" (abdominal cavity), which in TCM does not completely match the organ designated in Western Medicine from the standard of structure, location and function. Together with the stomach, it has the function of digestion, assimilation, and distribution of nutrients and water throughout the body. Some diseases of the digestive system, edema and chronic haemorrhagic diseases are usually attributable to malfunction of the spleen.

6.3.1. [pi zhu yun hua] 脾主运化 "The Spleen is responsible for Food digestion and Fluid transportation"

According to TCM, nutrients are obtained from food by the combined digestive activities of the spleen and stomach. The spleen assimilates the nutrients, which are the essence of food. Then it transports the food essence to the lung and heart to be disseminated through the body. When the spleen transports nutrient substances, it simultaneously distributes water to every part of the body carrying out its functions of nourishing and moistening. Water is absorbed first by the spleen and then transported along with the help of the lungs, heart, and urinary bladder to maintain normal water distribution. So the function of the spleen is to regulate the balance of the body fluids through the absorption and transportation and removal of excessive water.

6.3.2. [pi tong xue] 脾统血 "The Spleen controls the Blood Flow"

One of the functions of the spleen is to regulate blood flow inside the blood vessels. When spleen Qi is in deficiency, its function of controlling blood is lost, the blood flows outside the vessels, and then haemorrhagic diseases such as chronic uterine bleeding will occur.

6.3.3. [pi zhu si zhi ji rou] 脾主四肢肌肉 "The Spleen is responsible of Dominating the Four Limbs and Muscles"

One of the functions of the spleen is to transport and transform nutrient substances and energy to the extremities (the four limbs), in order to maintain their normal activities. And it also supplies nutrients to nourish the muscles to maintain their normal structures and functions. When the spleen is involved in diseases, the malnutrition of the muscles characterized by muscle atrophy, weakness of the four limbs, etc. may occur.

6.4. [fei] 肺 "The Lung"

The lung is situated in the chest and connected with the throat. Its main physiological functions are dominating Qi and controlling respiration, regulating water passage, and helping the heart in regulating blood flow, so as for provide the substances necessary for the physiological activities of the organs of the body. It also has an exterior and interior relationship with the large intestine.

6.4.1. [fei zhu qi] 肺主气 "The Lung dominates Qi and controls Respiration"

It refers to the air exchange through respiration-dominating the Qi (air) and controlling respiration. If the lung function is normal, there is an unobstructed circulation of Qi, with even and harmonious breathing. A deficiency of Qi will cause feeble respiration, uneven breathing, the abnormality of voice, lassitude etc.

6.4.2. [fei zhu su jiang] 肺主肃降 "The Lung dominates the function of Dispersion and Descent"

The function of dispersion and descent involves the distribution of Qi, blood, and body fluid to the Zang-Fu organs, the channels-collaterals, muscles, skin, and hair. For example, water and fluids travel throughout the body and are discharged along routes or passageways that rely on descending, which means the lung Qi is clear and descends. If the lung Qi fails to descend and instead ascends, then the Qi will accumulate in the lung, resulting in stuffy chest, cough, asthma etc.

6.4.3. [fei he da chang] 肺合大肠 "The Lung is connected with the Large Intestine"

The external organ associated with the lung is the large intestine. The lung and large intestine cooperate in their physiological functions and affect each other when diseased. When the descending function of the lung Qi is normal, the large intestine functions efficiently, eliminating smoothly. When the function is not normal, obstruction may occur in the large intestine. For example, lung-heat syndrome may result in constipation, and it can be relieved by relaxing the bowels.

6.4.4. [fei he mao pi] 肺合毛皮 "Skin and Hair are connected with the Lung"

The skin and hair represent the entire body surface including skin, sweat gland, and hair, together they perform the defensive function against the invasion of exogenous pathogenic factors. Through the dispersing function of the lung, the essentials of food and wastes are transported to the body surface in order to nourish the skin, hair and muscles. By regulating the respiratory function of the lung, the body temperature can be also adjustment by the skin, thus protecting the organic body against the invasion of external pathogenic evil factors.

6.5. [shen] 肾 "The Kidneys"

The kidneys are situated in the waist, one on either side of the spinal column. In TCM , the kidneys do not completely match with the Western Medicine from the standpoint of anatomy and physiology. They perform the functions of storing the congenital essence which is considered as the origin of Yin-Yang of Zang-Fu organs and the source of life of human body, promoting the growth and development of the body, controlling human production, water movement, regulating the flow of Qi. Together with the lung and spleen, they play an important part in the regulation of body fluids and perform the functions of urogenital system; hence they are called "The origin of congenital constitution". More specifically, they perform the following functions.

6.5.1. [shen zhu sheng zhi] 肾主生殖 "The Kidneys are in charge of Growth, Development and Reproduction"

One of the chief physiological functions of the kidney-essence is to promote the growth and development of the body. **[shang gu tian zhen lun]** 上古天真论 "Treatise on Innate Vital Essence in Ancient Times" of **[su wen]** 素问 "Plain Questions" (475-221 B.C.) points out that the birth, growth, full development, senility and death of man are closely related to the vicissitudes of the kidney-essence.

Another function of the kidney-essence is the reproduction power of the human body. When the essence in the kidney is replenished to a certain degree during youth, inside the body may be produced a kind of substance named **[tian gui]** 天葵 "Tian Gui" (sex-stimulating essence) which promotes the development and maturity of sex gland. When people get to their "Tian Gui ", a male begins to produce and ejaculate semen, while a female starts to have a regular menstruation with fertility. That is to say, he or she has possessed the ability of reproduction and reached puberty.

If the abundant kidney-essence changes into deficiency, the productive power of "Tian Gui" will slow down and the reproductive power is also reduced.

6.5.2. [shen zhu shui ye dai xie] 肾主水液代泻 "The Kidneys control Water Exchanges and Reception of Air"

One of the important functions of kidneys is to regulate the conveyance, distributing and discharging of body fluids, and maintain the balance of water transformation within the body by way of the functioning of the kidney-Qi.

Water is received by the stomach, transported and transformed by the spleen, the dispersing and descending functions of the lungs, and the steaming and ascending actions of the kidneys, all of which contribute more to the transformation of the body fluids. The body fluids are of two kinds: "clear fluid" and "turbid fluid", the former flows throughout the organs, parts, and muscles, and the latter is converted into sweat, urine and air then to be eliminated from the body by the steaming and ascending actions of kidney-Qi. The distribution of water is related to the functions of the stomach, spleen, small intestine, large intestine, lung, urinary bladder, and **[san jiao] 三焦** "Triple Energizers", but they also rely on the warming and ascending function of Kidney Yang. If there is an insufficiency of Kidney Yang, the retention of water resulting in scanty urination, retention of urine or frequent urination, enuresis, etc. may occur.

6.5.3. [shen zhu na qi] 肾主纳气 "The Kidney has the function of improving the Ability of Inspiration"

The function implies that the kidneys have the ability to help the body to receive and absorb the fresh air inhaled by the lungs. According to TCM, the lung dominates the respiratory function of the human body, but it must rely on the receiving action of the kidneys, which in fact demonstrates the storing function of the kidneys in the respiratory movement. If everything goes smoothly with the functioning of the kidneys, breathing would be even, moderate and harmonious. Hypo function of the kidneys, however, will give rise to a morbid condition marked by shallow breathing, liability to dyspnea on slight exertion, prolonged expiration and shortened inspiration. This kind of morbid condition in TCM is called "Failure of the kidneys in receiving air".

6.5.4. [shen zhu hua fa]肾主华发 "The Kidneys can show the growing condition of the Hairs on the Head"

The growth of the hair completely relies on the supply of essence and blood. The kidneys have the function of storing the essence, so the growing of the hair can be a symptom of the condition of the kidneys. The blood has also the function of nourishing the hairs, called "the remainder of blood". Generally speaking, the conditions of premature senility, dry and withered hairs and premature greying or loss of hairs are considered in TCM to be caused by the insufficiency of the kidney-essence or the deficiency of blood, thus the conditions of the kidney can be judged from the hair.

6.5.5. [shen kai qiao yu er yin] 肾开窍于二阴 "The Kidneys have their specific openings in Two Yin-orifices"

Two Yin-orifices refer to (1) anterior Yin-orifice, (including urethra and vagina) an organ for micturition and reproduction, (2) posterior Yin-orifice, (anus) an excretory opening for defecation. The excretion of urine involves in the functioning of the urinary bladder, but also depends on the functioning of the kidney-Qi for its accomplishment. Therefore dysfunction of the kidney-Qi often brings about frequent micturition, enuresis, oliguria or anuresis etc. And defecation is concerned not only with the transportation of the large intestine but also with the functioning of kidney-Qi. For instance, deficiency of the kidney-Yin may lead to constipation which is caused by dryness of the intestinal juice; insufficiency of the kidney-Yang may bring about constipation or diarrhea due to disturbance in Qi-transformation; and protracted diarrhea or incontinence of faeces are often caused by the failure of the kidneys to store essence and control urination and defecation.

6.7. [pang guang] 膀胱 "The Urinary Bladder"

The urinary bladder is situated in the center of the lower abdomen. It is an organ for storing urine with its chief function of storing and discharging it. According to TCM theory, the kidneys and the urinary bladder are interior-exteriorly related, which means that the kidneys as a Zang organ in the interior and the bladder as a Fu organ in the exterior are connected by meridians and coordinated in some of their functions. For instance, urine is formed from body fluids through the action of the kidney-Qi and then sent down to the urinary bladder, where it is retained to a certain amount, and finally automatically discharged from the body in time. The disorder of the urinary bladder usually manifests itself by frequency and urgency of urination, urodynia, oliguria, dysuria, dribbling urination, even anuresis, or incontinence of urine and so on. And the dysfunction of the kidney-Qi is mostly involved in these morbid conditions.

6.8. [san jiao] 三焦 "Tri-Jiao or Triple Energizer" (see Figure 16).

Tri-Jiao or triple energizer, a general term for the upper, middle and lower Jiao, as a passageway for ascending, descending in-going. out-going of Qi is regarded as water communications, such as regulating water changes, production and transformation of food essence. Generally the main functions of Tri-Jiao are to pass various kind of Qi and to control the movements of body fluids.

6.8.1. [shang jiao] 上焦 "The Upper-Jiao"

The upper-Jiao refers mainly to the thorax above the diaphragm, including the heart, lungs and head as well. Its physiological function is to distribute the vital essence throughout the body. In **[ling shu]** 灵枢 "Miraculous Pivot" (2589 B.C.) it is said that "The upper- Jiao resembles a sprayer". That is to say the upper-Jiao has the function to spread nutriments and vital energy throughout the whole body, and its functional state is compared to the natural fog-dew, which permeates throughout the earth to nourish all living things.

6.8.2. [zhong jiao] 中焦 "The Middle-Jiao"

The middle-Jiao refers usually to the epigastrium below the diaphragm and above the umbilicus, including such viscera as the spleen, stomach, liver and gallbladder. Its physiological functions are to digest foodstuff and to transport and transform the nutriments, just as the old saying goes: "The middle-Jiao works like a

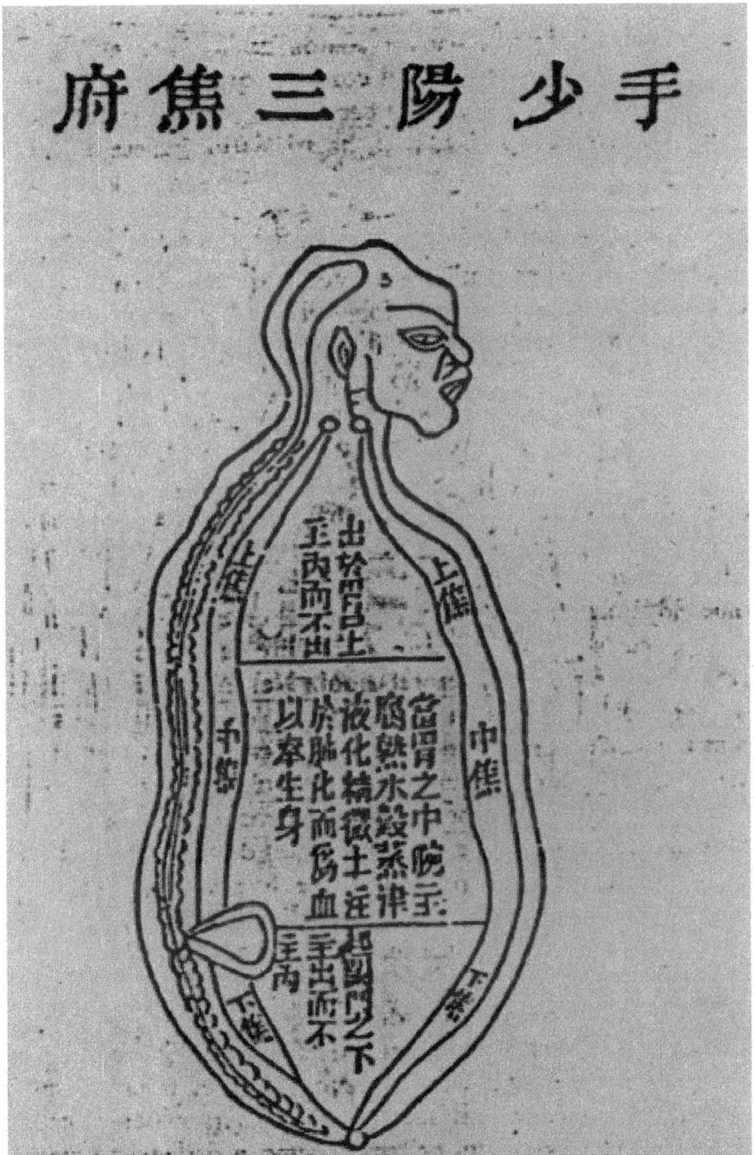

Figure 16: The "Three Energizers" ("Triple energizer") also called the "Three fire-sides".

fermentation tun", for the stomach and the spleen being housed in it are responsible for digesting food.

6.8.3. [xia jiao] 下焦 "The Lower-Jiao"

The lower-Jiao refers generally to the lower portion of the body cavity below the umbilicus, consisting of the small intestine, large intestine, kidneys, urinary bladder, etc. Its physiological function is to filter and drain off waste and surplus water. In fact, resembling water, it works like gutters.

7. [zang fu jian de guang xi] 脏腑间的关系 "Relationship between Zang-fu Organs"

7.1. [sheng yu pang guang xiang biao li] 肾与膀胱相表里 "The interior-exterior relationship between the Kidneys and the Urinary Bladder "

It is believed that "the kidneys and the urinary bladder are interior-exteriorly related" because of the interrelation between them through channels, for the kidneys play a very important role in the functions of the urinary bladder in storing and excreting urine. If there is a sufficiency of the kidney-Qi, the kidneys fulfill their reserving function normally and the urinary bladder functions to open and close at the right moment. However, in case of insufficiency of the Kidney-Qi, disturbance in Qi transformation will occur, followed by failure of the kidneys to fulfill their reserving function and by abnormal opening-closing of the urinary bladder, marked by oliguria or incontinence of urine, or enuresis, frequent urination, etc..

7.2. [xin yu shen de guan xi] 心与肾的关系 "Relationship between the Heart and the Kidneys"

The heart is situated in the upper part of the body, corresponding to fire according to TCM, while the kidneys are situated in the lower part of the body, corresponding to water. Therefore, the relation between the two is the "harmonious relationship between water and fire". That is to say, the heart-fire needs to go down to the kidneys while the kidney- water needs to go up to the heart. Only in this way can their functional activities be maintained in a harmonious rate. This is what is known as "coordination between the heart and the kidneys", or "mutual assistance of fire and water". The discordance between water and fire may bring about a morbid condition named "breakdown of the balance between the heart and the kidneys", marked by insomnia, palpitation, dysphoria, lassitude in the loins and legs, or nocturnal emission in men, orgasm during dream in women, ringing in the ears, muscular aching and so on.

7.3. [fei yu shen de guan xi] 肺与肾的关系 "Relationship between the Lung and the Kidneys"

We can understand the relationship between the lung and the kidneys through their mutual control of Qi and water. As for water transformation, the lung, as "the upper source of fluid", relies upon the kidney-Qi for support (especially its steaming activity). Conversely, the kidneys also require support from the lung (especially function in descending Qi and clearing water passages). As for respiratory activities, since the lung governs the exchange of air and the kidneys are in charge of the reception of air, sufficiency of the kidney-Qi helps the inhaled air sent down from the lung to be received in the kidneys, as the saying goes: " The lung is the dominator of Qi and the kidneys its root".

As for pathological changes, impairment of the dispersing and descending function of the lung and its failure to clear and regulate water passages must affect the kidneys, thus giving rise to oliguria and even edema; while disturbance in functioning of the kidney-Qi with the retained fluid overflowing upward results in dyspnea, or gasping cough with inability to lie flat. Either insufficiency of the kidney-essence or deficiency of the lungs with kidneys involved can bring about failure of the kidneys to receive air, marked by dyspnea or slight exertion between the lung (metal) and the kidneys (water). That is to say, the lung-Yin can replenish the kidney-Yin downward, which in turn can nourish the lung-Yin upward. Pathological deficiency of Yin fluid both of the lungs and the kidneys can frequently occur simultaneously, thereby giving rise to flushing of zygomatic regions, hectic fever like coming out from the bones, night sweat, dry cough with hoarseness, lassitude in the loins and legs. etc.

7.4. [gan yu shen de guan xi] 肝与肾的关系 "Relationship between the Liver and the Kidneys"

Since the liver stores blood and the kidneys store essence, blood and essence promote each other and transform themselves into each other. As the saying goes: "Essence and blood have a common source". That is to say the liver and the kidneys form a close relationship with each other because of the fact that they come from the same source. Pathologically speaking, they can affect each other, thus resulting in deficiency of both essence and blood.

From the physiological functions such as menstruation and seminal emission, we can see that the liver governs normal flow of Qi and the kidneys the storage of essence, so both of them restrain and oppose each other and get complement each other. For this reason, disorder of either may give rise to irregular menstruation in females and seminal emission or priapism without ejaculation in males. There is also a mutual restraining and coordinating relation between Yin-Yang of both the liver and the kidneys. Deficiency or excess of one will lead to excess or deficiency of the other.

7.5. [pi yu shen de guan xi] 脾与肾的关系 "Relationship between the Spleen and the Kidneys"

Physiologically, the spleen as the source of growth and development provides the material basis for the acquired constitution, while the kidneys as the origin of congenital constitution store vital essence and energy. Consequently, production of Qi-blood by the spleen depends on the warming-invigorating action of the kidneys. On the other hand, the essence stored in the kidneys relies on the replenishment of Qi-blood transformed from foodstuff. That is to say, the acquired nutriments take the congenital essence-Qi as their dominator, and the innate essence-

Qi takes the postnatal nutriments as its supplies. The function of the spleen in the transportation- transformation can't be accomplished without the warming-invigorating action of the kidney-Yang. Pathologically, the spleen and the kidneys or acquired essence and congenital essence influence each other, and act on each other as cause or effect alternatively. When one is diseased, the other too may easily become diseased; symptom complexes involving a deficiency of both kidney and spleen are common, often manifested as chilly sensation of the whole body, especially the limbs, pale complexion, cold sensation and pain of the loins and knees, morning diarrhea, general dropsy, dysuria, pale and tender tongue with whitish and moist fur, sunken and weak pulse, etc.

8. [jing luo xue shuo] 经络学说"The Theory of Meridians" (see Figures 17 and 18).

The theory of meridians is an important component part of traditional Chinese medicine, which is the theory to study the physiologic functions and pathologic changes of the meridian system - the system of the channels and collaterals and their relationship with the Zang-fu organs. Physiologically, the channels and collaterals are considered to be the specific passageways for the flow of Qi and the movement of blood throughout the body, and to maintain the interconnection between visceral organs and extremities, and keep the communication and the harmonization of the upper with the lower and of the interior with the exterior, and to regulate the mechanisms of the various parts of the body, hence making the human body an organic whole. Because it is the means of communication and regulation, the channels and collaterals are the pathways through which the exogenous pathological factors are transmitted. The onset of a disease in the internal organs will ultimately find expression in a given location on the body surface. Since channels and collaterals have certain running courses that connect with Zang-fu organs, therefore clinical diagnosis can be made according to symptoms that are related to those courses and their respective Zang-fu organs. In treatment, particularly in the practice of acupuncture, the theory of channels and collaterals is the basis of all treatment and clinical practice.

8.1. [jin luo] 经络"Channels and Collaterals"

Literally, the character **[jing]** 经 (channels), means the rout and [luo] 络 (collateral), the network. The channels, the cardinal conduits of the meridian system and the collateral its branch. The "meridian" is a general term for both the channel and collateral.

The channel system consists of several different types of pathways. The twelve principal Channels connect the internal organs to the surface of the body; each corresponds to either a Zang or a Fu organ. The main function of the Eight Extra Channels is to help reinforce the communication through the body, further assuring a steady flow of Qi and blood. The Divergent Channels also link the body surface to the internal organs, but in general they follow a more superficial course than the twelve principal Channels. The Tendon and Muscle Channels promote the flow of Qi on the body surface.

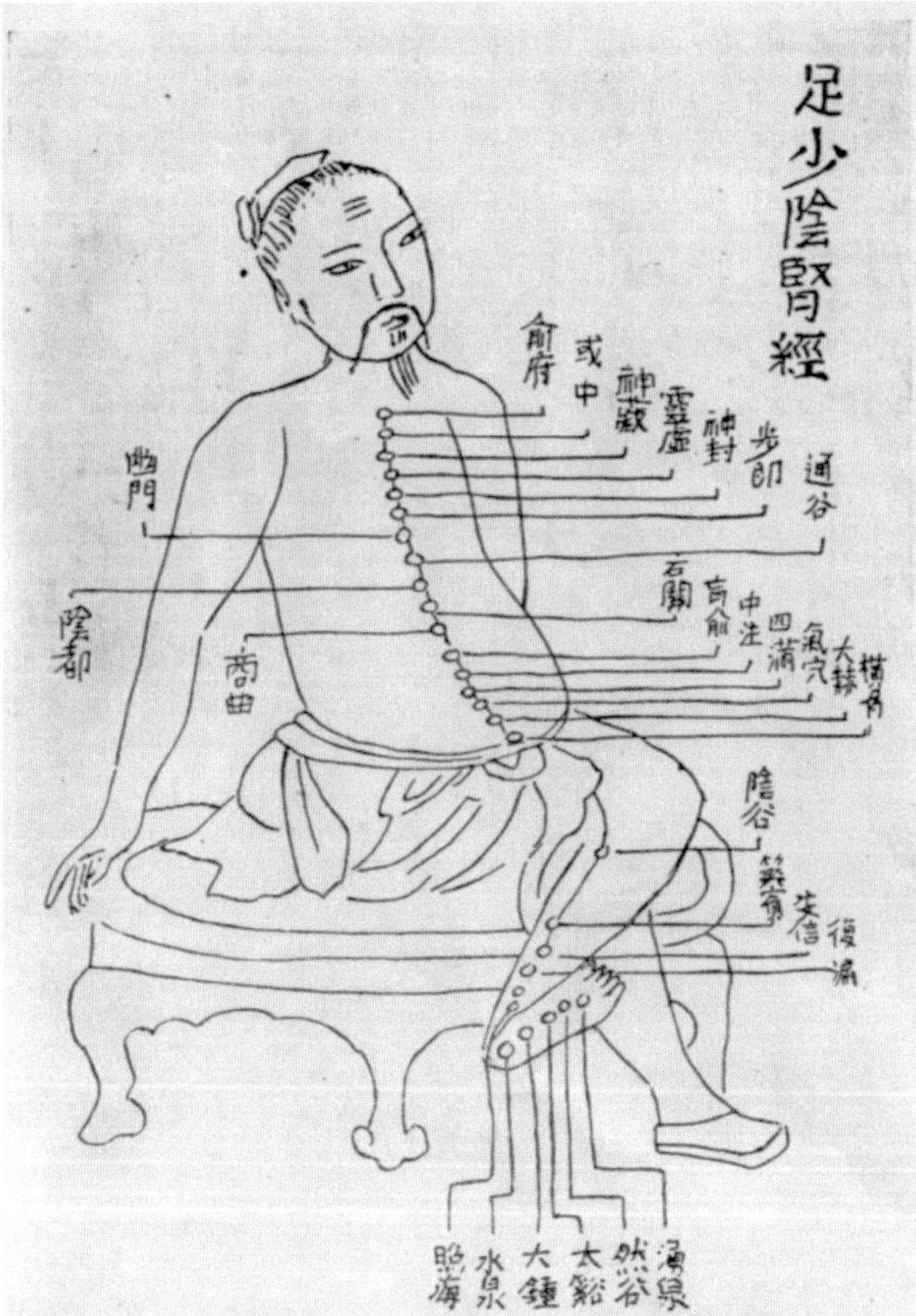

Figure 17: The meridian of the kidneys.

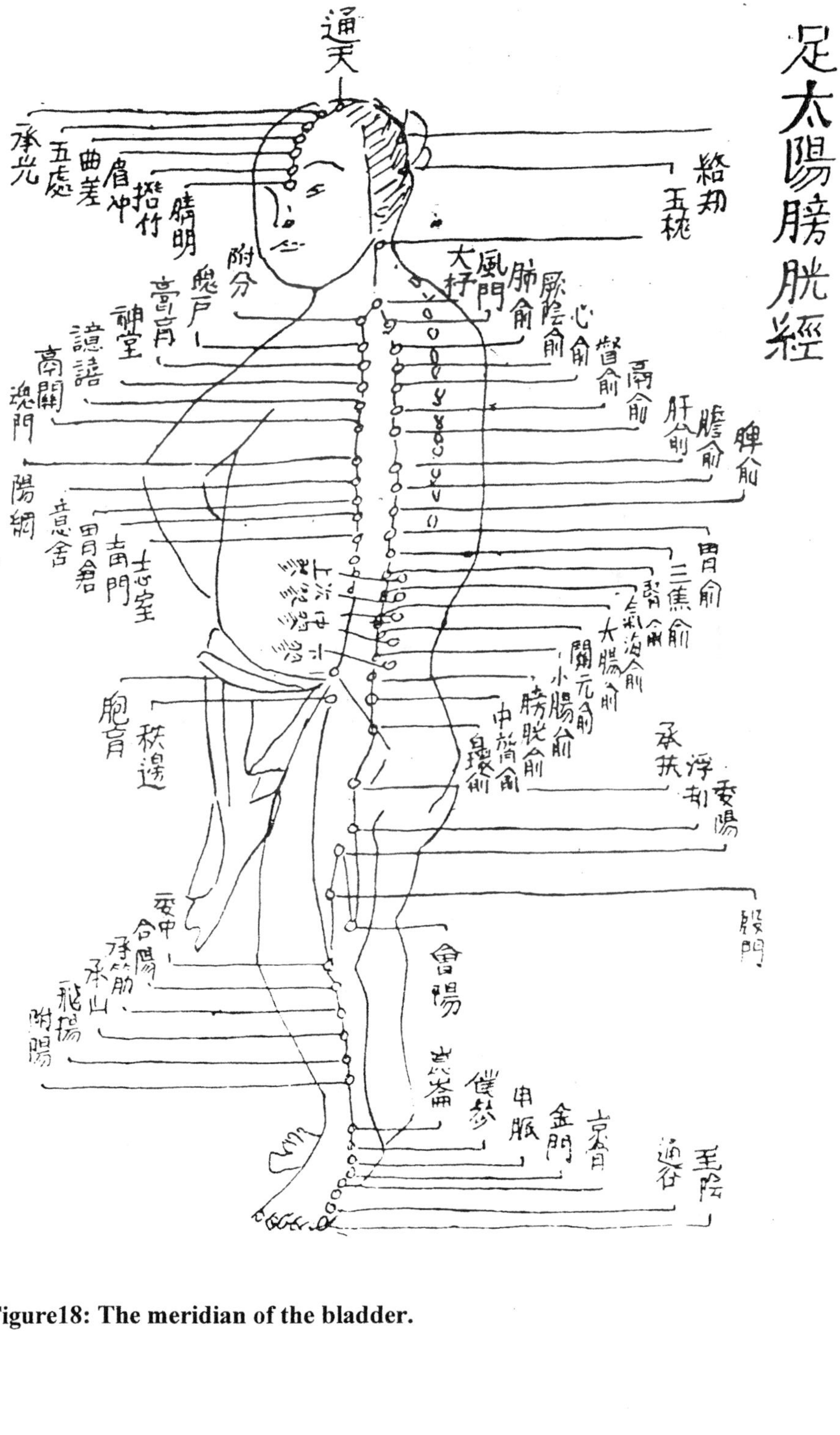

Figure18: The meridian of the bladder.

8.2. [zheng jing] 正经 "Principal Channels"

The main trunks of the channel system are the Twelve Principal Channels. These channels run lengthwise through the body and each channel is associated with Zang-fu organs. They are twelve channels of both hand and foot, and three Yin channels of both hand and foot, collectively known as " Twelve Principal Channels".

1. **[shou tai yin fei jing]** 手太阴肺经 "Lung Meridian of Hand Tai Yin" (LU).
2. **[shou yang ming da chang jing]** 手阳明大肠经 "Large Intestine Meridian of Hand Yangming" (LI).
3. **[zu yang ming wei jing]** 足阳明胃经 "Stomach Meridian of Foot Yangming" (ST).
4. **[zu tai yin pi jing]** 足太阴脾经 "Spleen Meridian of Foot Taiyin" (SP).
5. **[shou shao yin xin jing]** 手少阴心经 "Heart Meridian of Hand Shao Yin" (HT).
6. **[shou tai yang xiao chang jing]** 手太阳小肠经 "Small Intestine Meridian of Hand Tai Yang" (KI).
7. **[u tai yang pang guang jing]** 足太阳膀胱经 "Bladder Meridian of Foot Shaoyin" (BL).
8. **[zu shao yin shen jing]** 足少阴肾经 "Kidney Meridian of Foot Shao Yin (PC).

8.1. **[shou jue yin xin bao jing]** 手厥阴心包 "Pericardium Meridian of Hand Jue Yin (PC)

9. **[shou shao yang san jiao jing]** "Triple Energizer meridian of Hand Shao Yang" (TE).
10. **[zu shao yang dan jing]** 足少阳胆经 "Gallbladder Meridian of Foot Shao Yang" (GB).
11. **[zu jue yin gan jing]** 足厥阴肝经 "Liver meridian of Foot Jue Yin" (LR).

The Twelve Principal channels also play the roles of communication with the upper and lower parts of the body. Six of them communicate with the lower half of the body, passing through the legs and feet; these are known as the "Foot Channels". The remaining six travel through the upper half of the body, passing through the arms and hands; they are known as the" Hand Channels". The Yin channels are located on the medial (or inner) side of the extremities, while the Yang are located on the lateral (or outer) side. Each channel meets another channel. At the point where they meet, there is a transfer of channel Qi. In this way, the Twelve principal Channels help to smooth the orderly flow of Qi throughout the body.

8.2.1. [shi er jing mai de zou xiang gui li] 十二经脉的走向规律 "The Pathways of the Twelve Principal Channels"

The running direction and the interconjunction of the twelve regular channels consist of the following network: the three Yin channels of hand go from the chest to the hands, connecting with the three Yang channels of hand at the ends of the fingers; the three Yang channels of hand from the ends of the fingers to the head, joining with the three Yang channels of foot at the ends of the head to the feet; uniting with the three Yin channels of foot at the end of toes; and the three Yin channels of foot from feet to the abdomen, connecting with the three Yin channels of hand at the thoracic and abdominal cavities.

8.2.2. [qi liu zai shi er jing mai zhong de zhou xiang] 气流在十二经脉中的走向 "The order of the Qi flow in the Twelve Principal Channels"

The twelve principal channels have a connecting relationship with their pertaining Zang-fu organs and their exterior-interior relationship is the same as the exterior-interior relationship of the Zang-fu organs. With an exterior-interior relationship, channels run opposite each other on the lateral and medial aspects of the four limbs and connect with each other on the hand or foot, forming the six pairs of channels exteriorly-interiorly related with the Zang-fu organs. Qi flows continually, traveling throughout the channels in the following order:

The Lung Channel of hand Taiyin → The Large Intestine Channel of the Hand-Yangming → The Stomach Channel of the Foot-Yangming → The Spleen Channel of the Foot-Taiyin → The heart Channel of the Hand-Shaoyin → The Small Intestine Channel of the Hand-Taiyang → The Urinary Bladder channel of the Foot-Taiyang →The Kidney Channel of the Foot-Shaoyin → The Pericardium Channel of the Hand-Jueyin → The Sanjiao Channel of the Hand-Shaoyang → The Gall Bladder Channel of the Foot-Shaoyang → The Liver Channel of the Foot-Jueyin

8.3. [qi jing ba mai] 奇经八脉 "Eight Extra Channels"

The second group of channels is the Eight Extra Channels. They differ from the Twelve principal Channels in two ways: they are not directly related to any of the internal organs nor are they related to one another in the interior/exterior relationship. The Eight Extra Channels are interlaced with the Twelve Principal Channels, with the chief function of regulating the flow of Qi and blood of the Twelve principal Channels. When the Qi and blood is sufficient, they can be stored in the Eight Extra Channels for later use, when in insufficient, the channel can be replenished. They are described as follows:

1. **[du mai]** 督脉 "Du Mai- Governor Vessel" (GV).
2. **[ren mai]** 任脉 "Ren Mai-Conception Vessel" (CV).
3. **[chong mai]** 冲脉 "Chong Mai-Thoroughfare Vessel" (TV).
4. **[dai mai]** 代脉 "Dai Mai -Belt Vessel" (BV).
5. **[yin qiao mai]** 阴跷脉 "Yin Qiao Mai-Yin Heel Vessel" (Yin HV).
6. **[yang qiao mai]** 阳跷脉 "Yang Qiao Mai- Yang Heel Vessel" (Yang HV).
7. **[yin wei mai]** 阴维脉 "Yin Wei Mai-Yin Link Vessel" (Yin LV).
8. **[yang wei mai]** 阳维脉 "Yang Wei Mai- Yang Link Vessel "(Yang LV).

8.4. [shi wu luo mai] 十五络脉 "The Fifteen Collaterals"

They are connecting channels, diverging from the twelve principal channels and Eight Extra channels. There are fifteen collaterals in all, that is each of the twelve principal channels has a collateral, plus the **[ren]** 任 "Ren" and **[du]** 督 "Du" channels, and the great collateral of the spleen.

The fifteen collaterals strengthen the function of the twelve principal channels and closely connect the exterior- interior related channels. They also promote the transportation and distribution of Qi and blood so as for moisten and nourish the whole body.

8.5. [jin mai] 筋脉 "The Tendon and Muscle Channels"

The Tendon and Muscle Channels are located in the superficial parts of the body, they don't enter the internal organs, and so they mainly affect the muscles and tendons. When they are diseased, the manifestation may appear in the muscles of the extremities, head, and trunk rather than in the internal organs.

These channels do not circulate in a circular course and follow a course quite different fro that of the Twelve Principal Channels. They can reach the parts of the body the Twelve principal Channels cannot reach, thus supplementing the Twelve principal Channels.

8.6. [shi er jing bie] 十二经别 "The Twelve Divergent Channels"

The twelve principal channels have certain courses connecting with Zang-fu organs and thee four extremities respectively. Each channel also has a diverging branch penetrating the body cavity, and it is called " a divergent channel". The main function of the twelve divergent channels is to strengthen the exterior- interior relationship of the twelve principal channels, thus forming closer ties between all parts of the body.

Distribution of the Fifteen Collaterals*

Collateral	Location	Connection
Hand taiyin	0.5 cun above wrist	Hand yangming
Hand Shaoyin	1 cun above wrist	Hand Taiyang
Hand Jueyin	2 cun above wrist	Hand Shaoyang
Hand Yangming	3 cun above wrist	Hand Taiyin
Hand Taiyang	5 cun above wrist	Hand Shaoyin
Hand Shaoyang	2 cun above wrist	Hand Jueyin
Foot Yangming	8 cun above malleolus	Foot Shaoyang
Foot Taiyyang	7 cun above malleolus	Foot Shaoyin

Foot Shaoyang	5 cun above malleolous	Foot Jueyin
Foot Taiyin	1 cun proximal to phalanges joint of big toe	Foot Yangming
Foot Shaoyin	posterior to malleolus on heel	Foot Taiyang
Foot Jueyin	5 cun above malleolus	Foot Shaoyang
Ren Channel	Below xyphoid process	Over abdomen
Du Channel	at tip of coccyx	Over the head through spine
Great Collateral of Spleen	3 cun below axillary fossa	Overchest & hypochondriac region

* Abbreviations for the channels used in naming the points are as follows:

Lu-Lung	UB-Urinary Bladder
Li-Large Intestine	K-Kidney
St-Stomach	P- Pericardium
Sp-Spleen	SJ-Triple Burner
H-Heart	GB-Gall Bladder
Si-Small Intestine	Li-Liver

This nomenclature is based on *The Essential of Chinese Acupuncture* (Beijing: Foreign languages press, 1980)

9. [zhen fa] 诊法"Diagnostic Methods"

The diagnostic methods refer to the four basic techniques for diagnosis, namely inspection, auscultation and olfaction, interrogation and palpation. According to TCM, the human body is an organic entity, so local pathological changes may affect the whole body. TCM believes in a comprehensive analysis by four methods of examination, so the four diagnosis methods are indispensable and important steps of differentiation of symptoms and signs by an overall analysis and synthesis of data obtained from the practice pf the four methods in order to find the causes, nature, and interrelations of the disease and help to make a correct diagnosis.

9.1. [Wang hen] 望诊"Inspection"

Inspection is a method to examine the patient by observation of mental state, complexion, physical condition and behavior by the doctor's eye to gain clinical date concerning the disease. All visible signs related to disease are within the scope of inspection. The methods of observation are as follows:

(1) **[wang shen]** 望神 "Observation of Vitality"
(2) **[wang se]** 望色 "Observation of Complexion"
(3) **[wang xing ti]** 望形体 "Observation of Bodily Figure"
(4) **[wang zi tai]** 望姿态 "Observation of Behavior"
(5) **[wang yang]** 望眼 "Observation of the Eyes"
(6) **[wang er]** 望耳 "Observation of the Ears"
(7) **[wang bi]** 望鼻 "Observation of the Nose"
(8) **[wang chun]** 望唇 "Observation of the Lips"
(9) **[wang chi]** 望齿 "Observation of the Teeth"
(10) **[wang yan hou]** 望咽喉 "Observation of the Throat"
(11) **[wang pi fu]** 望皮肤 "Observation of the Skin"
(12) **[wang ban zhen]** 望斑疹 "Observation of Skin Eruption"
(13) **[wang bai bei]** 望白 "Observation of the Miliaria Alba"
(14) **[wang she]** 望舌 "Observation of the Tongue"
(15) **[wang pai chu wu]** 望排出物 "Observation of the Discharges"
(16) **[wang tan]** 望痰 "Observation of the Sputum"
(17) **[wang ou tu wu]** 望呕吐物 "Observation of the Vomitus"
(18) **[wang da bian]** 望大便 "Observation of the Stool"
(19) **[wang xiao bian]** 望小便 "Observation of the Urination"
(20) **[wang xiao er zhi wen]** 望小儿指纹 "Observation of Superficial Venules of the Infant's Index Fingers"

9.2. [ting zhen] 听诊 "Auscultation and Olfaction"

Auscultation and olfaction are the diagnostic method of detecting the clinical status of a patient by listening (to his voice, breathing, coughing) and smelling (odor of his secretion and excretion). According to TCM, all the sounds and odors from the human body, produced in the course of physiological and pathological activities of Zang-Fu organs, may reflect their physiological and pathological changes. There are several methods, e.g.

(1) **[ting sheng ying]** 听声音 "Listening to the Voice"
(2) **[ting yu ying]** 听语音 "Listening to the Speech Sounds"
(3) **[ting hu xi]** 听呼吸 "Listening to the Breath"
(4) **[ting ke sou]** 听咳嗽 "Listening to the Cough"
(5) **[wen qi wei]** 闻气味 "Smelling the Odors"

9.3. [wen zhen] 问诊 "Inquiring (Questioning)"

This is a diagnostic method of asking patients or their relatives about their trouble, which plays an important role in diagnosis. Through inquiring, doctors can know the patient's case history, subjective symptoms, family history, therapeutic measures already taken, and especially some kinds of diseases without signs which can only be detected by questioning. Here are several methods, e.g.

(1) **[wenhan re]** 问寒热 "Questioning about Chilliness and Fever"
(2) **[wen han]** 问汗 "Questioning about Perspiration"
(3) **[wen tong]** 问痛 "Questioning about Pain"

(4) **[wen yin shi kou wei]** 问饮食口味 "Questioning about Diet and Taste"
(5) **[wen da bian]** 问大便 "Questioning about Defecation"
(6) **[wen xiao bian]** 问小便 "Questioning about Urination"
(7) **[wen yue jing]** 问月经 "Questioning about Menstruation"
(8) **[wen dai xia]** 问带下 "Questioning about Leucorrhoea"
(9) **[wen xiao er]** 问小儿 "Questioning about the Condition of a Child"

9.4. [qie zhen] 切诊 "Palpation"

A method of physical examination by using hand to touch, feel, and press certain parts of body surface of the patient for the purpose of investigating the condition of pulse, chest, abdomen and extremities to establish a diagnosis.

9.5. [san bu jiu hou] 三部九候 "Three Regions and Nine Locations for Pulse Feeling"

Three regions refer to the head, upper and lower extremities in ancient times, and the sites of **[cun guan chi]** 寸, 关 尺 Cun, Guan and Chi along the radial artery at the wrist in modern times. One of the ancient methods for pulse feeling, i.e., to palpate the pulse located at different parts of the head, upper limbs and lower limbs in order to detect the disorders of the head, ear, eyes, mouth, thorax and the five viscera.
(1) Palpation of the Skin
(2) Palpation of the Extremities
(3) Palpation of Xuli
(4) Palpation of Epigastrium
(5) Palpation of Abdomen
(6) Palpation of Acupoints

10. [zhong cao yao] 中草药 "Chinese Traditional and Herbal Medicine"

It is difficult to make a clear-cut differentiation between medicinal herbs in folk medicine and regular traditional drugs and so Chinese drugs and herbal drugs are usually called " Chinese traditional and herbal medicines" in combination.

10.1. [xing wei] 性味 "Properties and Flavours of Drugs"

Drugs of different flavour have different effects and according to their therapeutic effects. The medicinal plants are categorised by their for properties and five flavours. The four properties are, cold, hot, warm and cool, and they indicate the basic effect of the herbs on the body. Among them, cold and cool medications belong to Yin (cool is next to cold), while warm and hot medications fall under the Yang (warm is next to cold. Drugs used to treat heat symptom-complexes and cure the causes of hot or Yang diseases are endowed with cold or cool properties or are classified as Yin drugs, while those effective for cold symptom-complexes are endowed with warm or hot properties and are classified as Yang drugs.

10.2. [wu wei] 五味 "Five Flavours"

The Five Flavours of herbal drugs have connections with the theory of the Five Elements. Five flavours are pungent, sweet, sour, bitter and salty. The flavours of drugs are different as their properties, e.g. most of the carminatives are pungent, tonifying drugs are usually sweet in taste and sour drugs have the property of astringency.

10.3. [wu wei suo ru] 五味所属 "Viscera on which Drugs of different tastes act selectively"

This is an ancient hypothesis in Chinese pharmacology based upon the theory of Five Evolutive Phases.

(1) Drugs bitter in taste act on the heart.
(2) Drugs sour in taste act on the liver.
(3) Drugs sweet in taste act on the spleen.
(4) Drugs pungent in taste act on the lung.
(5) Drugs salty in taste act on the kidney.

Flavour	Element	Related organ	Effects	Example
pungent	metal	lungs; large intestine	induce sweat; balance Qi; dispel stasis	fresh ginger
sweet	earth	stomach; spleen	digestive tonic; distribute nutrition	Chinese licorice
sour	wood	liver; gall bladder	binding; astringent; anti-pyretic	unripened plums
bitter	fire	heart; small intestine	drying; antidysenteric	back of amou cork tree
salty	water	kidneys; bladder	softening; laxative diuretic	weed

*pungent like ginger; sweet like sugar; sour like vinegar; bitter like lime; salty like salt

10.4. [sheng jiang fu chen] 升降浮沉 "Ascending and Descending, Floating and Sinking of the Drugs"

This is an important functional distinctions among herbal potions. The ascending and floating drugs have an upward and outward effect in the system tend to move vital-energy up and out, cause energy to rise in the body and can be used for activating vitality, inducing sweat and dispelling cold. They belong to Yang. While the descending and sinking drugs, having a downward and inward effect tend to move vital-energy down and in, can be used for tranquilizing, causing contraction, relieving cough, arresting emesis, and promoting diuresis or purgation. They belong to Yin.

10.5. [gui jing] 归经 "Classification of Drugs according to the Meridians"

The medications must depend on their natural affinities with various parts of the body, on which therapeutic action is manifested. For example, excess heat in the lungs and excess heat in the liver are both treated with Yin herbs, which cool, descend, and fall into the sour, bitter, or salty flavour categories. However, the specific items chosen for the lung prescription are not the same as those chosen for the liver prescription, because their organ affinities are different. So Radix Platycodi, Flos farfarae, Radix Asteris etc., are grouped under the drugs of the lung Meridian owing to their antitussive effect in lung diseases.

Herbal Drug		**Five Element Identity**		**Meridian**	
Color	**Flavour**	**Aroma**	**Element**	**Yin**	**Yang**
Blue/green	sour	pungent	wood	liver	gall bladder
Red	bitter	scorched	fire	heart	small intestine
Yellow	sweet	fragrant	earth	spleen	stomach
White	hot	rank/raw	metal	lungs	large intestine
Black	salty	rotten/putrid	water	kidneys	bladder

10.6. [da du, chang du, xiao du, wu du] 大毒, 常毒, 小毒, 无毒 "Extremely poisonous, moderately poisonous, slightly poisonous and non-poisonous drugs.
A classification of drugs according to their toxicity:

10.7. [san pin] 三品 "Three Grades of Drugs"

(1) High-grade drugs: which are supposed to be non-toxic, possessing rejuvenating properties and can be taken frequently and long periods of time without harm.
(2) medium grade drugs: which are said to have no or slight toxic effects and are used for treating deficiency syndromes.
(3) low grade drugs: which are toxic and should be taken for long period of time.

10.8. [yao wu fen lei] 药物分类 "The Classification of Drugs"

(1) Diaphoretics or drugs for treating exterior syndrome.
(2) Diaphoretics with pungent and warm properties.

(3) Phlegm-resolving drugs with warm properties.
(4) Phlegm-resolving drugs with cold properties.
(5) Antitussives and Antiasthmatics
(6) Antipyretics or Febrifuges
(7) Drugs for reducing intense heat.
(8) Drugs for eliminating pathological heat from blood
(9) Febrifugal and Antipyretic drugs; drugs for eliminating heat and dampness.
(10) Febrifugal and Detoxicant drugs; drugs for eliminating toxic heat.
(11) Antirheumatics: drugs for relieving rheumatic conditions
(12) Drugs for dispelling internal cold.
(13) Dampness-resolving drugs with fragrant odor.
(14) Diuretics and Hydragogues
(15) Carminatives; Drugs for regulating the flow of Qi (vital energy).
(16) Drugs for regulating blood conditions
(17) Haemostatic; drugs for arresting bleeding
(18) Blood-activating and stasis-removing drugs; drugs for invigorating blood circulation and eliminating blood stasis.
(19) Aromatic stimulants.
(20) Sedatives and tranquilizers
(21) Anticonvulsives drugs for subduing the hyperactivity of the liver and endogenous wind.
(22) Qi tonics
(23) Blood tonics
(24) Yang tonics
(25) Yin Tonics
(26) Astringents and Haemostatic
(27) Stomachics and evacuants
(28) Purgative; cathartics.
(29) Anthelmintics.

10.9. [ji xing] 剂型 "Preparation Form"

There are different dosage forms in TCM, e. g.

(1) pills such as watered pills, honeyed pills, pasted pills, concentrated pills, minute pills
(2) soft extract, ointment and adhesive plasters
(3) medical powder
(4) pepper powder
(5) distellate
(6) pastill
(7) medical wine
(8) decoction of medical ingredients
(9) cold decoction
(10) mecicinal herbs in small pieces or slices
(11) medical powder

(12) medical tea
(13) leaven
(14) glue
(15) tablet

10.10. [yao cai pao zhi] 药材炮制 "Processing of Crude Drugs"

The crude drugs are treated with cleaning , cutting, soaking, drying, calcining, baking, steaming, simmering, carbonizing, roasting, etc.

10.11. [fu yao fa] 服药法 "Method of Administration"

(1) to be taken after pouring liquid on it
(2) to be taken after mixing it with liquid
(3) to be swallowed
(4) to be taken away fro the mealtime
(5) to be taken with an empty stomach
(6) to be take at one draught
(7) to be taken in small portions at frequent intervals
(8) to be taken warm
(9) to be taken hot
(10) to be taken cold
(11) to be melt in mouth and then swallowed or spat out
(12) food taboo on patient's diet

11. [qi gong] 气功 "Qi Gong"

Qing Gong is a system of exercise performed by taking a proper posture, adjusting breathing and concentrating the mind and uniting vital essence and energy and mentality as a whole for physical training, health preservation and prevention and treatment of diseases, a psychosomatic therapy in traditional Chinese medicine.
There are several kinds of Qi Gong in TCM:
(1) static qigong -also-called **[nei gong]**内功 "internal exercise"
(2) dynamic qigong- also-called **[wai gong]** 外功 " external exercise"
(3) Qigong as martial arts- also-called **[ying gong]** 硬气功 " hard qigong"
(4) **[ruan qi gong]** 软气功 "soft qigong"
(5) **[zhi bing qi gong]** 治病气功 "medical qigong"

12. [yang sheng] 养生 "Health Care"

Health care has been highly appreciated and advocated by the physicians and experts of past ages. According to [nei jing] 内经 "Internal Classic" the techniques and methods of the health care should be based on the theory of Yin and Yang and should conform to the nature law. So there developed many concepts and principles of health preservation for people to follow.

12.1. [yang sheng zhi dao] 养生之道 "Principles of Health Care"

(1) Adaptation of the human body to the environment; ancient physicians thought that human beings and the natural environments are in unity. Consistent changes of climate of the four seasons and environments affect the body's physiological function of the human body. If people do not adapt to the geographical changes, they will develop diseases due to these changes. In order to gain and maintain health, people must adapt themselves to environmental changes and keep away from evil factors.

(2) Good character preserves one's soul, and good temperament preserves one's life; TCM pays great attention to the close relationship between mental activities and health. The theory of "integrating spirit with body" is just the guidance for people to follow. It holds that both the spirit and the body can make up an organic unity; that is to say , to strengthen the spirit, one must strengthen the body, and strengthen the body, one must strengthen the spirit. So mental health care - regulating the spirit and keepingi the balance of mind has always been highly valued and applied as a major means of maintaining good health and achieving longevity.

(3) One should keep an orderly life with proper and controlled diet and avoid overwork; dietetic health care plays an important in longevity. TCM medicine has developed systematic theories and come up with a series of principles and methods, which have contributed, a great deal to the health and longevity of the Chinese people. They are: choosing a simple and light diet, properly adjusting food and tastes, dining at regular times and controlling the amount of intake, regulating cold and heat of food, etc.

(4) Sexual desire should be controlled, and intemperance will bring harm; regulating sexual life is also important in health care. There are taboos for sexual life, the following three points must be kept in mind. sexual intercourse with no tipsiness, sexual intercourse with no anger, terror and tiredness, sexual intercourse in usual weather.

(5) Taking part in Physical Training, the ancient Chinese paid special attention to physical training and created many items unique, such as **[tai ji quan] 太极拳** "Tai Ji Quan", **[wu qin xi] 五禽戏** "Wu Qin Xi", **[ba duan jin] 八段锦** "Ba Duan Jin", and **[qi gong] 气功** "Qi Gong" etc.. Qing Gong is one of the particular systems of exercise performed by taking a proper posture, adjusting breathing and concentrating the mind and uniting vital essence and energy and mentality as a whole for physical training, health preservation and prevention and treatment of diseases, a psychosomatic therapy in TCM

.

12.2. [yang sheng chang jian yao] 养生常见药 "Commonly Used Chinese Medicines for Health Care"

These kinds of medicines are called tonics for their tonifying properties. They are classified as the following five kinds: Qi tonics, Blood tonics, Yang tonics, Yin tonics and the other tonics.

12.2.1.[bu qi yao] 补气药 "Qi Tonics"

Drugs that have the effects of rplenishing Qi and eliminating or relieving syndromes due to Qi deficiency are defined as Qi tonics. They are:

[ren shen] 人参 "Radix Ginseng",
[xi yang shen] 西洋参 "Radix panacis Quinquefolii"
[tai zi shen] 太子参 "Radix Pseudostellariae"
[ci wu jia] 刺五加 "Radix Acanthopanacis Senticosi"
[dang shen] 党参 "Radix Codonopsis"
[huang qi] 黄芪 "Radix Astragali"
[bai shu] 白术 "Rhizoma Atractylodis Macrocephalae"
[gan cao] 甘草 "Radix Glycyrrhizae"
[shan yao] 山药 "Rhizoma Dioscoreae"
[huang jing] 黄精 "Rhizoma Polygonati"
[da zao] 大枣 "Fructus Jujubae"
[yi tang] 饴糖 "Saccharum Granosum"
[feng mi] 蜂蜜 "Mel"

12.2.2.[yang xue yao] 养血药 "Blood Tonics"

[e jiao] 阿胶 "Colla Corii Asini"
[dang gui] 当归 "Radix Angelicae Sinensis"
[shu di huang] 熟地黄 "Radix Rehmanniae Praeparata"
[he shou wu] 何首乌 " Radix Polygoni Multiflori"
[bai shao] 白芍 "Radix Paeoniae Albae"
[long yan rou] 龙眼肉 "Arillus Longa"
[sang shen] 桑椹 "Fructus Mori"

12.2.3. [zhu yang yao] 助阳药 "Yang Tonics"

[lu rong] 鹿茸 "Cornu cervi pantotritum"
[ge jie] 蛤蚧 "Gecko"
[ba ji tian] 巴戟天 " Radix Morindae officinalis"
[du zhong] 杜仲 "Cortex Eucommiae"
[dong chong xia cao] 冬虫夏草 "Cordyceps"
[zi he che] 子河车 "Placenta Hominis"
[tu si zi] 菟丝子 "Semen Cuscutae"
[hu tao ren] 胡桃仁 " Semen Juglandis"
[yang qi shi] 阳起子 "Actinolitum"
[bu gu zhi] 补骨脂 " Fructus Psoraleae"
[yin yang huo] 淫羊藿 "Herba Epimedii"

12.2.4. [zi ying yao]滋阴药 "Yin Tonics"

[sha shen] 沙参 "Radix Adenophorae or Radix Glehniae"
[tian dong] 天冬 "Radix Asparagi"
[shi hu] 石斛 "Herba Dendrobii"
[mai dong] 麦冬 "Radix Ophiopogonis"

[yu zhu] 玉竹 "Rhizoma Polygonati Odorati"
[bai he] 百合 "Bulbus Lilii"
[gou ji zi] 枸杞子"Fructus Lycii"
[nu zhen zi] 女贞子 "Fructus Ligustri Lucidi"
[hei zhi ma] 黑芝麻 "Semen Sesami Nigri"
[bie] 鳖 "Trionycis"
[yin er] 银耳 "Tremella"

Chapter Three

The Visceral Manifestation of Urology, Andrology and Sexology

Part I.

[zhong yi qi guan ming cheng] 中医器官名称 "The Terms for Internal and External Organs of TCM"

[chan men] 产门
vaginal orifice

[er yin] 二阴
the two (front and back) privy parts, external genitalia, external urethral orifice and anus

[gang men] 肛门
anus

[gao] 睾
testicle

[hou yin] 后阴
back private parts; anus

[hui yin] 会阴
(1) perineum; (2) Huiyin a point just in the center of perineum

[jing] 茎
penis

[jing chui] 茎锤
penis and testes

[jing dao] 精道
including spermatic ducts, testis, and prostate gland in modern sense

[jing qiao] 精窍

external orifice of male urethra

[mao ji] 毛际
the area covered with pubic hair

[niao dao] 尿道
ureter

[qian yin] 前阴
Referring to external genitalia including external orifice of the urethra

[qi jie] 气街
the groin (inguen]

[shen nang] 肾囊
scrotum

[ting kong] 廷孔
external urethral orifice of the female

[yao] 腰
lumbus, loins

[yin hu] 阴户
external vaginal orifice

[yin qi] 阴器
external genitals

[yin jin] 阴筋
the spermatic cord.

[zi men] 子门
cervical orifice of the uterus

[zong jin] 宗筋
(1) the twelve Channels gathering in the genitalia; (2) male genitalia

[zong jing zhi hui] 宗筋之会
malc genitals

Part II [mi niao nan ke chang jian zhen zhuang] 秘尿男科常见症状主 "Symptoms Commonly Seen in Urology and Andrology"

1. [niao] 尿 "Urine"

The fluid discharged from the urethra, the formation and excretion of which is closely related to the functions of the kidney, spleen, triple energizer and bladder, and play an important role in the regulation of body fluid. Observation of the amount and color of the urine is helpful for diagnosis.

1.1. [xiao bian se tong] 小便涩痛 "Difficulty and Pain in Micturition"

Stranguria, slow and pain urination due to attack of the bladder by dampness-heat evil, usually seen in urinary infection, stones in the bladder, bladder cystitis and prostatitis.

1.2. [xiao bian bu li] 小便不利 "Dysuria"

Difficulty in micturition or deficient secretion of urine due to hypo function of vital energy, retention of wetness or consumption of body fluid and blood, usually referable to the dysfunction of the lung, spleen, kidney, triple energizer and bladder. The manifestations are bladder cystitis and prostatitis etc.

1.3. [xiao bian shi jin] 小便失禁 "Incontinence"

Failure of voluntary control of urination in adult or in continence of urine, caused by deficiency of spleen -, lung - and kidney-energy, usually seen in the aged, debilitated or comatose patients.

1.4 . [xiao bian huang chi] 小便黄赤 "Deep-colored Urine"

Discharge of dark urine mostly caused by the retention of heat-evil and wetness-heat, or occasionally by asthenia- heat.

1.5. [xiao bian lin li] 小便淋沥 "Stranguria"

Frequent, slow and difficult urination; usually caused by deficiency of kidney energy or asthenia of the spleen and kidney, and also by the stagnation or wetness-heat in the lower energizer.

1.6. [xiao bian duan chi] 小便短赤 "Oliguria with Reddish Urine"

A disorder seen in the patients afflicted with heat transformation from exogenous evils, retention of wetness-heat evil, or endogenous heat from Yin-deficiency.

1.7. [xiao bian pin shu] 小便频数 "Frequent Micturition"

A symptom due to attack of exogenous evil and dysfunction or debility of the internal organs, such as wetness-heat in the bladder, stagnation of liver-energy, deficiency of middle energizer energy, weakness of Kidney-Yang, insufficiency of Kidney-Yin, etc.

1.8. [niao xue] 尿血 "Haematuria"

Blood in the urine: that due to deficiency of Yin with hyperactivity of evil fire and manifested as bright red blood in the urine, soreness of the loins and legs, tinnitus, dizziness, restlessness, thirst, reddish tongue, and small, rapid pulse; that due to asthenia of both the spleen and the kidney is manifested as pink blood in the urine, sallow complexion, loss of appetite, lumbago, cold limbs, pale tongue, and weak, soft pulse.

1.9. [bai zhuo] 白浊"White and Turbid Urine"

A condition usually due to wetness-heat flowing downward and deficiency of both the spleen and kidney, and the attack of pathogenic damp-heat evil to the urinary bladder, causing turbid urine.

1.10. [jing ye niao] 精液尿"Spermaturia"

A morbid condition due to the deficiency of Kidney – Yang, accompanied by impotence, frequency of urination at night or even edema dyspnea.

1.11. [long bi] 癃闭"Dysuria"

Difficult urination or retention of urine caused by the stagnation of lung-energy, by the downward attack of evil wetness-heat or by the blockage of urinary tract, by blood stasis or stone in case of asthenia-syndrome, and by the deficiency of spleen-Yang and kidney-Yang leading to the retention of fluid in case of asthenia-syndrome.

2. [lin zheng] 淋症"Lin Symptom"

Frequency of urination, urgency of urination, painful micturition or incontinence of urination mainly manifest it. It may be classified into five types, such as **[shi lin]** 石淋 Stone Lin (dysuria caused by stone), **[qi lin]** 气淋 Qi Lin (dysuria caused by dysfunction of bladder), **[gao lin]** 膏淋 Milk Lin (chyluria), **[lao lin]** 劳淋 Consumptive Lin (chronic dysuria), and **[xue lin]** 血淋 blood Lin (haematuria with pain), and including such diseases as infection, calculus and tuberculosis of the urinary system, chyluria, and prostatitis, etc.

2.1. [shi lin] also [sha lin] 湿淋"Stranguria due to Urinary Stone"

One of the Lin Symptom Complexes, caused by urinary stone due to calculus in the urinary system. It results form the retention of wetness and heat-evil in the lower energizer; manifested by pain of one side of the lower back or intermittent colicky pain, radiating to the lower abdomen and genitalia, difficulty in urination, discharge of yellow turbid urine or haematuria.

2.2. [gao lin] also-called [nei lin] 膏淋"Stranguria with Chyluria"

A disease characterized by dysuria and presence of chyle in the urine, giving it a milky appearance. The condition is caused by the inability to control the chyle flow resulting form the asthenia of spleen and kidney in the asthenic type and from the accumulation of wetness-heat evil in the lower warmer in the sthenic type. The chief manifestation is cloudy urine.

2.3. [qi lin] 气淋"Stranguria due to Disorder of Vital Energy"

A disorder characterized by the distention and pain in the hypogastrium and the scrotum, difficulty of urination, pain in the hypogastrium and genitalia after micturition, caused by the stagnation of bladder-energy, and deficiency of spleen-energy and kidney- energy.

2.4. [lao lin] 劳淋"Stranguria Induced by Overstrain"

A disorder due to consumption of vital energy and blood, or deficiency of Yang and Yin, usually manifested as dribbling of urine, vague pain of the genitalia after micturition, lassitude, lower backache, superficial feverishness, spontaneous perspiration, restlessness, etc.

2.5. [xue lin] 血淋"Stranguria Complicated with Haematruria"

Stranguria is due to blood disorders, such as blood-deficiency, blood-cold, blood-heat blood-stasis, etc., manifested by haematuria with urethral pains, distention and pain of the hypogastrium.

2.6. [re lin] 热淋"Stranguria due to Heat Pathogenic Factor"

The chief manifestations are distention and pain of the hypogastrium, difficulty of urination, dark urine, burning pain of the urethra on micturition, sometimes accompanied by fever, etc. It is similar to infections of the urinary system.

2.7. [yi niao] 遗尿"Enuresis"

Involuntary urination during sleep. It is usually seen in children. Incontinence of urine, most of which appear as asthenia-cold syndrome and are attributable to asthenia-cold of the kidney and bladder; some appear as sthenia- heat syndrome, and are attributable to the stirring of fire-pathogenic evil in the bladder or retention of heat evil in the liver channel.

3. [teng tong] 疼痛"Pains"

Generally speaking, stagnant Qi and blood due to blockage of the meridians cause pains. In most cases, it is brought about by invasion of exogenous pathogens or Qi stagnancy and blood stasis. Different nature, location and intensity of pain reflect different nature of pathogens and affected portions of the body.

3.1. [fu tong] 腹痛"Abdominal Pain"

A symptom caused by attack of six exogenous evils, immoderate diet, emotional upsets, stagnation of vital energy, blood stasis, etc. Upper abdomen, situated above umbilicus, contains the liver, gallbladder, spleen and stomach. The lower abdomen, situated below umbilicus, comprises the kidneys, bladder, large and small intestines, and the uterus. The causes for the pains in these organs may be renal pelvis calculus, and stones in the ureter, stones in the kidney, etc.

3.2. [yao tong] 腰痛 "Lumbago"

Pain over the lumbar region due to deficiency of kidney-energy resulting from overstrains, or obstruction of vital energy and blood flow in the meridians, kidney calculus, and accumulation of body fluids. The symptoms manifested as edema over the lower limbs, lumbago and infected kidney, etc..

3.3. [wai gan yao tong] 外感腰痛 "Lumbago due to Exogenous Evil"

Lumbago due to involvement of meridians by exogenous evils, usually manifested as asthenia-syndrome.

3.4. [han shi yao tong] 寒湿腰痛 "Lumbago due to Cold-wetness Evil"

A symptom due to and stagnation of cold-wetness evil in the meridians leading to the poor movement of Vital energy and blood; manifested as feeling of cold and heaviness sensation, pain, stiffness over the lumbar region which can be relieved by heat and aggravated by cold especially on rainy days, sunken and tense pulse, etc..

3.5. [feng shi yao tong] 风湿腰痛 "Lumbago due to Wind-wetness Evil"

A disease with lumbago as the major symptom, caused by exposing to wetness or sleeping in a damp place, wind evils or asthenia of the kidney; manifested as pain and immobility of the waist and back, contracture, accompanied with fever, chilliness, edema, and aversion to wind, etc.

3.6. [shen xu yao tong] 肾虚腰痛 "Lumbago due to Kidney-asthenia"

A type of lumbago due to deficiency of the kidney essence and hypo function of the kidney, manifested as aching and debility of the loins and weakness of the legs which are aggravated by overstrain and exertion, etc.

3.7. [xue xu yao tong] 血虚腰痛 "Lumbago due to Deficiency of Blood"

A type of lumbago due to excessive bleeding and deficiency of blood leading to the failure of nourishing the tendons and vessels, usually occurring in women with metrorrhagia.

3.8. [qi zhi yao tong] 气滞腰痛 "Lumbago due to Energy-stagnation"

A condition with lumbar pain, stabbing in character but not fixed in location, caused by emotional upsets or contusion resulting in the stagnation of vital energy in the channel, often accompanied by distention of the abdomen.

3.9. [xue yu yao tong] 血瘀腰痛 "Lumbago due to Blood Stasis"

A variety of lumbago with fixed location, ameliorated at daytime and aggravated at night.

3.10. [hui yin sheng zhi qi tong] 会阴生殖器痛 "Pains in the Perineum and External Genitals"

They are usually caused by the diseases in the testicle, scrotum, sperm duct, and prostate gland, usually caused by the stagnation of damp-heat, coldness, stasis of Qi and blood. Pains in the testicle, often caused by testitis; pains in the perineum often caused by prostatitis, etc.

3.11. [niao tong] 尿痛 "Stranguria"

Slow and painful urination due to attack of the bladder by wetness-heat evil, caused by urinary infection, bladder or kidney stone and prostatitis, usually with manifestations of frequent urination, incontinence of urine, burning sensation during urination and difficulty and pain in micturition.

3.12. [fang shi jin tong] 房事筋痛 "Penis Pain in Sexual Intercourses"

Distention and painful sensation in the penis, fullness and pain in the hypochondria while having sexual intercourse due to the depression of the liver and Qi stagnation or coldness in the liver meridian or kidney-deficiency.

4. [jing bing] 精病 "Sperm Diseases"

4.1. [zao xie] 早泄 "Premature Ejaculation"

Emission of the seminal fluid too early during sexual intercourse. It is usually caused by weakness of the kidney, the impairment of the kidney-energy by excessive libido and excess of **[xiang huo]** 相火 Prime-minster Fire (a kind of Yang-energy originating from the fire in the gate of life and existing in the liver, gallbladder and triple energizers).

4.2. [yin jing] 遗精 "Nocturnal Emission"

Involuntary discharge of semen or the seminal fluid escapes in dream, also-called **[meng yi]** 梦遗 "Dreamy spermatorrhea", often accompanied with dizziness, tinnitus, lassitude and low-back soreness. And the seminal fluid involuntarily excreted without dream is called **[hua jing]** 滑精 "Slippery spermatorrhea" accompanied with palpitation and impotence, deep and weak pulse and pale tongue, due to imbalance between heart Yang and Kidney-Yin, deficiency of Kidney-energy, overabundance of Prime-minster fire, or local attack of wetness-heat evil, downward flow of dampness-heat into the lower portion of the body.

4.3 [jing leng] 精冷 "Cold Semen"

The thin seminal fluid and infertility caused by deficiency of the Kidney-Yang. It is similar to sexual neurasthenia and lack of spermatozoa, etc.

4.4. [jing shao] 精少 "Oligospermia" or "Defective Ejaculation"

4.5. [xue jing] 血精 "Haemospermia"

Reddish substance exists in the ejaculated sperm, usually caused by the hyperactivity of asthenic due to the consumption of Yin –essence, the deficiency of the spleen and the kidney and damp-heat accumulated in the lower energizer. Commonly seen in prostatitis, diseases in the testicles, tuberculocele, etc.

4.5. [bu she jing] 不射精 "Non-Ejaculation"

A morbid condition of being incapable of ejaculating during the sexual intercourses, usually caused by excessive sexual activities, the asthenia syndrome due to the consumption of the kidney-essence, deficiency of Kidney-Yang, deficiency of heart and spleen, stagnation of Qi and blood.

4.6. [shen xu yi jing] 肾虚遗精 "Nocturnal Emission due to Kidney-asthenia"

A disorder caused by insufficiency of Kidney-Yin or deficiency of kidney-energy.

4.7. [jing ye nang zhong] 精液囊肿 "Spermatocyst"

It is usually caused by improper diet, overstrain due to consumption of spleen-energy, accumulation of phlegm-wetness in the body which may further affect the activities of the lung, stomach, and even the Chong, and Ren channels. It usually causes sterility.

4.8. [tan yong yi jing] 痰痈遗精 "Nocturnal Emission due to accumulation of Phlegm"

A disorder due to attack of the chamber of seminal fluid by the accumulation of phlegm resulting from anxiety.

5. [xing gong neng zhang ai yu bu yu atitis] 性功能障碍与不育 "Sexual dysfunction and Sterility"

5.1. [yang wei] 阳痿 "Impotence"

Inability to have an erection of the penis or lack of copulative power in the male before climacteric; usually due to sexual excess or prostatitis. Kidney Yang deficiency: usually caused by worrying, lassitude and intemperance in sexual life, manifested as dizziness, tinnitus, aversion to cold and lassitude of the loins and legs. The pulse is deep and thready, the tongue pale with thin coating. The downward flow of damp-heat type: usually caused by greasy food and alcohol, accompanied red-hot urination, thirsty mouth with bitter taste. The pulse is vague and rapid, the tongue coating is yellow and greasy.

5.2. [qiang zhong] 强中 "Priapism-Persistent Erection"

A prolonged erection of the penis with involuntary emission of semen or swelling and flaccidity of the penis, also-called **[yin zong]** 阴纵 "priapism" in TCM, due to deficiency of kidney-yin, hyperactivity of life-gate fire or excessive libido, and the accumulation of wetness-heat evil in the liver channel.

5.3. [bu yu] 不育 "Sterility in Male"

A disorder in man with lack of reproductive function, caused by congenital malformations of the sexual organs, or decline of Kidney-energy, deficiency of both Qi and blood and asthenial-cold of essence-energy secondary to other diseases. The manifestations are impotence, premature ejaculation, nocturnal emission or non-ejaculation.

5.3.1. [xue xu bu yun] 血虚不育 "Sterility due to Blood-deficiency"

A condition usually accompanied with emaciation, sallow complexion and fatigue; due to asthenia of the spleen and stomach, or prolonged illness with bleeding and Yin-blood and dysfunction of **[chong ren]** 冲任 "Chong and Ren channels"(one of the eight extra channels related to infertility when diseased) with failure to nourish the **[bao]** 胞Bao channels (vessels of the uterus).

5.3.2. [gan qi yu jie bu yun] 肝气郁结不育 "Sterility due to Stagnation of Liver-energy"

Inability to conceive, usually accompanied with emotional depression, feeling of fullness and oppression over the chest and hypochondria, distending pain over the breasts and menoxenia caused by the stagnation of liver-energy and incoordination between vital energy and blood leading to the dysfunction of Chong, Ren and Bao channels.

5.3.3. [wu bu nan] 五不男 "Five Types of Male Sterility"

Sterility caused by the congenital malformations or acquired l defects of male external genitalia or only the testes, or a lack of the secondary sexual characteristics; **[lou]** 漏spermatorrhea; **[jian]** 犍surgical resection of the penis or the testes; **[qie]** 怯 impotence; **[bian]** 变also-called **[ren o]** 人"Ren O" hermaphrodism or hermaphrodite, or popularly known as the **[yin yang ren]** 阴阳人"Yin-Yang person" hermaphroditism.

5.4. [yang suo] 阳缩 "Yang Retraction"

A morbid condition of retraction of penis, testicle and scrotum, accompanied with acute pain in the lower abdomen, usually caused by the deficiency of Kidney-Yang, attack of cold pathogenic factor after sexual intercourses and weak and deficient of liver Yang.

6. [shan] 疝 "Shan"

(1) Hernia- a protrusion of a part of an organ in the cavity through an aperture in its wall; (2) a collective term for diseases of the external genitalia, testicles and scrotum; accompanied by painful swelling of testicle or scrotum; and (3) severe abdominal pain accompanied by difficulty of urination, ischuria and constipation.

6.1. [hu shan] 狐疝 "Inguinal Hernia"

A part of the small intestine intermittently into the inguinal canal, or down to the scrotum, disappears when the patient lies flat or when it is pushed by hand, and descends again when the patient stands up, usually caused by the dysfunction of liver-energy.

6.2. [han shan] 寒疝"Cold Shan"

(1) acute abdominal pain caused by the invasion of the pathogenic cold evil condition marked by colicky pain around the umbilicus, night sweat, chills, cold extremities, sunken and tense pulse, and even numbness of extremities and general aching; caused by the attack of cold –damp pathogenic evil to the liver channel.
(2) testalgia due to cold-evil; a disease similar to tuberculosis of epididymus, manifested as coldness of the scrotum with painful and indurated mass in it, loss of erective ability of the penis, and secondary to sterility; caused by the attack of cold-wetness to the liver channel-Jueyin Channel.

6.3. [tui shan] 癞疝"Tui Shan"

(1)The testicle is swollen and hardened with dragging pain or numb, insensible to pain and touch due to cold-wetness evil; (2) swelling of the lower abdomen in female; (3) prolapse of vagina.

6.4. [qi shan] 气疝"Colic due to Disorder of Vital Energy"

(1) pain caused by the stagnation of vital energy resulting from immoderate diet and inadaptability to the change of weather; (2) bearing-down pain in the scrotum, caused by the stagnation of vital energy resulting from fury, overfatigue, etc.

6.5. [xue shan] 血疝"Bloody Shan"

(3)swelling and stabbing pain of the scrotum due to accumulation of blood in the scrotum;
(4) carbuncle of the hypogastrium near external genitalia.

6.6. [jin shan] 筋疝"Penis Shan"

The penis is painful and markedly retracted, swollen, or ulcerated with purulent discharge, or accompanied by impotence and white mucoid urethral discharge.

6.7. [shan jia] 疝瘕"Shan Jia"

Burning pain in the hypogastrium with white mucoid discharge from urethra.

6.8. [tui long shan] 癞癃疝"Tui Long Shan"

Encapsulated abscess in the abdominal cavity together with difficulty of urination.

6.9. [fei shan] 肺疝"Pulmonary Shan"

Invasion of the Lung Channel by external pathogenic factor causes a loss of the pulmonary functions and retardation of flow of fluids, and results in accumulation of the pathogenic heat in the bladder. Its chief manifestations are distention and pain of the hypogastrium and testicles, uroschesis, etc.

6.10. [jue shan] 厥疝"Jue Shan"

Colicky pain around the umbilicus, pain in the hypochondrium, nausea, vomiting of frothy saliva, cold clammy extremities as the chief manifestations.

6.11. [yin hu shan] 阴狐疝"Inguinal Hernia"

A condition due to disorder of the liver-energy, manifested as intermittent swelling of the scrotum and distending pain in the abdomen.

6.11. [yin shan] 阴疝"Yin-type Testalgia"

Pain in the testicle accompanied with swelling, due to attack of liver channel by cold-evil.

6.12. [long shan] 癃疝"Dysuria-colic Syndrome"

A syndrome consisting of colicky pain over the lower abdomen radiating to tests, and difficulty in urination.

7. [gao wan yu yin nang lei ji bing] 睾丸与阴囊类疾病 "Diseases in Testicles and Scrotum"

7.1. [zi yong] 子痈"Orchitis with abscess Formation"

A morbid condition in testicle with the formation of abscess usually caused by wetness-heat evil attacking the lower energizer, heat -stasis in the Liver Channel, attacking of cold and dampness and traumatic injuries.

7.2. [zi tong] 子痛"Pains in the testicles and Scrotum"

Usually caused by cold-evil stasis in the Liver Channel, wetness-heat evil attacking the lower energizer, stasis of Liver Qi, stagnation of Vital Qi and blood stasis and deficiency of Vital Qi. The chief manifestations are red and swelling testis, solid and slightly painful sensation, difficulty in micturition with slippery and stringy pulse.

7.3. [zi tan] 子痰"Pyogenic Infection and Ulceration in Testis and Scrotum"

Usually caused by impairment of liver and kidney, stagnation of phlegm in lung-collaterals, retention of phlegm-heat, deficiency of Vital Qi and blood. Swelling and distention of testicle with painful sensation with by slightly pressure, marked by lower fever, sleepless during the night, constipation, burning sensation during urination, aching with weakness, heaviness and distension felt in the lower back, red tongue and rapid and frequent pulse.

7.4. [yin suo] 阴缩"Retraction of the Penis"

Retraction and softness of the penis usually caused by the attack of cold pathogenic evil, leading to the deficiency of the liver Yang. It is often accompanied by drastic abdominal pain and usually seen in children.

7.5. [gao wan wei suo] 睾丸萎缩 "Atrophy of Testis"

One side or both sides of testis, and epididymis are shrink and small, soft in property with no flexibility, usually caused by epidemic mumps with the complexity of testitis, prolonged spermophlebectasia and traumatic injuries of testis. Or congenital malformation of testis.

7.6. [gao wan zhong tong] 睾丸肿痛 "Painful and Swollen Testis"

It is a localized collection of pus in the scrotum, also-called **[nang yong]** 囊痈 "abscess of scrotum", caused by accumulation of wetness-heat evil from liver and kidney channels or invasion of exogenous evils; appearing as redness, swelling, heat and pain of the scrotum with tense and shiny appearance, and followed by pus formation, accompanied with fever, chilliness, dry mouth and desire for cold drink.

7.7. [pian zhui] 偏坠 "Unilateral Enlargement of Testis"

A disorder accompanied with bearing-down pain, caused by phlegm-wetness, blood stasis or hyperactivity of liver-fire.

7.8. [luan zi wen] 卵子瘟 "Swelling of Testis"

Usually appearing after the occurring of mumps- epidemic parotitis due to the attack of heat-evil leading to the accumulation of the heat-evil in the intestine and stomach and the stagnation of fire-evil in the liver and gallbladder involving Shaoyang channel.

7.10. [yin gao] 隐睾 "Cryptorchidism"

One or both the testicles are undescended from birth. usually with the disability of reproduction.

7.11. [nang yong] 囊痈 or [shen nang yong] 肾囊痈 "Scrotal Abscess"

The acute, localized, suppurative infection of the scrotum. (see 7.6.)

7.12. [yin zhong] 阴肿 "Edema in Prepuce of Penis"

Swelling pain and edema in the penis usually caused by the attack of wind-evil and accumulation of cold pathogenic evil, or insects bites, often seen in children under the age of five.

7.13. [yin jing yu jie] 阴茎郁结 "Stony Cellulitis in the Penis"

Cellulitis hard as a stone, gradually increasing in size, difficult to subside and break, usually caused by stagnation of liver and stasis of Vital Qi, overdrinking causes damages to spleen and stomach, exhaustion due to sexual indulgence etc.

7.14. [jin shuo jin mai qu zhang] 精缩静脉曲张 "Spermophlebectasia"

In TCM, it belongs to **[shan]** 疝"hernia" or **[jin liu]** 筋瘤"Varicosity of veins". It is a tumor-like mass formed by tortuous, engorged vein, caused by deficiency of liver and kidney, irregularity of meridians, stagnation of blood.

7.15. [shen nang feng] 肾囊风 "Dermatitis of Scrotum"

A condition caused by the attack of wetness-heat evil in the liver channel and the exposure to exogenous wind-evil; characterized by dryness and itching of the skin of the scrotum, miliary red rashes, profuse discharge after scratching, burning pain and its chronicity.

7.16. [nang suo] 囊缩 "Shrinkage of Scrotum"

A critical condition usually accompanied with curling-up of the tongue, caused by the evil heat in yang-ming channel attacking the Jueyin channel or the cold-evil attacking the Shaoyin channel directly.

7.17. [xiao muo ji ye] 霄膜积液 "Perididymitis"

Also-called **[shui shan] 水疝"Scrotal Hydrocele" a** collection of fluid in the scrotum caused by descending accumulation of fluid or exposure to wind-cold-wetness evils; marked by painful and swollen scrotum which is not red and hot, sweating in the genital area, or itching of the scrotum with discharge of yellowish discharge.

7.18. [bao pi yan] 包皮岩 "Posthitis"

An inflammation in the testis and on the surface of prepuce, usually caused unclean sexual activity, damp-heat accumulated on the lower part of the body, leading to the localized edema, ulcer accompanied with white, foul fluid.

7.19. [shen yan] 肾岩or [shen yan fan hua] 肾岩翻花or [fan hua xia gan] 翻花下疳 "Penile Carcinoma"

7.20. [shen yan fan hua] 肾岩翻花"Carcinoma of the Penis with Ulceration"

8. [qian lie xian ji bing] 前列腺疾病 "Prostatic Disorder"

8.1. [qian lie xian yan] 前列腺炎 "Prostatitis"

In TCM, there is no corresponding name for this. Generally speaking, it belongs to the disorders of "white and turbid urine", "spermaturia", "stranguria due to overstrain", etc.

8.2. [qian lie xian fei da] 前列腺肥大 "Prostatomegaly"

In TCM, it belongs to the field of **[long bi]** 癃闭"dysuria" (see 1.11. in this section)

8.3. [lin bing] 淋病"Stranguria"

A disorder characterized by frequent, difficult and painful discharge of urine, due to accumulation of wetness-heat evil in the bladder, or collapse of middle-energizer, or asthenia and hypo function of the kidney. It includes **[lin zhuo]** 淋浊 "Stranguria with turbid urine", **[bai zhuo]** 白浊 "Whitish and turbid urine" and "red and whitish urine" etc.

9. [xing bing] 性病 "Sexual Diseases"

9.1. [mei du] 梅毒 "Syphilis"

A contagious venereal disease caused by the spirochete "Treponema pallidum", transmitted through sexual intercourse or any direct contact. In TCM, it is called respectively as follows: **[yang mei chuang du]** 杨梅疮毒 "Syphilitic ulcer" and **[hua liu du lin]** 花柳毒淋 "venereal disease".

9.2. [yang mei chuang] 杨梅疮 "Strawberry Sores"

Skin lesions caused by syphilis manifested various forms of eruptions, such as erythema, maculae, papule, bulla, pustule, erosion etc. It is so-called because the lesions appear like strawberries.

9.3. [xia gan] 下疳 "Chancre"

The primary sore of syphilis; a painless, indurated papule occurring at the site of entry of the infection over the external genitals, called also hard chancre; while that ulcerates which is called soft chancre.

9..4. [heng xuan] 横痃 "Bubo"

An enlarged lymphonodus in the groin due to syphilis and various venereal diseases.

9..5. [chuang yang] 疮疡 "Pyogenic Infection and Ulceration of Skin"

A general term for the suppurative infection over the body surface and dermatosis, including carbuncle, deep-rooted carbuncle, furuncle, multiple abscess, tuberculosis of bones and joints, scrofula, etc., due to stagnation of vital energy and blood resulting from the attack of evil and consumption of blood by heat pathogenic evil.

9.6. [jian rui shi you] 尖锐湿疣 "Pyogenic Infection and Ulceration in External genitals"

9.7. [yin xuan] 阴癣 "Tinea Inguinalis"

A superficial fungal infection occurring in the medial side of the thigh or extending to the external genitals, buttock and around the anus, due to attack of wind, heat and wetness evil to the skin; appearing as papules or vesicles as onset, gradually spreading and forming well demarcated, red patches covered with thin desquamation, and intolerable itching.

10. [qi ta zhen zhuang] 其他症状"The Other Symptoms"

10.1. [qi shang] 七伤"Seven Injuries"

A collective term for seven manifestations of weakness of the kidney, e.g. cold genital organs, genital atrophy, inability of the penis to erect, spermatorrhea, thin semen, oligospermia, and moist genital organs, frequency or dribbling of urine.

10.2. [lao juan] 劳倦"Overstrain"

Two kinds of pathogens: excessive fatigue and indulgence in sexual activities due to consumption of spleen-energy, deficiency of vital energy and hyperactivity of fire-evil; manifested as lassitude, exertion dyspnea, superficial feverishness, spontaneous perspiration, restlessness.

10.3. [fang lao] 房劳"Fatigue due to Sexual Indulgence"

The fatigue syndrome resulting from impairment of the kidney from indulgence of sexual activities.

11. [fu ke] 妇科" Gynecology"

11.1. [chan hou xiao bian bu tong] 产后小便不 通"Postpartum Retention of Urine"

Retention of urine with hypogastric distention after delivery due to hyper function of the bladder resulting from impairment of the kidney by childbirth, or from stagnation of liver-energy caused by emotional upsets.

11.2. [chan hou xiao bian bu li] 产后小便不利 "Postpartum Dysuria"

Difficult urination in puerperium due to hyper function of the bladder resulting from impairment of the kidney by childbirth, or from stagnation of liver-energy caused by emotional upsets.

11.3. [chan hou xiao bian shi jin] 产后小便失禁 "Postpartum Incontinence of urine"

Incontinence of Urination after delivery due to asthenia and hypo function of the kidney, or injure of the bladder during labor.

11.4. [chan hou yu men bu bi] 产后玉门不闭 "Subinvolution of Uterine Cervix after Delivery"

A condition due to over consumption of vital energy and blood in puerperium leading to atony of the cervix.

11.5. [e lu] 恶露 "Lochia"

The vaginal discharge of decomposed blood and necrotic decidua during the puerperium, usually due to the stagnation of vital energy and blood stasis.

11.6. [yin ting] 阴廷 "Prolapse of Genitalia" or "Vaginal Hernia"

The prolapse of certain genital structures in or out of the vagina, usually of the uterus, but possibly of the bladder or rectum. A disorder caused by the deficiency of middle-energizer or insufficiency of kidney-energy. Usually seen in hysteroptosis, rectocele, cystocele etc.

11.7. [yin yang] 阴痒 "Pruritus Vulva"

Itching, sometimes unbearable itching, and pain of the vulva or vagina, caused by local infection or accumulation of wetness heat evil, or by Yin-deficiency and blood dryness.

11.8. [yin shi] 阴蚀"Vulvar Erosion"

A disorder due to retention of evil fire from emotional upsets impairing the liver and spleen, leading to local accumulation of wetness-heat evil; manifested as vulvar ulceration or erosion secondary to severe pruritus of the vulva or vagina after scratching with discharge of pus and blood, itching, pain and swelling, usually accompanied with whitish vaginal discharge and stranguria.

11.9. [shi nu] 石女"Stony Girl"

(1) female with congenital stricture of vagina;

(2) female with primary amenorrhea .

11.10. [luoo] 螺"The Spiral"

One of five congenital defects of female. (1) The vaginal has spiral striata or septa, which would embarrass coitus, or (2) an infertile woman.

11.11. [wen] 瘟" Atresia"

One of the five congenital defects of female. Congenital narrowing or other similar defects of the vagina.

11.12. [gu] 鼓" Drum "

One of five congenital defects of female. The introitus is tense like a drum, as if there were no opening such as with unperforated hymen.

11.13. [jiao] 角"Horn "

One of the five congenital defects of female. The clitoris is exceedingly long.

11.14. [mai] 脉"Sterility "

One of five congenital defects of female. Permanent amenorrhea or irregular menstruation and infertility.

11.15. [xuan yong] 癬痈 "Hanging Carbuncle"

(1) The acute, circumscribed, suppurative inflammatory lesion of the perineum; or (2) the acute, circumscribed suppurative inflammatory lesion of the palate.

11.16. [hai di yong] 海底痈 "Sea-Bottom Carbuncle"

The acute, localised, suppurative inflammatory lesion of the perineum.

11.17. [yin tuo] 阴脱 "Vaginal Hernia" "Atonia of Vagina"

A condition manifested as dilatation of the vaginal orifice with local swelling and pain, or even stranguria, due to impairment of Bao collaterals during labor, or excessive sexual intercourse.

12. [bu yun] 不育 "Infertility"

12.1. [shen xu bu yun] 肾虚不育 "Infertility due to Insufficiency of the Kidneys"

12.2. [gong leng bu yun] 宫冷不育 "Infertility due to Coldness of the Uterus"

A type of infertility due to hypo function of the kidney which fails to warm the uterus, usually marked by coldness in the lower abdomen, aversion to cold, cold limbs, retarded menstruation, and even frigidity.

12.3. [xue xu bu yun] 血虚不 育 "Infertility due to Deficiency of Blood"

A type of infertility caused by hypo function of the spleen and stomach or chronic loss of blood, marked by general weakness, lassitude, sallow complexion, and fatigue, or prolonged illness with leading to insufficiency of Yin blood and dysfunction of Chong and Ren channels with failure to nourish the Bao channel.

12.4. [gan yu bu yun] 肝郁不孕 "Sterility due to Stagnation of Liver-energy"

Inability to conceive, usually accompanied with emotional depression, feeling of fullness and oppression over the chest and hypochondria, distending pain over the breasts and menoxenia; caused by the stagnation of liver-energy and incoordination between vital energy and blood leading to the dysfunction of Chong, Ren and Bao channels.

12.5. [tan shi bu yun] 痰湿不孕 "Sterility due to Retention of Phlegm Wetness"

The sterility usually occurring in obese women who are fond of greasy foods, caused by the formation of phlegm-wetness evil in the interior involving the Chong, Ren and Bao channels; usually accompanied with leukorrhagia and irregular menstruation.

12.6. [fei pang bu yun] 肥胖不孕 "Infertility due to Obesity"

A type of infertility occurring in obese women who eat too much fat which turns to phlegm-damp blocking the Conception Vessel, often accompanied by palpitation, shortness and leukorrhagia.

Chapter Four

[Bing Yin Yu Bing Li] 病因与病理 "Aetiology and Pathology"

Part I 1. [bing yin] 病因 "Causes of Diseases"

The Chinese concept of aetiology has it origins in **[nei jing]** 内经 "Classic of Internal Medicine", in which the causes of diseases are classified into three kinds, so-called **[san yin]** 三因 "Three Groups of Aetiologic Factors of Diseases". They are: a) external cosmological factors that attack the human body from the outside, called **[wai yin]** 外因 "The External Aetiologic Factors"; b) internal emotional factors that weaken the human body or cause imbalance from the inside, called **[nei yin]** 内因 "The Internal Aetiologic Factor"; c) a small group of factors that are not classified as either external or internal, called **[bu nei wai yin]** 不内外因 "Factors Other than the Internal and External". These factors conform with and act according to the principles of **[yin yang]** 阴阳 "Yin and Yang" and **[wu xing]** 五行 "Five Elements". These pathogenic factors in Chinese medicine are literally translated as **[xie qi]** 邪气 "Evil Qi", which can cause diseases when it disturbs the "unity of opposites" in the body, leading to imbalance between Yin and Yang. When the balance of the body is disturbed by exogenous and endogenous pathogenic factors, different symptom-complexes appear.

1.1. [wai yin] 外因 "The External Aetiologic Factors"

The ancient Chinese categorized the external factors according to seasonal and climatic characteristics, and they are called **[liu yin]** 六淫 "six evils" or "six excesses": wind, cold, heat dryness, summer-heat, dampness, and fire (heat). Except for fire, they are accord with normal phenomena of the four seasons: spring-wind, summer-heat, midsummer-dampness, fall-dryness, and winter-cold. Wind, heat, and fire are Yang in nature, while cold, dampness and dryness are Yin in nature.

When there are abrupt and extreme changes in environmental conditions, they tend to have adverse effects on the body. So heat, damp, cold, dryness, and various combinations of the six evils accumulate in the weakened parts of the body with low resistance. The pathogenic factors will destroy the physiological equilibrium of human body and diseases appear.

1.2 [nei yin] 内因 "The Internal Aetiologic Factor"

In TCM, emotions are the principal endogenous source of diseases. There are seven emotional factors; joy, anger, melancholy, worry, grief, fear, and fright. TCM holds that the seven pathogenic emotions are physiological reflections of the human mental state. Emotional activities are closely related to the functioning of the internal organs thus diseases of the emotions are brought about when environmental factors excite the mind and caused undesirable changes. Under normal conditions, the seven emotional factors will not cause diseases. However, if the emotional excitation is too stressful and persistent and exceeds the normal endurance of the human body, they may produce functional disorder of Zang Fu organs, disturb the harmonious balance of Yin and Yang , Qi and blood, leading to diseases and organic lesions.

Different pathogenic emotional factors selectively damage certain Zang or Fu organs. For example: anger injures the liver, overjoy injures the heart, grief and melancholy injuries the lung, preoccupation injuries the spleen, fright and fear injure the kidney. However, the heart has a special role to play in the development of the diseases from the seven emotional pathogenic factors. **[su wen]** 素 问 "Plain Questions" says: "The heart is the monarch of the Five Zang and Six Fu organs", therefore extreme emotional stimuli will first attack the heart, and a disturbance of the heart leads to the affection of the internal organs.

1.3. [bu nei wai yin] 不内外因 "Factors that are Neither Internal nor External"

Traditionally, the causes of disease have been put into three categories: exogenous, endogenous, and neither exogenous nor endogenous. The third mainly refer to such pathogenic factors such as improper diet, fatigue, trauma, phlegm-humor, blood stasis, sexual indulgence, bites by insects and beasts, drowning, etc.

2. [mi niao nan ke fa bing de bing yin] 泌尿男科发病的病因 "The Causes of the Occurrence of Diseases in Urological Andrology"

The causes for the occurrence of diseases particularly in andrology are complicated. According to TCM, there are two respects. (1) the physiological dysfunction of the human body; (2) the external pathogenic factors. Wind, cold, summer-heat, dampness, dry and fire pathogenic factors are all responsible for the occurrence of the diseases of andrology, urology and sexology, among them dampness, (fire) heat and coldness are the chief pathogenic factors. In addition, abnormal sexual activities are also the cause of the related diseases, traumatic injuries, insects and beasts are also the causes of the diseases. In the internal pathogenic factors, besides extremely emotional reasons, excessive sexual indulgence and over-strain are the principal pathogenic factors for the diseases. The followings are the chief pathogenic factors causing the diseases.

2.1. [shi] 湿 "Dampness"

As an external factor, dampness generally refers to fog, dew, rain, or humidity. Diseases of pathogenic dampness can occur when the weather has been wet and rainy for several days. They may also attack a person who has been dwelling in a damp place. The dampness pathogenic evil is heavy, impure, sticky, viscous and difficult to dissolve.

Generally speaking, dampness is a Yin pathogenic factor and is apt to disturb the normal flow of Qi, especially it impairs Yang Qi, with spleen Yang as its chief impairment. If the Yang-Qi in male is damaged, there will be deficiency of vital essence, thus causing diseases with manifestation of heaviness of the body, fullness sensation in the chest and abdomen, sticky loose stools, turbid urine, oliguria with reddish urine, massive, foul-smelling vaginal discharge, oozing eczema or even ulcers, yellow and greasy fur on the tongue, floating and rapid pulse. Symptom-complexes of pathogenic dampness are:

2.1.1. [shi du] 湿毒 "Toxic material produced by Wetness-evil"

Toxins produced after prolonged stagnation of the pathogenic damp factor in the body, which causes disease characterized by its chronicity, intractability and copious exudation. For example, the stagnation may cause haematochezia, while the wetness-evil permeates downward and accumulates in the skin, the muscle of the leg, external genitalia, often causing local erosion, exudation, and even ulcerations.

2.1.2. [shi zu zhong jiao] 湿阻中焦 "Dampness stagnated in Zhong jiao"

A morbid condition due to retention of pathogenic dampness in the spleen and stomach. The main manifestations are anorexia, heaviness of the head, fatigue, vomiting, epigastric distress, oliguria with deep-colored urine, thick and whitish fur on the tongue, slow pulse.

2.1.3. [shi yu re fu] 湿郁热伏 "Stagnation of dampness causing Heat Retention"

As the damp pathogen is stagnated internally, the thermal pathogen can not be easily dissipated outwards, leading to fatigue, feeling of oppression over the chest, fullness of the abdomen, poor appetite, deep-colored urine etc.

2.1.4. [shi du dai xia] 湿毒带下 "Leukorrhagia due to Dampness"

Profuse leukorrhea caused by the impairment of Chong, Ren, resulting from attack of dampness evil during the menstrual period or puerperium; characterized by whitish or greenish yellow or multicolored vaginal discharge with foul odor; accompanied with itching and pain of the vulva, or fever and abdominal pain, or oliguria with reddish urine, etc.

2.1.5. [shi re xia zhu] 湿热下注 "Downward flow of Dampness-heat"

The pathologic changes due to downward flow of dampness-heat evil pathogens into the lower portion of the body, manifested as oliguria with reddish urine, dribbling of urine, wet and itching genitalia, hurting-pain in penis, leucorrhoea in pelvic infection, etc.

2.1.6. [shi re xia zhu pang guang] 湿热下注膀胱 "Accumulation of Dampness and Heat in the Bladder"

The pathologic manifestation caused by downward flow and stagnation of the dampness and heat factors in the urinary bladder. The main symptoms are frequency of an urgency of urination, painful urination with scanty urine, brownish red or bloody urine, fullness and distension of the hypochodrium, reddish tongue with yellowish fur, rapid pulse, etc.

2.2. [re xie] 热邪 "(Fire) Heat Pathogen" or "Heat Evil"

Fire-heat, brought about by an excess of Yang is Yang pathogenic factor and is interchangeable called fire or heat. The features characteristic of fire-pathogen are summarized as follows (1) Fire pathogen burns vital essence, producing dryness and is scorching in nature and its manifestation are high fever, scorching heat, dysphoria, thirst, sweating, red tongue with yellow coating , full pulse, etc. (2) Fire-pathogen is apt to consume Qi and body fluid, clinically manifested by thirst with an inclination for drink, dry mouth and throat, constipation and concentrated urine, etc. (3) Fire-pathogen is liable to stir up wind-evil and disturb blood flow in the body. This is known as "extreme heat stirring up wind". Its clinical manifestations are high fever accompanied by coma and deliriumtic of limbs, convulsion, and leading to various types of haemorrhage. (4) It tends to consume Yin fkuid and cause painful swelling on the body surface. When an invasion of the pathogenic heat factor or hyperactivity of the Yang Qi is possible to have pathogenic symptoms such as oliguria with deep-colored urine, painful stranguria, reddish, swelling and pain in the testicle. Fire-evil also causes itching and pain in the penis, penis pain during the sexual intercourses, frequent, painful and dripping urination. Sore of syphilis may occur due to the stagnation of fire-heat., etc.

2.2.1. [re xie] 热邪 "Heat-evil"

A collective term for external pathogenic factor that produce severe febrile diseases, such as fever, noisy breathing, local redness, swelling, heat and pain, constipation, etc.

2.2.2. [re yu] 热郁 "Stagnation of Heat-evil"

The pathogens of heat-syndrome resulting from emotional upsets and the stagnation of liver- energy; manifested as headache, dry mouth and bitter taste, quick temper, feeling sensation in the hypochondrium, constipation, oliguria with deep-colored urine, red tongue with yellowish fur, wiry and rapid pulse, etc.

2.2.3. [re sheng ze zhong] 热胜则肿 "Overbundance of Heat-evil may bring about local swelling"

A morbid condition of overabundance of Yang-heat in the body, leading to local congestion with redness and swelling such carbuncle, dermatitis, manifested as swelling, heat, pain particularly in external genitalia, etc.

2.2.4. [re jie xia jiao] 热结下焦 "Heat- evil accumulating in the Lower Jiao"

A morbid state manifested as distending pain in the lower abdomen, constipation, dysuria, even haematuria, etc.

2.2.5. [re jie pang guang] 热结膀胱 "Accumulation of Heat in the Urinary Bladder"

A morbid condition in which the pathogenic factor of an acute febrile disease transformed into heat and accumulated in the urinary bladder. When heat pathogens stagnate in the intestines and urinary bladder, etc. The symptoms are mainly manifested by distension and fullness of the lower abdomen, stranguria, difficult and painful urination, frequent urination, and even haematuria.

2.2.6. [re li] 热痢 "Heat-type Dysentery"

A disease due to an invasion of the Pathogenic heat factor into the large intestine and retention of heat-evil and indigested food in the intestine. The chief symptoms are diarrhea with very foul mucoid discharge, fever, and abdominal pain. tenesmus, extreme thirst urination with burning sensation and reddish urine, scanty and dark urine, yellowish and greasy fur on the tongue, smooth and rapid, strong pulse, etc.

2.3. [han xie] 寒邪 "Cold Pathogen"

Cold is a Yin pathogenic factor. Pathogenic cold therefore tends to suppress the defensive Yang of the body . If pathogenic cold invades the interior of the body, the Yang function of the spleen and stomach is impaired, leading to cold-syndromes. The characteristic features of cold pathogen are as follows: (1) the pathogenic cold affects the kidney for the kidney is the organ most closely associated with pathogenic cold. Exogenous pathogenic cold and dampness usually bring about pathological changes in the kidney, leading to all kinds of diseases. At the same time, insufficiency of Kidney Yang is the source of endogenous or internal pathogenic cold. (2) Impairing Yang-Qi because cold is a pathogenic agent of Yin nature. The continuous smooth flow of Qi, blood, and body fluid throughout the body depends on the warming, impelling influence of Yang Qi. If the pathogenic cold impairs Yang Qi, producing stagnation and retardation of flow of Qi and blood and block of channels and collaterals, from which pain results. So the symptoms and signs caused by pathogenic cold factor, or a deficiency of Yang-Qi are manifested as subnormal temperature, pale complexion, listlessness, intolerance to cold, epigastric and abdominal pain which is relieved by hot compress, loose stools, copious pale urine, spasmodic pain in the testes and low abdomen, painful and cold feeling in the testicles, impotence, nocturnal emission, cold semen, shrinkage of scrotum, pale tongue with whitish mucoid coating, deep slow pulse etc.

2.3.1. [han shen ze fu] 寒胜则浮 "Excess of Cold-evil may bring about Edema"

A morbid condition of Yang Qi becomes deficient, Qi and blood flow sluggishly, and water and moisture are retained in the of body due to insufficiency of

Yang-Qi and stagnation of vital energy and blood resulting from the excessive cold pathogens, resulting in the pathological manifestations of edema and swelling.

2.3.2. [han jie] 寒结 "Cold-type Constipation"

Constipation due to retention of Yin-cold evil, accompanied with pale lips, flat taste in the mouth, abdominal distention and pain, discharge of large amount of light colored urine, white and smooth fur on the tongue, etc.

2.3.3. [han zhi gan mai] 寒滞肝脉 "Retention of Cold-evil in the Liver Channel"

A morbid condition due to cold-evil attacking the liver channel; manifested as distending pain over the lower abdomen radiating to testis, intolerance of cold, cold limbs, dragging pain of the testicles, whitish and smooth fur on the tongue, sunken and wiry pulse, etc.

2.4. [du xie] 毒邪 "Noxious Evil"

It includes **[shi du]** 湿毒 "Noxious Dampness" and **[re du]** 热毒 "Noxious Heat". The former is a noxious pathogenic factor formed by stagnation of dampness, which causes disease characterized by its chronicity, intractability and copious exudation. That stagnates in the intestines may cause haematochezia while that distributes to the skin may cause local erosion and exudation. The latter is a noxious pathogenic factor formed by accumulated heat or fire, which causes boils, ulcers and other purulent inflammations. Syphilis, stranguria, abscess of scrotum are often seen in man's diseases.

2.5. [nei shang] 内伤 "Internal Impairment"

The pathologic changes of the viscera Qi, blood and body fluids caused by emotional disturbances (see 2.6. "seven emotions"), improper diet, fatigue, excessive sexual activities, etc.

2.6. [qi qing] 七情 "Seven Modes of Emotions"

Emotional activities acting as the responses of human mentality to the environment. An intense and prolonged emotional upset may act as a pathogenic factor, i.e., overjoy, anger, melancholy, anxiety, sorrow, terror and fright causing the dysfunction of vital energy, blood and viscera and resulting in various diseases.

In TCM, It is generally considered that anger injuries the liver, and rage causes adverse smooth flow of the liver-Qi; joy impairs the heart, and excessive joy tends to cause unsteadiness of the heart-Qi and mental derangement; anxiety impairs the spleen. Among them anxiety, sorrow anger and terror have a great influence to the man's diseases. For instance; terror impairs the kidney, causing the collapse of vital energy. As a result, incontinence of urine, stool, nocturnal emission and seminal discharge may occur. An impaired kidney may lead to impotence, emission, involuntary seminal discharge, premature ejaculation, etc.

2.7. [yin shi bu yi] 饮食不宜 "Improper Diet"

Improper diet is an important pathogenic factor. Underfeeding, overeating, insanitary food or food preference, is often the factor predisposing to disease, causing injure to the spleen and stomach, leading to their inability to receive, digest, transport, and transform food. For example, insufficient nourishment intake due to underfeeding brings about malnutrition and insufficiency of Qi and blood, which gives rise to deficiency of the spleen and the kidney (Vital Qi), lower the body resistance, thus symptoms such as edema, oligospermia and sterility may occur. On the hand, excessive nourishment intake due to overeating, which exceeds the transporting and transforming capacities of the spleen and the stomach, if the food is too cold, causing damage to the spleen and the kidney Yang, thus sterility due to cold semen may occur, if the food is too hot, spicy, wetness-heat may form, causing multiple abscess in the lower energizer, impotence may occur.

In book **[lu shi chun qiu]** 吕氏春秋 "The History of Lu Shi", it says: "One should refrain from heavy, spicy food and strong wine". Wine is the most harmful factor that causes male diseases. Immoderate drinking gives rise to the accumulation of wetness-heat in the liver and spleen, leading to impairment of the spleen and stomach, which is often manifested as abdominal flatulence, oliguria, haematochezia, etc.

2.8. [lao yi shi du] 劳逸失度 "Imbalance between Work and Rest"

It means overwork or undue leisure, which may turn to be a pathogenic factor. Overwork can be classified into three types: (1) undue physical exertion; (2) undue mental exertion; (3) intemperance in sexual life.

Excessive sexual activity and overexertion are also endogenous pathogenic factors. **[zhang jing yue]** 张景岳 Zhang Jingyue said: "Sexual activities must be restricted, otherwise the primordial energy is bound to be exhausted; if so, the vital energy will be distracted. Primordial energy can transform into Qi which can in turn transform into spirit, thus nourishing the body". Excessive sexual activities consume the primordial energy (Kidney-essence), injure the spirit, thus leading to a deficiency condition and destroying the basis of life. The consumption of kidney essence may be accompanied by lassitude in the loins and knees, aching and weakness in the lumbar region, dizziness, ringing in the ears, vertigo, tinnitus, and listlessness. In men, night sweats, nocturnal emissions, spermatorrhea, and impotence often accompany the condition. In women, menstrual irregularities and foul-smelling vaginal discharges, etc.

3. [die pu chuang shang] 跌扑创伤 "Traumatic Injury"

Generally speaking, traumatic injury refers to gunshot injuries, incised wounds, contusions, sprains, scalds and burns, cold injury and injury inflicted by animal stings or bites. All of the above may lead to blood stasis and painful swelling on the skin and muscles and external genitalia, if not promptly treated, it may cause impairment to Chong, Ren channels and give rise to male diseases, such as haematuria, uroschesis, incontinence of urine, even impotence.

Part II [bing jing te dian] 病机特点 "The characteristics of the Pathogenesis"

Pathogenic mechanism of a disease includes its aetiology, location, manifestations, and the changes of the viscera, vital energy and blood. The diseases in urological field relate closely to the viscera, Qi and blood and channels and collaterals.

[zang fu gong neng shi chang] 脏腑功能失常 "Dysfunction of Zang-fu Organs"

1. [shen] 肾 "The Kidney"

1.1. [shen jing kui sun] 肾精亏损 "Insufficiency of the Kidney-Essence"

It is either due to the congenital deficiency, or lack of proper care after birth, or intemperance in sexual life. Insufficiency of the kidney-essence may delay the beginning of menstrual function and impede the development and maturity of sexual glands at puberty, or lead to senility and hypo sexuality among the middle-aged, manifested as sterility due to spermacrasis in males and due to amenorrhea in females, impotence and spermatorrhea, etc.

1.2. [shen yin xu] 肾阴虚 [shen shui bu zu] 肾水不足 "Deficiency of Kidney-Yin"

The pathologic manifestations due to insufficiency of the Yin Fluids of the kidney with the accompanying heat syndrome. The main symptoms are lumbago, lassitude, dizziness, tinnitus, spermatorrhea and premature ejaculation, or frequent erection of the penis and emission, dry mouth and sore throat, night sweat, malar flush, hot palm and soles, red tongue with little coating, faint and rapid pulse, etc.

1.3. [shen yang xu] 肾阳虚 or [shen huo bu zu] 肾火不足 "Deficiency of Kidney-Yang"

The pathologic manifestations due to the impairment of the renal function, kidney-deficiency in the aged, injury of the kidneys due to chronic disorders and intemperance sexual life, with the accompanying cold syndrome. The main symptoms are chilliness, cold limbs, lumbago, aversion to cold, speratorrhea, premature ejaculation, impotence, frequency of nocturia, sterility in females, pale tongue, deep and formicant pulse, etc.

1.4. [shen qi bu gu] 肾气不固 [xia yuan bu gu] 下元不足 "Unconsolidation of Kidney-Qi"

The pathological manifestations of incontinence of urine and spermatorrhea duc to decreased renal functions. The main symptoms are frequent micturition with light-colored urine, continuous dripping after urination, or enuresis, urinary incontinence, nocturia, spermatorrhea, premature ejaculation, clear leukorrhea or spontaneous abortion in women, pale tongue with whitish fur, and deep weak pulse.

1.5. [shen jing bu zu] 肾精不足 "Insufficiency of Kidney-Essence"

This refers to a syndrome due to consumption of the kidney-essence. It is caused mainly by congenital defects, improper care after birth, or intemperance in sexual life an injury of the kidneys due to chronic disorder. Its clinical manifestations are sterility due to spermacrasis in males and due to amenorrhea in females.

1.6. [long huo nei fan] 龙火内燔 or [shen huo pian kang] 肾火偏亢 "Hyperactivity of Kidney-fire"

The pathological change due to the deficiency of kidney-yin and a relative excess of the kidney-fire. The chief manifestations are excessive libido, frequent dreams, nocturnal emission, spermatorrhea, premature ejaculation, lumbago, dizziness, malar flush, hot palms and soles, etc.

1.7. [ming men huo wang] 命门火旺 or [shen huo pian kang] 肾火偏亢 "Hyperactivity of Kidney-fire"

The pathologic manifestations of the deficiency of Kidney-yin and hyperactivity of asthenic fire. The chief symptoms are excessive sexual libido, frequent erection of penis, nocturnal emission, precocious ejaculation, frequent dreams and insomnia, etc.

1.8. [xiang huo wang dong] 相火妄动 "Prime Minister-fire upsetting in the body"

The pathological manifestations of the "Liver fire" and burning of asthenic fire of the kidney caused by deficiency of both kidney-yin and liver-Yin. The chief symptoms are dizziness, headache, blurring of vision, tinnitus, deafness, irritability, feverish sensation of the palm, soles and chest, excessive sexual libido, nocturnal emission, premature ejaculation, etc.

2. [gan] 肝 "The Liver"

2.1. [gan qi yu jie] 肝气郁结 "Liver Stasis"

The stagnation and depression of the Hepatic Qi. When the dispersing function of the liver is disturbed, there may appear various symptoms, such as fullness or burning pain of the hypochodrium, chest distress, mental depression or anxiety, feeling of a lump in the throat, occasional epigastric distention and pain, hiccup, regurgitation of acid, suppressed appetite, occasional abdominal distension and pain, diarrhea, occasional irregular menstruation etc.

2.2. [han zhi gan mai] 寒滞肝脉 "Accumulation of Cold in the Liver Channel"

The pathologic changes in which the pathogenic cold factor is accumulated and stagnant in the Liver Channel. The main symptoms are distension, fullness, cold and pain of the hypogastrium, dragging pain of the testicles, cold chilly limbs, whitish and glossy coating of the tongue, deep, stringy or slow pulse, etc.

2.3. [gan shen kui sun] 肝 肾 亏 损 [gan shen yin xu] 肝 肾 阴 虚 "The Impairment of the Liver and the Kidneys"

The pathologic changes in which the Yin (Vital essence) Fluids of both the liver and the kidneys are simultaneously impaired. The main symptoms are dizziness, feeling of distension of the head, blurred vision, tinnitus, fever, bitter taste, hot palms and soles, insomnia, soreness of the waist and knees, spermatorrhea, stringy, faint, and rapid pulse, or faint and weak pulses, etc.

3 [xin] 心 "The Heart"

3.1. [xin shen bu jiao] 心肾不交 "Disharmony between Heart and Kidneys"

The pathologic manifestations due to abnormalities of the physiologic relationship between the Heart-Yang and the Kidney-Yin. The main symptoms are dysphoria, insomnia, palpitation, frequent dream, spermatorrhea, etc.

3.2. [xin pi liang xu] 心脾两虚 "Weakness of both Heart and Spleen"

The main symptoms are palpitation, amnesia, insomnia, frequent dream, reduced appetite, loose stools, abdominal distension and fullness, fatigue and weakness, sallow complexion, emaciation, pale tongue with whitish coating, faint and weak pulse.

3.3. [xia ji shen shui] 下及肾水 "Drawing the Kidneys Fluid from below"

The heart fire becomes excessive and exhausts the Kidney-Yin. The main symptoms are dysphoria, insomnia, palpitation, and restlessness, dry mouth and throat, increased sexual libido, spermatorrhea, premature ejaculation, faint and rapid pulse, etc.

3.4. [xin yi re yu xiao chang] 心移热于小肠 "The Heart transfers its Fire to the Small Intestine"

Excessive Heart Fire affects the small intestine. The main symptoms are dysphoria, ulcers of the mouth and the tongue, red tip of the tongue, scanty dark colored urine, or stabbing pain with urination, haematuria, etc.

3.5. [xin huo kang sheng] 心火亢盛 "Hyperactivity of Heart-Fire"

It refers to a morbid condition due to hyperactivity of the heart-fire in the interior, usually resulting from production of fire due to emotional upsets and stagnancy of Qi, or invasion of the interior by the pathogenic fire, or excessive intake of hot- natured food of acrid taste or warm- natured tonics, and manifested as dysphoria with feverish restless sensation in the thorax insomnia, flushed face, thirst, ulcers of the mouth and tongue, or difficult and painful urination with dark urine, haematuria or mania and delirium, redness of the tip of the tongue and rapid forceful pulse.

4. [pi] 脾 "The Spleen"

4.1. [pi shi jian yun] 脾失运输 "Spleen fails to transport and convert"

A morbid condition of dysfunction of the spleen; manifested as flatulence, poor appetite, diarrhea, emaciation, sallow complexion, general debility, or edema, etc.

4.2. [pi yang xu] 脾阳虚 "Deficiency of Spleen-Yang"

A morbid condition of marked hypofunction of the spleen and stomach with manifestations of asthenia-cols syndrome, such as cold feeling and pain of the upper abdomen, flatulence, hiccup, vomiting, poor appetite, chronic diarrhea, fatigue, oliguria, edema, emaciation, pale tongue, weak pulse, etc.

4.3. [pi shen liang xu] 脾肾两虚 "Deficiency of both Spleen and Kidneys"

A morbid condition due to deficiency of Kidney-Yang which fails to nourish spleen-Yang, or vice versa; manifested as chilly sensation of the whole body, especially the limbs, pale complexion, cold seasation and pain of the loins and knees or lower abdomen, lienteric diarrhea or morning diarrhea, dysuria or polyuria, pale and tender tongue with whitish and moist fur, sunken and weak pulse, etc.

4.4. [zhong qi xia xian] 中气下陷 "Descent of Qi in Zhong Jiao" (The Middle Energizer)

The pathologic manifestations due to visceroptosis as a result of relatively severe deficiency of the spleen and gastric-energy. The main symptoms are anorexia, loose stools, abdominal distension after eating, shortness of breath, lassitude, perspiration, sallow complexion, heavy and dragging feeling in the abdomen, frequent urination, prolapse of uterus, prolapse of rectum, etc.

5. [pang guang] 膀胱 "The Bladder"

5.1. [pang guang qi bi] 膀胱气痹 "Obstruction of the Bladder Qi"

The pathologic manifestations of distension and fullness of hypogastruim, dysuria or uroschesis, as a result of impaired functions of the urinary bladder.

5.2. [pang guang xu han] 膀胱虚寒 "Insuficiency and chills of the Urinary Bladder"

The pathologic manifestations of the cold syndrome accompanying the impairment of the urinary bladder functions. The major symptoms are frequency of urination, enuresis, light urine or dribbling of urine, cold feeling in hypogastrium, whitish moist coating of the tongue, faint pulse etc.

5.3. [pao qi bu gu] 脬气不固 "Deficiency of Bladder Energy"

The pathologic manifestations of inability to control the discharge of urine with enuresis or incontinence of urine and stranguri as a result of impaired function of the urinary bladder.

5.4. [pang guang shi re] 膀胱湿热"Damp-heat in the Urinary Bladder"

A morbid condition due to retention of pathogenic damp-heat in the urinary bladder usually due to the accumulation of exogenous damp-heat evil in the bladder or downward flow to the urinary bladder deriving from the improper diet. Its chief manifestations are: frequent and urgent micturition, scanty urine and dysuria, brownish red cloudy urine or haematuria, urine and dysuria, brownish red cloudy urine or haematuria, urinary calculus, often accompanied with fever and lumbago, red tongue with yellowish and greasy fur, and slippery rapid pulse.

6. [san jiao] 三焦"Triple Energizer"

6.1. [san jiao zhu jue du] 三焦主决渎 "Triple Energizer manages the dredging of Water Pathway"

The triple energizer has the function of clearing up passages and keepingi the fluid flowing freely. Whenever this function is in disorder, uropenia and edema may cause.

6.2. [san jiao xu han] 三焦虚寒"Cold and feebleness in San jiao"

The pathogenic changes of the chilly-feeble syndromes of the triple energizers. The chilly-feeble syndrome of the Upper Jiao are those of the heart and lungs; of the Middle Jiao, those of the spleen and stomach; of the Lower Jiao, those of the kidney and urinary bladder.

6.3. [xie liu san jiao] 邪留三焦"Retention of Pathogens in San jiao"

The pathologic manifestations due to retention of pathogens (the damp, heat, or damp heat factors) in the Upper, Middle and Lower Energizer respectively. For example, such retention in the Upper Jiao may cause chest distress; in the Middle, abdominal distention; and in the lower, dysuria; etc.

Part III. [yu sheng zhi qi xiang guan de jing luo] 与生殖器相关的经络 "The Channels and Collaterals connected with External Genitalia" (including the external orifice of the urethra)

1.1. [shou tai yin fei jing] 手太阴肺经"Lung Channel of Hand Tai yin , or simply Lung Channel"

One of the twelve channels, it is related to the lungs and connected with the large intestine, and communicates with the stomach and throat. It begins internally in the [zhong jiao] 中焦"middle energizer", descends to connect with the large intestine, then ascends to the lung and throat, courses laterally and exits superficially at [zhong fu] 中府"Zhongfu" (LU), then descends along the lateral side of the arm and forearm, ends at [shao shang] 少商"Shaoshang " (LU), with 11 points on either side.

Their indications are cough, bloody sputum, thirst, dypsnea, restlessness, full feeling of the chest, pain of the shoulder and upper back, perspiration, frequent urination and urine of dark color, and pain and numbness of the local symptoms along the path of this channel.

1.2. [zu tai yang pang guang jing] 足太阳膀胱经"Bladder Channel of Foot Tai yang, or simply Bladder Channel" (BL)

One of the twelve regualr channels. Inside the body, it is related to the urinary bladder and connected with the kidney and brain. On the body surface, it runs from [jing ming] 睛明"Jingming" (BL) at the medial canthus of the eyes, ascends the forehead to the vertex and then enters the brain and exits at the nape of the neck where it divides into two parallel branches: the first branch descends the back at a distance of 1.5 CUN from the spinal column, and during its course it connects with the kidney and urinary bladder, and continues along the posterior side of the thigh to the popliteal fold; the second branch descends the back at a distance of 3 CUN from the spine, continues along the latero-posterior side of the thigh to popliteal fold where it meets the first branch. Then the channel continues to descend along the posterior side of the calf to the lateral malleolus, terminating at [zhi yin] 至阴"Zhiyin" (BL) on the lateral side of the tip of the small toe. There are 67 points on either of the body.

Indications are malaria, mania, yellowish sclera, epiphoria, epistaxis, stiffness and pain of the neck and head, pain of the lower back, haemorrhoids, frequent urination, painful micturition, dysuria, etc., as well as local symptoms along its pathway.

1.3. [zhu dhao yin shen jing] 足少阴肾经" Kidney Channel of Foot Dhao yin, or simply Kidney Channel" (KI)

One of the regular twelve channels. Inside the body, it is related to the kidney and connected with the urinary bladder, spinal cord, liver, diaphragm, throat, the root of the tongue, lungs, heart, chest, etc.; on the body surface, it runsform the plantar tip of the small toe and travels to [yong quan] 涌泉"Yongquan" (KI) in the center of the sole, continues along the inner side of the lower limb to the symphsis pubis, turns internally to the kidney and urinary bladder, and back to the symphyasis pubis, descending along the abdomen and chest up to [shu fu] 俞府"Shufu" (KI) in the depression between the first rib and the lower border of the clavicle, with 27 points on either side. The kidney branch travels through the liver and diaphragm, enters the lungs and follows the trachea and larynx to the base of the tongue.

Indications are dryness of the tongue, sore throat, enuresis, spermatorrhea, frequent urination, impotence, menstruous complaints, asthma, edema, lumbago, and weakness of the lower limbs.

1.4. [zu jue yin gan jing] 足厥阴肝经"Liver Channel of Foot Jue yin, or simply Liver Channel"

One of the twelve regular channels. Inside the body, it is related to the liver and connected with gallbladder, genital organs, stomach, diaphragm, throat, and eyeball; on the body surface, it runs from **[da dun]** 大敦 "Dadun" (LR) on the big toe just behand the nail, through the inner side of the lower limb, external genitalia and abdomen, to **[qi men]** 期门 "Qimen" (LR), a point about 2 CUN below the nipple, with 14 points on either side. From Qimen (LR), the channel enters the abdomen, travels thre stomach para-laterally to connect with the liver and gallbladder. From the liver, the channel ascends past the diaphragm along the trachea, larynx, sinus cavity, connecting with the eyes, and then ascends to the vertex where it meets **[du mai]** 督脉 "Governor Vessel".

Indications are feeling fullness in the chest, hiccup, lumbago, diarrhea, hernia, incontinence of urine, dysuria, abnormal mestruation, metrorrhagia, dryness of the mouth and throat, dusky complexion etc., as well as the local symptoms along its pathway.

2. [du ren chong san mai] 督, 任, 冲三脉 "Du, Ren, Chong Three Channels"

2.1. [du mai] 督脉 "Du Mai or Governor Vessel" (GV)

One of the eight extra meridians, which begins at **[chang qiang]** 长强 "Changqiang" (GV1), a point at the back of the anus, sending one branch forward to **[hui yin]** 会阴 "Hui yin" (CV). The main portion of the meridian runs upward along the middle of the spinal column, to the back of the neck, turns anteriorly over the top of the head down the face to **[yin jiao]** 阴交 "Yinjiao" (GV), a point between the upper lip and the upper gum in the labia frenulum, with 28 points. During this corse, it is connected with the spinal cord, the brain, and governs all the Yang channels of the entire body. It is the reins of all Yang channels.

Indications are usually, febrile diseases, mental disorder, epilepsy and hysteria, stiffness and pain in the neck and back, dryness of the throat, dysuria, haemorrhoids, enuresis, porlapse of rectum, hernia, infertility, and debility, etc.

2.2. [ren mai] 任脉 "Ren Mai or Conception Vessel "(CV)

One of the eight extra meridians which runs from **[hui yin]** 会阴 "Huiyin" (CV 1), a point in the center of perineum, it arises out of the perineum, runs to the mons pubis, upwards along the midline of the abdomen, via the umbilicus, to the chest, neck and middle of the lower lip, **[cheng jiang]** 承浆 "Chengjiang" (CV), midpoint of the mentolabial sulcus, with 24 points. The internal portion of this meridian ascends from **[cheng jiang]** 承浆 "Chengjiang" (CV), encircling the mouth and traveling to the eyes. Another branch travels internally from the pelvic cavity to the throat. In the course of its circulation, it connects with all the Yin channels. It is the reins of the Yin channels. The character Ren also means pregnancy. As the saying goes: "The Ren meridian is responsible for the supply to fetus in the uterus".

Indications are menstrual disorders, leukorrhea, hernia, bloody leucorrhea, mass in the abdomen, dysfunction of the viscera in the chest and abdomen, deficiency of **[yuan qi]** 原气 "Yuan Qi " (primordial vital energy).

2.3. [chong mai] 冲脉"Chong Mai or Thoroughfare Vessel" (TV)

One of the eight extra meridians which originates from the uterus, runs upwards along the interior of the vertebra, coming into confluence with the Kidney Meridian. At the same time, it starts from the sides of the genitalia and passes by both sides of umbilicus, and ends at the chest. It is said Chong Mai to be "The sea of the twelve regular channels", because it can regulate the Qi-blood of the twelve regular channels. The Chong Mai is also known as "The reservior of blood", since it is closely related to menstruation in female.

Its pathological manifestations are abdominal pain, irregular menstruation, abnormal uterine bleeding and infertility.

Part IV. [bian zheng] 辨证"Differential Diagnosis"

1. [ba gang bian zheng] 八纲辨证"Differential Diagnosis in Accordance with the Eight Principal Syndromes"

The eight principal syndromes are: Yin or Yang, exterior or interior, cold or heat, and deficient or excessive. **[ba gang bian zheng] 八纲辨证 "Differential Diagnosis in Accordance with the Eight Principal Syndromes"** is a method of differetial diagnosis used to determine the nature and location of the pathological changes, and the conflict between body resistance and pathogens in terms of the eight principal syndromes, which are utilized clinically for analysis, deduction and diagnosis of diseases. In the fields of urology, andrology and sexuology, the chief syndromes are as follows:

1.1. [yang zheng] 阳症"Yang-syndrome"

The superficies-syndrome, heat-syndrome and sthenia-syndrome all belong to Yang syndrome. The syndromes are usually acute, febrile, active, exacerbated, excited, hyperfunctional, hypermetabolic, progressive, outward, and upward in nature. It is marked by such manifestations as fever, chilliness, flushed face, headache, desire for cooling of the body, irritability, dry mouth and lips, thirst, heavy breathing, constipation, foul stool, abdominal pain and tenderness, scanty and deep-coloured urine, red tongue with dry and yellowish fur, floating and full rapid pulse, etc.

1.2. [yin zhen] 阴症"Yin-syndrome"

The interior-syndrome, cold-syndrome and asthenia-syndrome are all belong to Yin-syndrome.The syndromes are usually chronic, cold, inactive, weak, depressed and downward in nature. It is marked by such manifestations such as pale or lusterless complexion, cold extremities, desire for lying quietly, low voice, weak breathing, lassitude, poor appetite, flat taste in mouth, loose stools, discharge of large amount of watery urine, abdominal pain which can be relieved by pressure, pale, enlarged and tender tongue with moist and smooth fur, sunken and slow, weak pulse, etc.

1.3. [biao zheng] 表症 "Superficies-syndrome"

It refers to a syndrome caused by an attack of the superficies by six exogenous pathogens through the skin, hair, mouth and nose, usually seen in the primary stage of diseases; manifested as chilliness, fever, headache, stuffy nose, cough, thin and whitish fur on the tongue, floating pulse, etc.

1.4. [li zheng] 里症 "Interior Syndrome"

It is a syndrome contrary to the exterior one and is characterized by pathological changes of the internal organs caused by pathogens. For example, heat-syndrome of the interior is chiefly manifested as fever without chilliness thirst, restlessness, bitter taste in the mouth, oliguria with reddish urine; asthenis-syndrome in the interior, manifested as fatigue, listlessness, dizziness, palpitation, insomina, nocturnal emission; cold-syndrome in the interior, manifested as intolerance of cold, cold limbs, loose stools or diarrhea, polyuria with watery urine, etc.

1.5. [han zheng] 寒症 "Cold Syndrome"

It is the syndrome caused by invasion of the pathogenic cold, or hypofunction of the body due to insufficience of Yang and excess of Yin, marked by aversion to cold, pale complexion, no thirst, loose stools, copious pale urine, pale tongue with whitish mucoid coating, deep slow pulse, etc. It is frequenctly seen in chronic and hypofunctional diseases.

1.6. [re zheng] 热症 "Heat Syndrome"

It is a syndrome caused by invasion of pathogenic heat or hyperactivity of the body due to deficiency of Yin and excess of Yang, marked by fever, aversion to heat, restlessness, flushed face, dry mouth and throat, thirst with a predilection for cold drink, red and dry lips, constipation scanty dark urine, red tongue with brownish or blackish coating and rapid pulse, etc. It is usually seen in infectious diseases and those due to hyperfunction of Yang.

1.7. [xu zheng] 虚症 "Deficiency Syndrome"

It refers to a morbid condition manifested by deficiency of vital energy and essence, which weakens the resistance to diseases and impaired physiologic functions including deficiencies of Blood, Qi, Yin and Yang. The chief manifestations are pale or yellowish complexion, listlessness, shortness of breath, emaciation, fatigue and weakenss, lassitude in loins and knees, spontaneous perspiration, night sweat, incontinence of stool and urine, thick and tender tongue, feeble pulse, etc.

1.8. [shi zheng] 实症 "Excess Syndrome"

It refers to a morbid condition marked by exuberant pathogens, occurring in a relatively strong patient exposed to exirulent evil or dysfunction of the viscera, leading to the Qi stagnation, blood stasis, phlegm obstruction, stagnancy of water. The chief manifestations are coarse breathing, irritability, pain and distention in the chest and abdomen, constipation, oliguria with deep-colored urine, red tongue with rough, dry and yellowish fur, forceful pulse.

3. [zang fu bian zheng] 脏腑辨证 "Differentiating Syndromes according to the Zang-fu Organs"

One of the basic methods of differential diagnosis, involving analyzing and identifying the diseases through the observation of the physiological and pathological characteristics of the viscera. There are differentiating syndromes of the heart, the liver, the spleen, the lung, the kidney, the small intestines and the large intestines, the urinary bladder, the stomach, etc.

3. [liu jing bian zheng] 六经辨证 "Differentiating Syndromes According to Six Channels Theory"

This is one of the methods of differential diagnosis first appearing in **[shang han lun]** 伤寒论 "The Treatise on Febrile Diseases" by **[zhang zhong jing]** 张中景 of the **[dong han]** 东汉 "Eastern Han Dynasty" (25-220 AD). Six channels are Taiyang, Yangming, Shaoyang, Taiyin, Shaoyin, and Jueyin, and various clinical manifestations of febrile diseases caused by exogenous pathogenic factors are involved in theses channels, which are used to determine the nature and site of pathological changes, the confliction between body resistance and evil, and the tendency of disease development, as a guide for clinical treatment.

4. [wei qi ying xue bian zheng] 卫气营血辨证 "Differential Diagnosis by the Analysis of Wei, Qi Ying and Xue"

This is diagnostic method for epidemic febrile diseases according to the theory of four stages in the development of an epidemic febrile disease. It is used to identify the location, the nature, the variation of the four stages of the clinical courses of an acute febrile diseases due to external affection. The theory was first put forward by **[ye tian shi]** 叶天氏 a **[qing]** 清 Qing Dynasty physician. In his book, he classified the clinical manifestations of febrible diseases into four stages: Wei (outer defensive) stage, Qi (inner defensive) stage, Wei (outer defensive) stage, and Xue (blood) stage, hence (superficial, deep, mild or serious) stages of the diseases , which are used to guide the clinical treatment.

5. [san jiao bian zheng] 三焦辨证 "Differentiating Syndromes According to the San jiao Theory"

This method of differential syndromes was advocated by **[wu ju tong]** 吴鞠通 a physician in Qi Dynasty (1551-1836). He summarized clinical manifestations of epidemic febrile diseases as having the three areas: the upper, middle, and lower portions of the body cavity. For example, if pathogenic damp and heat spread through all the upper, middle and lower- the triple energizers to obstruct the circulation of Qi, and block the smooth transportation and transformation of water and fluid, it is difficult to differential damp-heat diseases only by using the theory of Wei, Qi Ying and Xue, the theory of San Jiao is used to analyze the diseases, thus it is a further supplement to the differential diagnosis by the analysis of Wei, Qi Ying and Xue.

Part V. [zhi ze] 治则 "Therapeutic Principles"

1. [bian zheng lun zhi] 辨证论治 "Selection of Treatment Based on the Differential Diagnosis"

In TCM, **[bian zheng]** 辨证 "Differential Diagnosis" means that the patient's symotoms and signs are analyzed and summarized in order to identify the aetiology, the location of the lesion, the pathological changes and body condition by the comprehension of the clinical data by the four methods of examination. **[lun zhi]** 论治 "Selection of the treatment" means the proper therapeutic program is determined according to the result of the diagnosis. There are different therapeutic methods in TCM, **[biao ben]** 标本 "Branch and Root" are two important concepts in clinical practice.

2. [biao ben] 标本 "Branch and Root"

They are contrasting concepts used to indicate the primary and secondary relationship of contraditory sides in various kinds of diseases and syndromes.Clinically, it implies the follows:

Between the human body and the pathogenic factor, the primordial Qi is Ben (the primary) and the pathogenic factor, Biao (the secondary); so far as the diseases is concerned, the aetiology is Ben and the symptoms are Biao; as for the course of the disease, the original or the primary condition is Ben while the complication or the secondary condition, Biao; for the location of a lesion, the internal portion is Ben while the external, Biao. The differentiation between them would be helpful to determine the therapeutical principle in clinical practice.

3. [ba fa] 八法 "Eight Therapeutic Methods"

It refers to the eight comprehensive principles of therapy, including diaphoresis, inducing emesis, purgation, reconciliation (regulation of the functional relationship between the internal organs), warming, heat-clearing, resolution and invigoration. Here are some of the methods commonly used in treating the diseases.

4. [jie biao fa] 解表法 "Expelling Superficial Evils"

A therapy commonly used in treating the exterior syndrome by dispelling pathogenic factors from the exterior of the body by using diaphoretics. The methods of dispelling pathogenic factors from the exterior of the body with drugs of pungent and warm-nature and drugs of pungent and cold-nature can be both applied.

5. [qu feng] 祛风 "Dispelling Wind-evil"

A therapy for treating the stagnation of wind-evil in the body surface, meridians, muscles and joints by using the drugs effective for dispelling the wind-evil.

The drugs of expelling wind and removing dampness; expelling wind to relieve pain; expelling wind and nourishing blood, expelling wind and removing obstruction of the meridians, etc. are often used.

6. [qing fa] 清法 "Heat-clearing away Therapy"

A method by administering drugs of cool or cold nature to treat acute febrile diseases and other diseases with internal heat. Different drugs are applied according to the location of heat-evil.

6.1. [qing re li shi] 清热利湿 "Clearing Away the Heat-evil and Promoting Diuresis"

The method is to treat the symptom complex caused by wetness-heat evil accumulated in the lower energizer (lower Jiao) by using the heat - clearing drugs and the drugs for inducing the diuresis. The chief manifestations are distension of the lower abdomen, cloudy urine, oliguria, dysuria, yellowish and greasy fur on the tongue.

6.2. [qing shu li shi] 清暑利湿 "Clearing Away Summer-heat Evil and promoting Diuresis"

The method to treat the syndrome caused by the attack summer-heat and damp by using the drugs with effects of clearing pathogenic summer-heat and dispelling damp. The chief manifestations of the case are fever, bodily heaviness, restlessness, thirst, difficult urination, etc.

7. [wen fa] 温法 "Warming Therapy"

A method by dispelling internal cold by applying drugs with warming effect to treat cold syndrome.

7.1. [wen yang li shi] 温阳利湿 "Warming Yang to Eliminate Wetness Evil"

The method to treat cold and damp symptom complex and edema and dysuria due to the attack of cold-wetness evil, etc. by using the drugs with the effect of warming Yang, activating energy, invigorating the spleen and eliminating the accumulated fluid to promote diuress.

7.2. [wen shen li shui] 温肾利水 "Warming the Kidney to Promote Diuresis"

The method to treat edema due to deficiency of kidney Yang and the retention of wetness-evil in the body by using the drugs for warming and reinforcing Yang energy and promoting diuresis. It is applicable to various disorders such as edema, pale complex, dizziness, vertigo, lumbago, cold accumulated in the extremities, pale tongue with whitish fur, deep and thready pulse, etc.

7.3. [wen shen zhu yang] 温肾助阳 "Warming the Kidney and Supporting Yang"

A method to treat Yang deficiency of kidney by using the drugs with the action of warming and reinforcing kidney Yang, applicable to various disorders, such as morning diarrhea, nephrotic syndrome of chronic nephritis, etc.

7.4. [wen bu ming men] 温补命门 "Warming and Recuperating the Gate of Life" or [bu huo sheng tu] 补火生土 "the Fire to Produce the Earth"

To recuperate Spleen Yang and the Kidney Yang by invigorating vital function of the kidney with warming tonics, applicable to the case with declining of the fire in the vital gate, manifested as morning diarrhea, aversion to cold, chilliness of abdomen, cold limbs, chills and pain of the waist and knees, or sexual impotence, etc.

8. [bu fa] 补法 "Therapy for Invigoration"

A therapy for treating various types of asthenia-syndrome due the deficiency of Yin, Yang, vital energy and blood by reinforcing and nourishing the deficiencies of Yin, Yang Vital and blood.

8.1. [bu yang] 补阳 "Invigorating Yang" or [fu yang] 扶阳 "Tonifying Yang"

A therapy for treating syndrome of Yang-deficiency of the heart, spleen and kidney with Yang tonics. The chief manifestations are soreness, cold feeling in the loins and knees, lassitude, impotence, emission, frequent micturition, sterility in female due to cold womb, edema more serious in lower part of the body, pale tongue with whitish coating, sunken and weak pulse, etc.

8.2. [bu yin] 补阴 "Invigorating Yin"

Using the Yin tonics with sweet and cold-nature to treat the syndromes due to Yin deficiency, applicable to various diseases caused by Yin-deficiency and fluid consumption. The chief manifestations are weakness of the loins and knees, dizziness, tinnitus, insomnia, dreminess, frequent erection of the penis or emission in mae, scanty menstruaturin or amenorrhea in women.

8.3. [bu shen gu jing] 补肾固精 "Invigorating the Kidney to arrest Spontaneous Emission"

A therapy to arrest spontaneous by invigorating the kidney, usually classified into invigoration of kidney Yin and kidney Yang.

8.4. [zi yin li shi] 滋阴利湿 "Nourishing Yin and Eliminating the Wetness-evil"

The method to using drugs of nourishing Yin and also the drugs of supplementing blood to treat the disturbance of urinary excretion due to the consumption of Yin caused by the attack of wetness-heat evil and dysuria. It is commonly used in treating edema due to Yin deficiency.

8.5. [zhuag yang] 壮阳 "Strengthening Yang"

A therapy of invigorating Yang by applying warm-natured tonics to promote vital function, especially virility in the treatment of sexual impotence.

9. [shou se] 收涩 "Causing Contraction and Arresting Discharge" or [gu se] 固涩 "Inducing Astringency and arresting Discharge"

A therapy by applying tonics of styptic and astringent agents to treat excessive loss of essence-energy and body fluid, manifested as spontaneous sweating, seminal emission, chronic diarrhea, or haemorrhage, etc.

9.1. [gu shen se jing] 固肾涩精 "Strengthening the Kidney to Restore its Astringent Function"

A method to treat nocturnal emission, frequent micturition due to the deficiency of kidney energy, manifested as night sweat, soreness, of loins, tinnitus, lassitude, seminal emission, etc.

9.2. [gu shen suo niao] 固肾缩尿 "Strengthening the Kidney to reduce urination"

A method to treat frequent urination or enuresis due to the debility of kidney-energy.

10. [tiao he fa] 调和法 "Mediation Method"

A therapy of applying drugs with regulating or intermediating action to restore normal correlation between the internal organs or eliminate the pathogenic factors. E.g. regulating the Yin and Yang to restore relative equilibrium between the two; regulating the relationship amomg all the Zang-fu organs, enabling them to coordinate each other in normal functioning; regulating Qi and blood to promote natural flow of vital energy and keep blood circulation smooth, etc.

Chapter Five

[dian xiang bing li] 典型病例 "Typical Diseases"

[mi niao xi tong ji bing] 泌尿系统疾病 "Diseases of the Urinary System"

1. [mi niao xi gan ran] 泌尿系感染 "Urinary Infection"

Urinary infection is defined as the infections of the urethra, bladder, pelvis and renal parenchyma, of which pyelitis is the most common. It is commonly seen in female and especially in pregnant women. This disease belongs to the category of **[lin zheng]** 淋症 "stranguria", **[yao tong]** 腰痛 "lumbago" and **[shen re]** 肾热 "heat in the kidney". As for the chronic urinary infection, it has more complex pathogenesis and different clinical manifestations, such as frequent, difficult and painful discharge of urine due to the accumulation of wetness-heat in the bladder, asthenia and hypofunction of the kidney. The one with remarkable symptoms due to deficiency such as edema, acratia and emaciation should be included in the syndromes of **[shui zhong]** 水肿 and **[xu lao]** 虚劳 "consumptive disease" of TCM.

1.1. [bing yin bing ji] 病因病机 "Aetiology and Pathogenesis"

It is usually caused by the deficiendy of the kidneys and the invasion of the external pathogenic factors.Too much food pungent and sweet in flavor and hot and fatty in nature or too much drink also cause damp-heat flowing downward into the urinary bladder, so damp-heat is accumulated which is also due to unclean orifices, dirty and turbid pathogens invading the urinary bladder; the Qi in the urinary bladder fails to perform its normal function due to the accumulation of damp-heat. In this case, urgent urination, frequent micturition, and oliguria or haematuria will appear.

1.2. [bian zheng lun zhi] 辨症论治 "Differentiation and Treatment"

1.2.1. [pang guang shi ren] 膀胱湿热 "Damp-heat in the Urinary Bladder"

(1) **[zhu zheng]** 主症 "Symptoms":

Aversion to cold, fever, urgent and frequent micturition, dripping discharge of urine with burning sensation and stabbing pain, distending pain in the lower abdomen, frequent micturition, oliguria, dysuria, haematuria, lumbago, restlessness with frequent crying in infants, reddish tongue with yellowish fur and slippery rapid pulse.

(2) **[zhi fa]** 治法"Therapeutic Method":

Clearing away and purging pathogenic heat-fire, remoiving toxic material and inducing diuresis to treat stranguria.

(3) **[chu fang]** 处方"Prescription":

[shi wei tong lin fang] 石苇通淋方 "Pyrrosia Leaf recipe for Treating Stranguria"

Ingredients:

[shi wei] 石苇	Folium Pyrrosiae	30g
[pian xu] 扁蓄	Herba Polygoni Avicularis	12g
[qu mai] 瞿麦	Herbal Dian thi	9g
[da huang] 大黄	Radix Rhei	6g
[dan zhu ye] 淡竹叶	Herbal Lophatheri	9g
[bai mao gen] 白茅根	Rhimaogen Imperatae	30g
[che qian zi] 车前子	Semen Plantaginis	15g (decocted after being wrapped in a piece of cloth)
[hua shi] 滑石	Talcum	30g
[kun cao] 坤草	Harba Leonuri	150g
[gan cao] 甘草	Radix Glycyrrhizae	3g

Decocted in water for oral use, 1 dose daily.

(4) **[jia jian]** 加减"Modification"

In case of more severe chills and fever, bitter taste, nausea and vomiting, the drugs added are **[chai hu]** 柴胡Radix Bupleuri15g, **[ban xia]** 半夏Rhizoma Pinelliae 9g and **[huang qin]** 黄芩Radix Scutellariae 12g.

If the number of pus cell fails to be reduced and the tongue coating is yellow and greasy, the drugs added are **[pu gong ying]** 蒲公英Herba Taraxaci 30g, **[tu fu lin]** 土茯苓Rhizoma Smilacis Glabrae 12g.

In case of haematuria, the drugs added are **[xiao ji]** 小蓟Herba Cirii 30g, **[sheng di]** 生地 Radix Rehmanniae 30g, and **[ou jie]** 藕节 Nodus Nelumbini Rhizomatis.

1.2.2. [shen yin bu zu shi re liu lian] 肾阴不足 湿热留恋"Retention of damp-heat due to Insufficiency of Renal Yin-fluid and the Kidney-Yin"(usually seen in chronic urinary infection)

(1) **[zhu zheng]** 主症"Symptoms":

Manifested as lumbago, fatigue, dizziness, tinnitus, dry throat and lips, low fever, mild or severe frequent and urgent urination and urodynia, feverish sensation of the palms, and soles and chest, reddish tongue with thin coating, and taut thready rapid pulse.

(2) **[zhi fa]** 治法 "Therapeutic Method":

Nourishing Yin, invigorating the kidney, clearing away heat and descending fire-evil.

(3) **[chu fang]** 处方 "Presription":

[zhi bai di huang tang jia wei] 知柏地黄汤加味 "Modified Decoction of Anemarrhena, Phellodendro and Rehmannia"

Ingredients:

[sheng di] 生地	Radix Rehmanniae	15g
[shan yao] 山药	Rhizoma Dioscoreae	10g
[shan yu rou] 山萸肉	Fructus Corni	9g
[dan pi] 丹皮	Cortex Moutan	12g
[fu ling] 茯苓	Poria	9g
[ze xie] 泽泻	Rhizoma Alismatis	15g
[zhi mu] 知母	Rhizoma Anemarrhenae	12g
[huang bai] 黄柏	Herba Pyrrosiae	9g
[shi wei] 石苇	Herba Pyrrosiae	15g
[dan zhu ye] 淡竹叶	Herba Lophatheri	9g

1.2.3. [pi shen liang xu] 脾肾两虚 "Deficiency of both Spleen and Kidney" (usually seen in chronic pyelonephritis)

(1) **[zhu zheng]** 主症 "Symptoms":

A morbid condition due to deficiency of kidney-Yang which fails to nourish spleen-Yang, or vice versa; manifested as chilly sensation of the whole body, especially the limbs, difficulty and pain in micturition and dripping urination, short breath, listlessness, disinclination to speak, edema of the face and feet, anorexia and abdominal distention, soreness and weakness of the loins and knees, loose stool, dysuria or polyuria, pale tongue with thin and white fur, and deep, thready and weak pulse.

(2) **[zhi fa]** 治法 "Therapeutic Method":

Strengthening the spleen and tonifying the kidney to eliminate dampness.

(3) **[chu fang]** 处方 "Prescription"

[si jun zi tang he ji sheng shen qi wan jia jian] 四君子汤合济生肾气丸加减 "Modified Decoction of Four Noble Drugs with Life Preserving Pill for Rplenishing the Kidney Qi".

Ingredients:

[dang sheng] 党生	Radix Codonopsis Pilosulae	9g
[fu ling] 茯苓	Poria	9g
[bai shu] 白术	Rhizoma Atracylodis Macrocephalae	9g
[shan yao] 山药	Rhizoma Dioscoreae	9g
[shan yu rou] 山萸肉	Fructus Corni	9g
[che qian zi] 车前子	Semen Plantaginis	9g (dococted after being wrapped in a piece of cloth)
[niu xi] 牛膝	Radix Achydranthis Bidentatae	9g
[sheng yi ren] 生苡仁	Semen Coicis	12g

All the above drugs are to be decocted in water for oral administration, 1 dose daily.

(4) **[jia jian]** 加减"Modification":

For those with sore waist, add **[ji sheng]** 寄生 Ramulus Loranthi 9g; in case of edema, add **[dong gua pi]** 冬瓜皮 Exocarpium Benincasae 15g, [ze xie] 泽泻 Rhizoma Alismatis 9g.

2. [mi niao xi jie shi] 泌尿系结石 "Calculus in the Urinary System"

It includes kidney stone, ureteral calculus and vesical calculus resulting from the retention of wetness and heat-evils in the lower warmer. In TCM it belongs to the syndromes of **[niao jie shi]** 尿结石 "stranguria from urolithiasis", **[yao tong]** 腰痛 "lumbago" and "stranguria caused by the passage of urinary stone" called **[shi lin]** 石淋" Stone Lin".

2.1. [bing yin bing ji] 病因病机 "Aetiology and Pathogenesis"

[shi lin] 石淋 "Stone Lin" syndrome is due to stones formed in a long time of damp-heat accumulation. It is marked by pain or colics in the lower abdomen, loins and urethra, difficulty in urination, discharge of yellow turbid urine or haematuria caused by sandy stones obstructing the urethra and irritative pain during urinary discharge. Prolonged stranguria will lead to insufficiency of Qi and blood and impairment of Yin-fluid.

2.2. [bian zheng lun zhi] 辩症论治 "Differentiation and Treatment"

Clinical manifestations are characterized by symptoms of infection such as fever, vomiting, diarrhea, pallor and loss of appetite. In infants, jaundice may be present. The typical symptoms of urinary infection may include urodynia, urgency and frequency of urination, dysuria, dripping urine, pin in the lumbar region, occasionally with transient haematuria and enuresis. Chronic recurrent infection may be accompanied with intermittent fever, lumbar soreness, fatigue and anemia, or with renal failure in severe cases.

2.2.1. [shi re xing] 湿热型 "Type of Damp-heat"

(1) **[zhu zheng]** 主症 "Symptoms":

Urine sometimes with sand and stone, difficulty in urinary or sudden stop of urination, stabbing pain in urethra, rigidity of the lower abdomen or intolerable colicky pain in the loins and abdomen, even haematuria, reddish tongue with thin yellow coating, and slightly rapid pulse.

(2) **[zhi fa]** 治法"Therapeutic Method":

Clearing away heat, including diuresis, and treating stranguria through removing urinary calculus.

(3) **[chu fang]** 处方"Prescription":

[si jin pai shi tang] 四金排石汤 "Decoction of Lysimachia, Climbing Fer Sporn, Chicken's-skin and Curcuma Root"

Ingredients:

[jing qian cao] 金钱草Herba Lysimachiae	45g
[hai jin sha] 海金砂Spora Lygodii	15g
[jin ne jin] 鸡内金Endothelium Corneum Gigeriae	15g
[yu jin] 郁金Radix Curcumae	18g
[bai shao] 白芍Radix Paeoniae Albae	30g
[hua shi] 滑石Talcum	30g
[qu mai] 瞿麦Herba Dianthi	9g
[dong qui zi] 冬葵子 Semen Malvae	15g
[da huang] 大黄Radix et Rhizoma Rei	6g
[guang mu xiang] 广木香Radix Aucklandiae	6g
[niu xi] 牛膝Radix Achranthis Bidentatae	30g
[gan cao]甘草 Radix Glycyrrhizae	3g

Decocted in water for oral use, 1 dose daily.

(4) **[jia jian]** 加减"Modification":

For haematuria, the drugs added are **[xiao ji]** 小蓟Herba Cirsii 30g, **[sheng di]** 生地Radix Rehmanniae, **[ou jie]** 藕节 Nodus Nelumbinis Rhizomatis 15g.

For fever, the drugs added are **[pu gong ying]** 蒲公英Herba Taraxaci 30g, **[huang qin]** 黄芩 Radix Scutellariae.

For severe colicky pain in the kidney, the drugs added are **[zhi ru xiang]** 制乳香 Olibanum Praeparata 6g, **[zhi mo yao]** 制没药 Myrrha Praeparata 6g., in addition, the following two kinds of powder are mixed evenly and taken after being infused in water.

[san qi fen] 三七粉Notoginseng 3g (in the form of powder) **[chen xiang fen]** 沉香粉 Lignum Aquilariae Resinatum 1g (in the form of powder).

2.2.2. [qi yin liang kui xing] 气阴两亏型"Type of Insufficiency of Qi and Yin"

(1) **[zhu zheng]** 主症"Symptoms":

Stone formed long ago, difficulty in urination, urodynia, ache of the loins and abdomen, haematuria, shortness of breath, acratia, emaciation or edema, dry mouth, pale tongue with white coating, and deep weak pulse.

(2) **[zhi fa]** 治法 "Therapeutic Method":

Invigorating Qi, nourishing Yin, and clearing the channels todischarge urinary calculus.

(3) **[chu fang]** 处方"Prescription":

[ren shen pai shi tang] 人生排石汤 "Ginseng Decoction for Removing Urinary Calculus"

Ingredients:

[xi yang shen] 西洋参 Radix Panacis Quinquefolli (decocted first of all)	6g
[sheng mu li] 生牡蛎Concha Ostreae (decocted first)	30g
[chuan shan jia] 穿山甲Squama Manitis	9g
[shi hu] 石斛Herba Dendrobii	15g
[qu mai] 瞿麦Herba Dianthi	12g
[dong qui zi] 冬葵子 Semen Malvae	9g
[xue yu tan] 血余碳Crinis Carbonisatus	6g
[chuan lian zi] 川楝子Fructus Toosendan	9g
[fu ling] 茯苓Poria	12g
[ze xie] 泽泻Rhizoma Alismatis	15g
[shi wei] 石苇Folium Pyrrosiae	15g
[jing qian cao] 金钱草Herba Lysimachiae	15g
[jin ne jin] 鸡内金Endothelium Corneum	9g
[gan cao] 甘草Radix Glycyrrhizae	6g

Decocted in 1500 ml of water until 500 ml of decoction can be got. The decoction is divided into two portions, one portion is taken each time, twice a daily. One dose is used every other day.

3. [yi niao zheng] 遗尿"Enuresis"

Clinically it falls into two kinds. One refers to frequent spontaneous urination with dribbling urine; the other spontaneous urination during sleep. Enuresis of children is defined as involuntary emptying of bladder during the daytime or at night when the children are above the age of 3.

3.1. [bing yin bing ji] 病因病机"Aetiology and Pathogenesis"

Insufficiency and weakness of Qi of the lung, spleen and kidney weaken the function of the urinary bladder in storing urine so that urination can not be controlled and enuresis results. It is called **[yi niao]** 遗尿"bed wetting".

3.2. [bian zheng lun zhi] 辩症论治 "Differentiation and Treatment"

Clinical features are controlled diurnal or nocturnal enuresis without dysuria. Careful examination should be made on the life habit and mental status of the children to make sure if there are infections of the urinary tract or organic disorders.

3.2.1. [xia yuan xu han] 下元虚寒 "Deficiency-cold of the Kidney"

(1) **[zhu zheng] 主症** "Symptoms":

Frequent urination during sleep, difficult in being waken up from sound sleep, frequent light-colored urine, pallor, cold limbs, fear of cold, weakness of the lower extremities, lassitude of the loins and legs, mental retardation, pale tongue with thin and white fur, and deep, slow and weak pulse.

(2) **[zhi fa] 治法** "Therapeutic Method":

Warming and recuperating the Kidney-Yang to treat enuresis.

(3) **[chu fang] 处方** "Prescription":

[sang piao xiao san he gong di wan jia jian] 桑螵蛸散合巩堤丸加减 "Modificated Prescription of Mantis Egg-case Powder and Enuresis Power"

Ingredients:

[sang piao xiao] 桑螵蛸 Ootheca Mantidis	15g
[tu si zi] 菟丝子 Semen Cuscutae	9g
[yi zhi ren] 益智仁 Fructus Alpinize Oxyphtllae	15g
[bu gu zhi] 补骨脂 Fructus Psoraleae	15g
[fu pen zi] 覆盆子 Fructus Rubi	15g
[shu fu zi] 熟附子 Radix Aconiti Praeparata	6g
[rou gui] 肉桂 Cortex Cinnamomi	4.5g
[huang qi] 黄芪 Radix Astragali	15g
[dang sheng] 党生 Radix Codonopsis Pilosulae	15g

Decocted in water for oral administration.

3.2.2.[pi fei qi xu] 脾肺气虚 "Deficiency of the Spleen and Lung"

(1) **[zhu zheng] 主症** "Symptoms":

Frequent urination with less amount of urine, often spontaneous urination, usually accompanied by tenesmus and distension in the lower abdomen, shortness of breath, acratia, poor appetite, emaciation, pale tongue with thin white coating, and weak pulse.

(2) **[zhi fa] 治法** "Therapeutic Method":

Supplementing Qi to prevent the sinking of it.

(3) **[chu fang]** 处方 "Prescription": **[bu zhong yi qi tang jia jian]** 补中益气汤加减 "Modified decoction for reinforcing the Middle-Jiao and Rplenishing Qi"

Ingredients:

[huang qi] 黄芪Radix Astragali	15g
[dang gui] 当归Radix Angelicae Sinensis	12g
[chen pi] 陈皮Pericarpium Citri Reticulatae	9g
[chai hu] 柴胡Radix Bupleuri	6g
[sheng ma] 升麻Rhizoma Cimicifugae	6g
[yi zhi ren] 益智仁Fructus Alpinize Oxyphyllae	9g
[wu wei zi] 五味子Fructus Schisandrae	9g
[bu gu zhi] 补骨脂Fructus Psoraleae	12g
[sang piao xiao] 桑螵蛸Ootheca Mantidis	15g
[gan cao] 甘草Radix Glycyrrhizae	6g

Decocted in water for oral use, 1 dose daily.

(4) **[jia jian]** 加减"Modification":

In case of abundant cold due to deficiency of Yang and slow pulse, the drugs added are **[rou gui]** 肉桂 Cortex Cinnamomi 6g, **[fu zi]** 附子 Radix Aconiti Lateralis Praeparata 9g.

4. [ru mi niao] 乳糜尿 "Chyluria"

Chyluria is usually due to bancroftosis but occasionally due to tuberculosis of urinary system or tumors. Its main clinical manifestations are intermittent recurrence of cream white urine, haematuria with urethral pain in most patients, difficult in urination, swelling of testicle, hydrocele of tunica vaginalis, elephantiasis of crus, distention and pain of the hypogastrium, etc., TCM names it as **[chi bai zhuo]** 赤白浊 "reddish and whitish turbid urine" or **[gao lin]** 膏淋 "Milky Lin" according to the color of urine.

4.1. [bing yin bing ji] 病因病机 "Aetiology and Pathogenesis"

This disease is caused by downward flow of damp-heat due to over-intake of fatty and sweet food or by downward flow of refined nutritious substances due to exhaustion of Qi and blood resulting from deficiency of the spleen, deficiency of Yin with hyperactivity of evil fire and failure to astringe resulting from deficiency of the kidney.

4.2. [bian zheng lun zhi] 辩症论治 "Differentiation and treatment"

In the early stage, this disease is mainly due to downward flow of damp-heat. So, mainly clearing away heat and inducing diuresis should conclude the treatment. When it becomes protracted and recurrent, the spleen and kidney have been made weak. At this time, the treatment should be, accordingly, concentrated on invigorating the spleen-Qi and reinforcing the kidney. Simultaneous, the symptoms and cause should be treated together.

4.2.1. [shi re xia zhu]湿热下注"Downward flow of Damp-heat"

(1) **[zhu zheng]** 主症 "Symptoms":

Turbid and cream white urine sometimes with coagula which becomes evident whenever fish or meat is eaten, no pain during urinating, full and choking sensation in the chest and epigastrium, thirst without desire for drinking, yellow thick greasy tongue coating, and soft rapid pulse.

(2) **[zhi fa]** 治法"Therapeutic Method":

Eliminating damp-heat as the main means.

(3) **[chu fang]** 处方"Prescription":

[ru mi niao tang] 乳糜尿汤 "Decoction for Treating Chyluria"

Ingredients:

[bi xie] 萆Rhizoma Dioscoreae Hypoglaucae	30g
[hai jin sha] 海金砂Spora Lygodii	30g
[shi wei] 石苇Folium Pyrrosiae	30g
[fu ling] 茯苓Poria	12g
[sheng di] 生地Radix Rehmanniae	15g
[bian xu] 蓄Herba Polygoni Avicularis	15g
[nu zhen zi] 女贞子Semen Ligustri Lucidi	12g
[hong hua] 红花Flos Carthami	9g
[huang bai] 黄柏Cortex Phellodendri	6g

Decocted in water for oral use, 1 dose daily.

(4) **[jia jian]**加减"Modification":

In case of lassitude, poor appetite and edema, the drugs added are

[dang sheng] 党生Radix Codonopsis Pilosulae	15g
[bai shu] 白术Rhizoma Atracylodis Macrocephalae	15g
[qian shi] 芡实Semen Euryaleaee	30g

In case of haematuria, the drugs added are

[mao gen] 茅根Rhizoma Imperatae	30g
[yi mu cao] 益母草Herba Leonuri	30g
[xian he cao] 仙鹤草 Herba Agrimoniae	15g
[zhong lu tan] 棕榈炭 Petiolus Trachycarpi carbomisatus	9g

4.2.2. **[shen xu bu gu]** 肾虚不固 "Failure of the Deficient Kidney to perform its Astringing Function"

(1) **[zhu zheng]** 主症"Symptoms":

Turbid urine, restlessness, fever, thirst, soreness and weakness of the loins and knees, fatigue, acratia, dizziness, blurred vision, reddened tongue with little coating, and deep thready or thready rapid pulse.

(2) **[zhi fa]** 治法 "Therapeutic Method":

Reinforcing the Kidney for Consolidation.

(3) **[chu fang]** 处方 "Prescription":

[liu wei di huang tang he tu shi zi wan jia jian] 六味地黄汤和兔丝子丸加减 "Modified Decoction of Six Ingredients with Rehmannia and Pill of Dodder Seed"

Ingredients:

[shu di] 熟地 Radix Rehmanniae Praeparata	30g
[shan yu rou] 山萸肉 Fructus Corni	12g
[shan yao] 山药 Rhizoma Dioscoreae	15g
[tu si zi] 菟丝子 Semen Cuscutae	24g
[gou qi] 枸杞 Fructus Lycii	15g
[lian zi rou] 莲子肉 Seman Nelumbinis	12g
[sheng qian shi] 生芡实 Semen Euryales	15g
[duan long gu] 段龙牯 Forged Os Draconis Fossilis	30g
[wu wei zi] 五味子 Fructus Schisandrae	9g

Decocted in water for oral use, 1 dose daily.

(4) **[jia jian]** 加减 "Modification":

In case of remarkable deficiency of the spleen, the drugs added are

[bai shu] 白术 Rhizoma Atractylodis Macrocephalae	12g
[huang qi] 黄芪 Radix Astragali	15g
[dang sheng] 党生 Radix Codonopsis Pilosulae	15g

In case of deficiency and weakness of the kidney-Yang marked by cold limbs, loose stools, pale tongue with white coating, and deep weak pulse, the drugs added are

[lu rong] 鹿茸 Cornu Cervi Pantotritum	9g
[bu gu zhi] 补骨脂 Fructus Psoraleae	12g
[zhi fu zi] 制附子 Radix Aconiti Lateralis Praeparata	9g
[rou gui] 肉桂 Cortex Cinnamomi	6g

[pi qi xia xian] 脾气下陷 "Downward flow of the Spleen-Qi"

(1) **[zhu zheng]** 主症 "Symptoms":

Turbid urine which becomes more evident due to overstrain, sallow complexion, lassitude, weakness, pale tongue with thin white coating, and weak pulse.

(2) **[zhi fa]** 治法"Therapeutic Method":

Supplementing Qi to send up the lucid Yang.

(3) **[chu fang]** 处方"Prescription":

[bu zhong yi qi tang] 补中益气汤 "Decoction for reinforcing the Middle-Jiao and replenishing Qi"

Ingredients:

[huang qi] 黄芪Radix Astragali	15g
[dang sheng] 党生Radix Codonopsis Pilosulae	12g
[bai shu] 白术Rhizoma Atractylodis Macrocephalae	12g
[dang gui] 当归Radix Angelicae Sinensis	9g
[chen pi] 陈皮Pericarpium Citri Reticulatae	9g
[chai hu] 柴胡Radix Bupleuri	6g
[sheng ma] 升麻Rhizoma Cimicifugae	6g
[zhi gan coa] 炙甘草Radix Glycyrrhizae Praeparata	6g
[da zao] 大枣Fructus Jujubae	5 dates

Decocted in water for oral use, 1 dose daily.

(4) **[jia jian]** 加减"Modification":

In case of poor appetite, abdominal distention, emaciation and insufficiency of Qi of the Middle-Jiao, the drugs added are

[shan yao] 山药Rhizoma Dioscoreae	15g
[qian shi] 芡实Semen Euryaleaee	12g
[bai guo] 白果Fructus Ginkgo	9g

5. [ji xing shen yan] 急性肾炎 "Acute Nephritis"

Acute nephritis is a diseases with edema, especially of face and head as the major sign, usually caused by the attack of wind-evil resulting in the failure to keepthe lung-energy dispersive and descendant, and retention of fluid in the body. It occurs mostly in children with males predominating. Its main manifestations are sudden onset, arthralgia, edema, oliguria, haematuria, high blood pressure, nausea, vomiting or fever, etc.. This disease pertains to the category of **[feng shui]** 风水"edema" in TCM.

5.1. [bing yin bing ji] 病因病机 "Aetiology and Pathogenesis"

Attack of exogen ous wind, cold and dempness, improper diet and daily life or internal injury due to overstrain lead to dysfunction of the lung in clearing and regulating, of the spleen in transporting, of the kidney in opening and closing, of the urinary bladder in transforming Qi, and of the tri-Jiao in clearing water passage, and cause retention of water in the muscles and abdomen, resulting in edema.

5.2. [bian zheng lun zhi] 辨症论治 "Differentiation and Treatment"

A vast majority of patients have the symptoms 1-3 weeks prior to the onset of acute nephritis such as tonsillitis angina, scarlet fever or purulent infection of the skin.

The onset is sudden. Edema, hypertension, albuminuria, dropsy of face and four limbs, dysuria are the major manifestations accompanied with haematuria. In mild cases, only slight edema of eyelids and urinary changes may be present. In severe cases there may be heart failure, and even renal failure.

5.2.1. [feng shui] 风水 "Type of Wind-water"

(1) **[zhu zheng]** 主症 "Symptoms":

Sudden onset, fever and chill characterized by higher fever and slight chill, dry mouth, sore throat, scanty and deep colored urine, facial edema at the beginning followed by edema all over the body especially face and head, thin white tongue coating, floating pulse or deep pulse seen if edema is severe.

(2) **[zhi fa]** 治法 "Therapeutic Method":

Dispelling pathogenic wind, removing pathogenic heat and ventilating the lung to promote the flow of fluid.

(3) **[chu fang]** 处方 "Prescription":

[yue bi jia shu tang jia jian] 越婢加术汤加减 "Decoction for Relieving Edema with Bighead Atractylodes Modified"

Ingredients:

[ma huang] 麻黄 Herba Ephedrae	9g
[sheng shi gao] 生石膏 Gypsum Fibrosum	30g
[bai shu] 白术 Rhizoma Atractylodis Macrocephalae	9g
[sang bai pi] 桑白皮 Cortex Mori	9g
[gan cao] 甘草 Radix Glycyrrhizae	6g
[fu ling pi] 茯苓皮 Extra Poria	15g
[fu ping] 浮萍 Herba Spirodelae	12g
[sheng jiang] 生姜 Rhizoma Zingiberis Recens	3g
[da zao] 大枣 Fructus Jujubae	5 dates

Decocted in water for oral use, 1dose daily.

(4) **[jia jian]** 加减 "Modification":

For sore throat, the drugs added are **[ban lan gen]** 板兰根 Radix Isatidis 15g, **[lian qiao]** 连翘 Fructus Forsythiae 12g, **[niu pang zi]** 牛子 Fructus Arcii 12g.

5.2.2. [re du] 热毒 "Noxious-heat"

(1) **[zhu zheng]** 主症 "Symptoms":

Boils and carbuncles on the skin, edema of the body and limbs, dry mouth, dysphoria, scanty and deep-closured urine, dry stool, red tongue with yellowish fur, slippery and rapid pulse.

(2) **[zhi fa]** 治法 "Therapeutic Method":

Clearing away pathogenic heat and toxic materials and inducing diuresis to reduce edema.

(3) **[chu fang]** 处方 "Prescription":

[wu wei xiao du yin jia jian] **五味消毒饮加减** "Modified Antiphlogistic Decoction of Five Drugs"

Ingredients:

[jin yin hua] 金银花 Flos Lonicerae	30g
[lian qiao] 连翘 Fructus Forsythiae	15g
[pu gong ying] 蒲公英 Herba Taraxaci	30g
[di ding] 地丁 Herba Violae	15g
[da huang] 大黄 Rhizoma Rhei	6g
[huang qin] 黄芩 Radix Scutellariae	10g
[bai mao gen] 白茅根 Rhizoma Imperatae	30g
[chen qian cao] 车前草 Herba Plantaginis	12g

Decocted in water for oral use, 1 dose daily.

5.2.3. [shui shi] 水湿 "Retention of Water"

(1) **[zhu zheng]** 主症 "Symptoms":

General edema, which is sometimes so severe that there appear pits on the body surface when pressed, fatigue and bodily heaviness, distension in the stomach, anorexia, oliguria, white and greasy coating of the tongue, deep and slow pulse.

(2) **[zhi fa]** 治法 "Therapeutic Method":

Invigorating the spleen for excreting dampness and activating Yang to induce diuresis.

(3) **[chu fang]** 处方 "Prescription":

[wu lin sangwu pi yin jia jian] 五苓散五皮饮加减 "Modified Prescriptions of Powder of Five Drugs with Poria and Decoction of Peel of Five Drugs"

Ingredients:

[gui zhi] 桂枝 Ramulus Cinnamomi	10g
[bai shu] 白术 Rhizoma Atractylodis Macrocephalae	10g
[zhu ling] 猪苓 Polyporus Umbrellatus	10g
[fu ling] 茯苓 Poria	12g
[ze xie] 泽泻 Rhizoma Alismatis	10g
[da fu pi] 大腹皮 Pericarpium Arecae	12g
[fu ling pi] 茯苓皮 Extra Poria	15g
[dong gua pi] 冬瓜皮 Exocarpium Benincasae	15g
[chen qian cao] 车前草 Herba Plantaginis	12g

Decocted in water for oral use, 1dose daily.

(4) **[jia jian]**加减"Modification":

In case of stagnation of dampness-heat manifested as edema of the whole body, bitter taste in the mouth, dry throat, fullness in the chest, distension in the abdomen, scanty dark urine, yellow and greasy coating of the tongue, smooth and rapid pulse, the treatment is aimed at clearing up pathogenic heat and dampness. The preferable recipe is **[er miao san he shu zuo yi zi jia jian] 二妙散合**凿饮**子加减** "Two Wonderful Drugs Powder and Decoction for Diuresis".

Ingredients:

[chang shu] 苍术Rhizoma Atractylodis	10g
[huang bai] 黄柏 Cortex Phellodendri	10g
[fang yi] 防已 Radix Stephiae	10g
[zhu ling] 猪苓 Polyporus Umbrellatus	10g
[ze xie] 泽泻Rhizoma Alismatis	10g
[da fu pi] 大腹皮 Pericarpium Arecae	12g
[fu ling] 茯苓 Poria	12g
[mu tong] 木通 Caulis Clematidis Armandii	10g
[chi xiao dou] 赤小豆Semen Phaseoli	30g
[bai mao gen] 白茅根 Rhizoma Imperatae	30g

Decocted in water for oral use, 1 dose daily.

6. [man xing shen yan] 慢性肾炎"Chronic Nephritis"

Chronic nephritis is a disease caused by a wide variety of aetiological factors. Chronic nephritis is common in young adults and middle aged people, marked by edema, abdominal distention, soreness of the waist, oliguria, haematuria, high blood pressure, white and greasy coating of the tongue, deep and slow pulse, etc. and decreased renal function in different levels. In TCM, it is categorized as **[shui zhong]** 水肿"edema", **[xu lao]** 虚劳, "consumptive diseases", **[yao tong] 腰痛**"lumbago", etc.

6.1. [bing yin bing ji] 病因病机"Aetiology and Pathogenesis"

Attack of exopathogens, weakness of the spleen and kidney, and disturbance in both distribution of body fluid and functioning of Qi lead to edema. Long-term edema results in insufficiency of the liver, spleen and kidney, weakness of the spleen in the function of transportation and transformation, inability of the kidney to separate the clear from the turbid, and gradual failure of the whole body to perform its Qi function.

6.2. [bian zheng lun zhi] 辩症论治"Differentiation and Treatment"

There are three types of chronic nephritis according to the clinical features.1) Common type: the course of this type is persistent. 2) Nephrotic type and 3) Hypertensive type.

6.2.1. [pi shen yang xu] 脾肾阳虚 "Deficiency of Kidney-Yin and Kidney-Yang"

(1) **[zhu zheng] 主症**"Symptoms":

Pale complexion, lassitude, listlessness, aversion to cold, cold limbs, high-grade edema, abdominal distension, anorexia, soreness of the waist, oliguria, thin and whitish coating of the tongue, deep and fine pulse.

(2) **[zhi fa]** 治法"Therapeutic Method":

Warming Yang of the spleen and kidney to promote diuresis.

(3) **[chu fang]** 处方"Prescription":

[shi pi yin] 实脾饮"Decoction for reinforcing the Spleen"

Ingredients:

[huang qi] 黄芪Radix Astragali	15g
[dang sheng] 党生Radix Codonopsis Pilosulae	15g
[bai shu] 白术Rhizoma Atractylodis Macrocephalae	15g
[fu zi] 附子Radix Aconiti	15g
[rou gui] 肉桂Cortex Cinnamomi	6g
[da fu pi] 大腹皮Pericarpium Arecae	12g
[ze xie] 泽泻Rhizoma Alismatis	10g
[che qian zi] 车前子Semen Plantaginis	30g
(decocted after being wrapped in a piece of cloth)	

Decocted in water for oral use, 1 dose daily.

(4) **[jia jian]**加减"Modification":

If the edema is mild but persistent, it suggests the deficiency of spleen-Qi. The treatment should be aimed at replenishing Qi and invigorating the spleen to induce diuresis. **[fang yi huang qi tang jia jian]** 防已黄芪汤加减 "Modified Tetrandra and Astragalus Decoction"

Ingredients:

[fang yi] 防已Radix Stephiae	10g
[huang qi] 黄芪Radix Astragali	15g
[bai shu] 白术Rhizoma Atractylodis Macrocephalae	15g
[dang sheng] 党生Radix Codonopsis Pilosulae	15g
[fu ling] 茯苓Poria	15g
[zhu ling] 猪苓Polyporus Umbrellatus	12g
[ze xie] 泽泻Rhizoma Alismatis	12g
[chen pi] 陈皮Pericarpium Citri Reticulatae	10g
[zhi gan cao] 炙甘草Radix Glycyrrhizae Praeparata	3g

Decocted in water for oral use, I dose daily.

6.2.2. [yin xu yang kang] 阴虚阳亢 "Hyperactivity of Yang due to Deficiency of Yin"

(1) **[zhu zheng]** 主症"Symptoms":

Indistinct edema, headache, dizziness, tinnitus, dry mouth, irritability, feverish sensation in the palms and soles, palpitation, insomnia, red tongue, taut and ready pulse.

(2) **[zhi fa]** 治法"Therapeutic Method":

Nourishing Yin and suppressing hyperactive Yang.

(3) **[chu fang]** 处方"Prescription":

[qi ju di huang wan] 杞菊地黄丸 "Bolus of Six Drugs with Wolfberry, Chrysanthemum and Rehmannia in"

Ingredients:

[sheng di] 生地Radix Rehmanniae	15g
[shan yao] 山药Rhizoma Dioscoreae	12g
[shan yu rou] 山萸肉Fructus Corni	9g
[dan pi] 单皮Cortex Moputan	9g
[ze xie] 泽泻Rhizoma Alismatis	9g
[gou qi] 枸杞Fructus Lycii	15g
[fu ling] 茯苓Poria	9g
[ju hua] 菊花Flos Chrysanthemi	12g

Decocted in water for oral use, 1 dose daily.

(4) **[jia jian]** 加减"Modification":

In case of severe emission, the drugs added are **[jin ying zi]** 金樱子Fructus Rosae Laevigatae 9g, **[qian shi]** 芡实Semen Euryalae 12g.

6.2.3. [shi re ne wen] 湿热内 "Retention of damp-heat in the Body"

(1) **[zhu zheng]** 主症"Symptoms":

Flushed face, obesity, edema, distention of head, headache, dry mouth, irritability, constipation, heaviness of the body, lassitude, thin and yellowish or yellowish and greasy coating of the tongue, taut and rapid or slippery and rapid pulse.

(2) **[zhi fa]** 治法"Therapeutic Method":

Clearing away pathogenic heat and dampness.

(3) **[chu fang]** 处方"Prescription":

[long dan xie gan tang jia jian] 龙胆泻肝汤加减 "Modified Decoction of Gentian for purging Liver Fire"

Ingredients:

[long dan cao] 龙胆草Radix Gentianae	10g
[huang qi] 黄芪Radix Astragali	10g
[zhi zi] 栀子Fructus Gardeniae	10g
[mu tong] 木通Caulis Clematidis Armandii	10g

[ze xie] 泽泻Rhizoma Alismatis 10g
[che qian zi] 车前子Semen Plantaginis 10g
(decocted after being wrapped in a piece of cloth)
[sheng di] 生地Radix Rehmanniae 12g
[huang bai] 黄柏Cortex Phellodendri 10g
[pu gong ying] 蒲公英Herba Taraxaci 20g
[bai mao gen] 白茅根Rhizoma Imperatae 30g
Decocted in water for oral use, 1 dose daily.

7. [yang wei] 阳痿"Impotence"

Impotence refers to weakness of penis erecting during sexual intercourse, characterized by poor erecting or erection that lasts only for seconds. Impotence is a main symptom due to sexual neurasthenia or some other chromic diseases.

7.1. [bing yin bing ji] 病因病机"Aetiology and Pathogenesis"

Impotence is often the consequence of the deficiency of the essential Qi and decline of life gate fire due to over sexual indulgence or juvenile masturbation. Over consumption of Qi of the heart, spleen and kidney due to fear, fright or worry can also cause impotence. Internal damp-heat retention affecting the liver and kidney with looseness of penis accounts for another factor to cause impotence.

7.2. [bian zheng lun zhi] 辨症论治"Differentiation and Treatment"

7.2.1. [shen yang kui xu ming men huo shuai] 肾阳亏虚命门火衰 "Kidney-Yang Insufficiency and Life gate Fire Decline"

(1) **[zhu zheng]** 主症"Symptoms":

Poor erecting of penis or erection that lasts only for seconds, pallor complexion, cold limbs, dizziness, blurring of vision, poor spirit, soreness in the lumbar region and knee joints, frequent urination, pale tongue proper with white coating, and deep thready pulse. There will also be palpitation and insomnia if the impairment of heart and spleen involved.

(2) **[zhi fa]** 治法"Therapeutic Method":

Warming the kidney to invigorate Yang.

(3) **[chu fang]** 处方"Prescription":[zan yu dan] 赞育丹"Fertility-Promoting Pill" (from **[jing yue quan shu]** 景岳全书"Jing yue's Complete works" **[ming]** 明Ming Dynasty.

Ingredients:
[shu di] 熟地Rhizoma Rehmanniae Praeparata 240g
[bai shu] 白术Rhizoma Atractylodis Macrocephalae 240g
[gou qi] 枸杞Fructus Lycii 180g

[dang gui] 当归Radix Angelicae Sinensis	180g
[du zhong] 杜仲Cortex Eucommiae	120g
[shan zhu yu] 山茱萸Fructus Corni	120g
[xian mao] 仙茅Rhizoma Curculiginis	120g
[jiu zi] 韭子Semen Allii Tuberosi	120g
[ba ji rou] 巴戟肉Radix Morindae Officinalis	120g
[rou cong rong] 肉苁蓉Herba Cistanchis	120g
[yin yang huo] 淫羊藿Herba Epimedii	120g
[she chuang] 蛇床Frutus Cnidii	60g
[fu zi] 附子Radix Aconiti Praeparata	60g
[rou gui] 肉桂Cortex Cinnamomi	60g

Make pellets by mixing the mixture-powder of these drugs with honey, to be taken twice a day, 9 grams each time.

(4) **[jia jian]**加减"Modification":

In severe and completed cases with syndrome of Qi deficiency, the above recipe may be added with **[ren shen]** 人参 Radix Ginseng 60g, **[lu rong]** 鹿茸 Cornu Cervi Pantotritum 60g.

(5) **[zhen jiu zhi liao]** 针灸治疗"Treatment of Acupuncture"

Prescriptions:

The 1st group-:

[ming men] 命门"Mingmen" (DU)
[shen shu] 肾俞"Shenshu" (BL)
[shang laio] 上髎 "Shangliao" (BL)

The 2nd group:

[guan yuan] 关元"Gyanyuan" (RN)
[da he] 赫 "Dahe" (KI)
[san yin jiao] 三阴交"Sanyinjiao" (ST}

Perpendicularly needle Mingmen (Du), Shenshu (BL) and Shanglao (BL) with the twisting and reducing method and retain the needles; by warming the handle of the needles with two cones of moxa, moxibustion is administered. The treatment is given once a day or every other day. A course of the treatment consists of 15 times. During the treatment the patient should refrain from sexual activity and relax as much as possible.

7.2.2. [shi re xia zhu] 湿热下注"Downward flow of Damp-heat"

(1) **[zhu zheng]** 主症"Symptoms":

The chief manifestation includes inability of the penis to erect and wet scrotum with foul smell. It can be accompanied by bitter taste in the mouth, thirst, short scanty urine, soreness in the lower limbs, greasy tongue coating, and rapid pulse.

(2) **[zhi fa]** 治法"Therapeutic Method":

Clearing away heat and promoting diuresis.

(3) **[chu fang]** 处方"Prescription":

[long dan xie gan tang] 龙胆泻肝汤"Decoction of Gentian for purging Liver-Fire" (from the **[yi zong jin jian]** 医宗金鉴 "The Golden Mirror of Medicine")

Ingredients:

[long dan cao] 龙胆草Radix Gentianae	9g
[huang qin] 芩Radix Scutellariae	6g
[shan zhi] 山栀Fructus Cardeniae	6g
[ze xie] 泽泻Rhizoma Alismatis	6g
[mu tong] 木通Caulis Clematidis Armandii	10g
[che qian zi] 车前子Semen Plantaginis	9g
(decocted after being wrapped in a piece of cloth)	
[dang gui] 当归Radix Angelicae Sinensis	3g
[chai hu] 柴胡Radix Bupleuri	6g
[sheng di] 生地Radix Rehmanniae	6g
[gan cao] 甘草Radix Glycyrrhizae	3g

Decocted in water for oral use, 1dose daily.

(4) **[jia jian]**加减"Modification":

When the damp-heat gets alleviated, change to using **[zhi bai di huang wan]** 枝柏地黄丸"Pill of Anemarrhena, Phyllodendron and Rehmannia"

Ingredients:

[zhi mu] 知母Rhizoma Anemarrhenae	9 portions
[huang bai] 黄柏Cortex Phellodendri	6 portions
[shu di] 熟地Rhizoma Rehmanniae Praeparata	24 portions
[shan yu rou] 山萸肉Fructus Corni	12 portions
[chao shan yao] 炒山药Rhizoma Dioscoreae Praeparata	12 portions
[ze xie] 泽泻Rhizoma Alismatis	9 portions
[fu ling] 茯苓Poria	9 portions
[dan pi] 丹皮Cortex Moutan Radicis	9 portions

Make pellets by mixing the powder of these drugs in the above propotion with honey, to be taken with warm boiled water or light salt water, twice a day, 6-9 grams each time.

(4) **[jia jian]** 加减"Modification":

For cases with stagnation of liver-Qi caused by emotions, depression, the principle of soothing the liver and regulating the circulation of Qi should be followed in its treatment. **[xiao yao san]** 逍遥散(from **[he ji ju fang]** 和剂局方 "Formularies of the Bureau of the People's Welfare pharmacies")

Ingredients:

[chai hu] 柴胡Radix Bupleuri	9g
[dang gui] 当归Radix Angelicae Sinensis	9g
[bai shao] 白芍Radix Angelicae Sinensis	9g
[bai shu] 白术Rhizoma Atractylodis Macrocephalae	9g
[fu ling] 茯苓Poria	12g
[zhi gan coa] 炙甘草Radix Glycyrrhizae Praeparata	5g
[bo he] 薄荷Herba Menthae	2g
[wei jiang] 煨姜Rhizoma Zingiberis Recens Praeparata	2 slices
[wu gong] 蜈蚣Scolopendra	1pc.

Decocted in water for oral use, 1 dose daily.

(5) **[zhen jiu zhi liao]** 针灸治疗"Treatment of Acupuncture"
Prescriptions:
[zhong ji] 中极"Zhongji" (RN)
[yin ling quan] 阴灵泉"Yinglinquan" (SP)
[san yin jiao] 三阴交"Sanyinjio"(SP)
[nei ting] 内庭"Neiting" (ST)

First needle Zhongji (RN) with the reducing method by lifting and thrusting for half a minute and retained until Qi spreads. Then needle Yinlingquan (SP), Sanyinjiao (SP), Neiting (ST) with the twisting and reducing method for half a minute and retained for 20 minutes. The treatment is given once a day. A course of the treatment consists of 12 times. If the disease is accompanied with spleen, stomach, Qi and blood deficiency, add some points such as **[pi shu]** 脾俞"Pishu" (BL), **[zu san li]** 足三里"Zusanli" (ST) with the twisting and reinforcing method for half a minute, and moxibustion is adopted by warming the handle of the needles with moxa-stick for 15 minutes.

8. [yi jing] 遗精"Emission"

Seminal emission refers to the involuntary seminal discharge that takes place often apart from sexual intercourse. Specially, nocturnal emission happens during dreams in sleep while spermatorrhea happens when the patient has no dreams. However, occasional seminal emission in adult males, married or unmarried, is not considered as disease condition.

8.1. [bing yin bing ji] 病因病机"Aetiology and Pathogenesis"

Nocturnal emission in dreams is mainly due to overstrain or stress, or excessive sexual indulgence that leads to flaring up of heart fire that does not descend to control the kidney water while the kidney water can not ascend to cool the heart fire, thus appearing the disharmony between heart and kidney. The hyperactive heart fire disturbs the sperms, causing nocturnal emission in dreams. Also functional impairment of the spleen and stomach due to over eating of sweat, greasy, fatty or pungent food can cause damp-heat accumulation in the middle-jiao. The downward flowing of such a damp-heat can induce dreams and disturb the sperm, resulting in nocturnal emission. Spermatorrhea is often due to damage of the kidney after prolonged illness, over indulgence in sex or habitual masturbation. Exhausted kidney essence due to stubborn nocturnal emission causes the deficiency of kidney Qi, which fails to consolidate sperm. The kidney cannot store sperm because the spermatic gate is not firm.

8.2. [bian zheng lun zhi] 辩症论治 "Differentiation and Treatment"

(1) **[zhu zheng]** 主症 "Symptoms":

1) **[meng yi]** 梦遗 "Nocturnal Emission"

This kind of seminal emission takes place at night when the sleep is not profound. There can be several emission a night or one emissions every several nights with dreaming of penis erecting or with premature ejaculation. The accompanying symptoms and signs include dizziness, vertigo, restlessness, poor sleep, lumbar soreness, tinnitus, lassitude, poor spirit, yellow urine, red tongue, and thready rapid pulse.

(2) **[zhi fa]** 治法 "Therapeutic Method":

Nourishing the kidney-Yin and clearing away heart-fire.

(3) **[chu fang]** 处方 "Prescription":

[san cai feng sui dan] 三才封髓丹 "Essence-preserving Pill" (from **[wei sheng bao jian]** 卫生宝鉴 "The Precious Mirror of Hygiene").

Ingredients:

[tain dong] 天冬 Radix Asparagi	150g
[shu di huang] 熟地黄 Radix Rehmenniae Praeparata	150g
[dang shen] 党参 Radix Codonopsis Pilosulae	150g
[huang bai] 黄柏 Cortex Phellodendri	90g
[sha ren] 砂仁 Fructus Amomi	45g
[zhi gan cao] 炙甘草 Radix Glycyrrhizae Praeparata	23g
[huang lian] 黄连 Rhizoma Coptidis	60g
[long gu] 龙骨 Os Draconis	150g
[mu li] 牡蛎 Concha Ostreae	150g
[chao zao ren] 炒枣仁 Semen Ziziphi Spinosae Praeparata	150g

Make pellets by mixing the powder of the drugs with starch paste or honey, to be taken with decoction of 15 g. Of **[rou cong rong]** 肉从蓉 Desert living Cistanche or herba Cistanchis twice a day, 9 g. each time. Or decoct one tenth of each of the above-mentioned herbal medicines in water for oral use, 1 dose daily.

(5) **[zhen jiu zhi liao]** 针灸治疗 "Treatment of Acupuncture"

Prescriptions:

The 1st group- **[xin shu]** 心俞 "Xinshu"(BL)

[shen shu] 肾俞"Shenshu"(BL)
[zhi shi] 志室"zhishi" (BL)
[tai xi] 太 "Taixi"(KI)
The 2nd group-**[guan yuan]** 关元"Guanyuan"(RN)
[da he] 大赫"Tahe"(KI)
[shen men] 神门"Shenmen"(HT)
[tai xi] 太 "Taixi"(KI)

These two groups of points can be alternately punctured to clear the heart fire, invigorate the kidney and stop emission.

Slightly needle Xinshu (BL) towards spinal column with the twisting and reducing method for one minute and withdraw. Zhizhi (BL), Shenshu (BL) and Taixi (KI) are perpendicularly needle with the twisting and reducing method by lifting and thrusting, the needles are retained for 20 minutes. The treatment is given once a day or every other day. Acourse of the treatment consists of 8 times.

8.3. [hua jing] 滑精 "Spermatorrhea"

This kind of emission may happen without any dreams at any time during the day or the night. There may be emission on sexual thoughts in severe cases. The accompanying symptoms and signs include emaciation, pallor complexion, soreness and cold sensation in the lumbar region, pale tongue with white coating, and deep thready pulse.

(2) **[zhi fa]** 治法"Therapeutic Method":

Tonifying the kidney-Qi to arrest spontaneous emission.

(3) **[chu fang]** 处方"Prescription": **[jiu suo gu jing wan]** 金锁固精丸"Golden Lock Pill for keeping the Kidney Essence"(from **[yi fang ji jie]** 医方集解 "A Collection of Prescriptions with Notes")

Ingredients:

[qian shi] 芡实Semen Euryaleae	90g
[tong ji li] 潼蒺藜Semen Astragali Complanati	90g
[lian xu] 莲须Stamen Nelumbinis	90g
[long gu] 骨Os Draconis	30g
[mu li] 牡蛎 Concha Ostreae	30g
[jin ying zi] 金樱子Fructus Rosae Laevigatae	60g
[huai shan yao] 淮山药Fructus Dioscoreae	90g
[tu si zi] 菟丝子Semen Cuscutae	90g

All the above herbal medicines are pulverised first and , then prepared into pills with the addition of **[lain rou fen]** 莲肉粉 "Semen Nelumbinis" powder. 9 g of pills are taken with lightly salty water each time, twice a day.

(4) **[jia jian]** 加减"Modification":

In case of symptoms with coldness of genitals and impotence, the drugs added are **[suo yang]** 锁阳 Herba Cynomorii 60g, **[jiu zi]** 韭子 Semen Allii Tuberosi 60g, **[lu jiao shuang]** 鹿角霜 Cornu Cervi Degelatinatum 60g for the purpose of warming and recuperating Kidney-Yang.

(5) **[zhen jiu zhi liao]** 针灸治疗 "Treatment of Acupuncture"
Prescriptions:
The 1st group-**[ming men]** 命门 "Mingmen" (DU),
[yao yang guan] 腰阳关 "Yaoyangguan" (DU), combined with
[shen shu] 肾俞 "Shenshu"(BL)
[zhi shi] 志室 "Zhishi" (BL)
[tai xi] 太 "Taixi" (KI)
The 2nd group-**[qi hai]** 气海 "Qihai" (RN)
[san yin jiao] 三阴交 "Shayinjiao" (SP)
[guan yuan] 关元 "Guanyuan" (RN)
[da he] 大赫 "Dahe" (KI)
[tai xi] 太 "Taixi" (KI)

These two groups of points can be alternately punctured to invigorate the kidney and stop emission.

Shenshu (BL), Yaoyangguan (DU) and Taixi (KI) are perpendicularly punctured with the twisting and reinforcing method by lifting and thrusting for half a minute, and the needles are retained. Moxibustion is taken to Mingmen (DU) and Zhishi (BL) with moxa-stick for about 20 minutes. The treatment is given once a day or every other day. A course of the treatment consists of 10 times. Exhort the patient to relieve stress, give up reading pornographic books, stop masturbation and sexual life. It is necessary to give up smoking and drinking liquor and coffee.

Chapter Six

External Treatment and the others

1. [wai zhi fa] 外 治 法 "External Treatment"

The methods to treat various diseases and symptoms consist of other than oral use of drugs. It is the application of drugs and manipulations (even together) with proper instruments on the body surface, such as acupuncture, plaster, stem bath, massage etc.

2. [fu yao fa] 敷 药 法 "Topical Application of Drugs"

Fresh medicinal herbs are smashed or dried drugs ground into fine powders and made into a paste with wine, honey, vinegar, etc, which are applied over the affected parts and changed periodically, so as for maintain their effectiveness for a comparatively long time. It is applicable to local infections, ulcers, swellings, pains and injuries.

3. [yan fa] 罨 法 "Compress"

It includes hot compress and cold compress. 1) The hot compress: a towel (or clean cloth) twisted dry after soaking in hot water is applied to the painful part. It may relieve pain. 2) The cold compress: a towel (or clean cloth) after soaking in cold water is applied to the head, nose, etc. It may relieve pain and stop bleeding.

4. [yun fa] 熨 法 "Ironing"

Topical application of heated drugs; drug powders or granules are heated and packed in a cloth by gauze over the affected part, applicable to the painful disorders of cold type.

5. [xun zheng fa] 熏 蒸 法 "Fuming and Steaming"

To treat certain skin diseases, pain and immobility of the joints or swelling by making use of the smoke produced by burning drugs, or steam produced by boiling the drugs with water.

6. [xi ru fa] 吸 入 法 "Inhalation"

To treat diseases by inhaling smoke or steam produced by a drug, e.g., cough caused by chronic bronchitis may be treated by smoking certain drugs, or postpartum haemorrhagic shock may be treated by inhaling the stem produced by putting a piece of burning iron into vinegar, so as for revive unconsciousness.

7. [re hong] 热 烘 "Warming by Fire"

The affected parts of the body are painted with drugs and toasted with heat, a treatment particularly applicable to certain skin diseases.

8. [luo fa] 烙 法 "Cauterization"

to cauterize the affected part with certain red-hot iron apparatus, so as for get rid of the putrid parts.

9. [ta yu] 溻 浴 "Herbal Decoction Bath"

A treatment by using the decocted juice of drugs to bathe the body. It may be used for skin diseases, measles, urticaria, and arthritis, etc.

10. [fa pao] 发 泡 "Vesiculating"

Irritative drugs are smashed or ground and applied on the skin to raise vesicles.

11. [fa pao jiu] 发 泡 灸 "Vesiculation Moxibustion"

A therapy by applying irritant drugs to acu-point or directly cauterizing the skin over an acu-point with moxa cone to produce vesiculation.

12. [chui yao] 吹 药 "Insufflations of Medicinal Powder"

To blow the fine-drug-powders mechanically into the mouth and throat with an insufflator or a tube for the treatment of oral and throat diseases.

13. [pu fen] 扑 粉 "Powder Spreading"

The fine powders of drugs are spread over the skin for the treatment of persistent sweating in febrile diseases, hyperhydrosis and itching.

14. [dao fa] 导 法 "Moving the Bowels by topical Applications of drugs"

A treatment for constipation by introducing a solution of drugs or inserting a suppository made of some lubricant into the rectum.

15. [mi jian dao fa] 蜜 煎 导 法 "Honey Suppository"

One of enema and supositories. The honey is heated and concentrated. While warm, it is made into a small suppository, 6 cm. long like the little finger in diameter, and then inserted into the rectum for lubricating the bowel and inducing defecation.

16. [zhu dan zhi dao] 猪 胆 汁 导 "Pig-bile Enema"

One of enemas and supositories. The pig-bile is mixed thoroughly with a small amount of vinegar and then injected into the rectum for the treatment of constipation due to the serious heat-syndrome in the interior.

17. [sai fa] 塞 法 "Plug-in Method"

The dry powder (or suppository) packed into cotton or gauze as a plug for the diseases of the nose, vagina and rectum.

18. [gua xian fa] 挂 线 法 "Thread-drawing therapy"

One of the therapies for anal fistula. Under local anesthesia, a silver probe is inserted into the external opening of the anal fistula and into the rectum through its internal opening under the guidance of the left index finger in the anal canal by inserting a medicated thread into the fistula and tightening to block the blood flowing, Drugs are applied locally on the wound and changed periodically until the wounds healed. Its principle is to block Qi and blood and to erode the muscle for the purpose of promoting tissue necrosis and expose the fistula.

19. [ku zhi fa] 枯 痔 法 "Necrotizing therapy for haemorrhoids"

A method to apply drugs of necrotization locally on the haemorrhoid to rend it dry and necrotic, and dropping finally.

20. [jie zha fa] 结 扎 法 "Ligation Method"

A treatment for haemorrhoid, nevus, etc. by ligating a certain part of a superficial mass tightly to block the blood movement and to cause it necrotizing and dropping.

21. [yao xiang yin liu] 药 线 引 流 "Drainage with Medicated Strip"

Medicated strands of mulberry paper or silk wool socked with oil and impregnated with medication are inserted into the abscess cavity to facilitate the drainage of pus, especially for the treatment of fistula by removing the necrotic parts, drain the pus and promoting granulation.

22. [yao tong ba fa] 药 筒 拔 法 "Drainage by Medicated Cupping"

A treatment for drainage of pus or snake venom by local application of hot cupping with bamboo cup soaked in the boiled medicinal decoction.

23. [gu wei yao] 箍 围 药 "Encircling the lesion with Drugs"

At the early stage of a suppurative infection, a drug paste is applied around the affected area, so as for localize the infection and prevent it from spreading, and also to hasten suppuration and rupture of the abscess.

24. [chan yao] 掺 药 "Topical Application of Medicinal Powder"

A kind of external application of drugs for subsidence of swelling, pus drainage, clearing of necrotic parts, promotion of granulation, analgesia, hemostasis, etc., by scattering the medicinal powder directly on the lesion or dusting it onto a medicated plaster and applying the plaster on the abscess or ulcer.

25. [jiu fa] 灸 法 "Moxibustion Therapy"

A therapeutic method of applying heat produced by ignited moxa wool or roll over the skin surface. There are different kinds of moxibustion, e.g. moxibustion with moxa stick, pecking moxibustion with moxa stick, moxibustion with ignited moxa cone, direct moxibution, scar-drying moxibution, etc.

26. [ba huo guan] 拔 火 罐 "Cupping Therapy"

A treatment inducing local congestion by placing a heated cup or jar or glass (usually by fire) on to the affected or any part of the body surface for treating purpose.

27. [xue wei zhu she liao fa] 穴 位 注 射 疗 法 "Point Injection Therapy" "Hydro-acupuncture"

A therapy by which liquid medicine is injected into the point to obtain therapeutic results by needling stimulation and pharmaceutical reaction. This method is mostly used in treating asthma, neurosis, gastralgia, facial paralysis vomiting and sciatica.

28. [xue wei feng bi] 穴 位 封 闭 "Point-blocking Therapy"

A therapy with injection of anaesthetic and analgesic into the acu-points for treating pains of various kinds.

29. [zhen ci ma zui] 针 刺 麻 醉 "Acupuncture Anaesthesia"

An anaesthetic method developed on the basis of acupuncture analgesia. It is performed by inserting the filiform needle into the selected points and inducing analgesic effect by needle manipulation to cause relaxation of muscles and surgical operation may be carried out while the patient is perfectly conscious.

30 [zhen fa] 针 法 "Acupuncture Therapy"

A therapy by applying metal needles such as filiform needle, three edged needle, intradermal needle and plum-blossom needle to stimulate certain superficial parts for the treatment of diseases.

31. [mai xian liao fa] 埋 线 疗 法 “Thread Imbedding Therapy"

A form of acutherapy in which catgut is imbedded in the point to bring prolonged constant stimulation for treating purpose. Indications are gastric and duodenal ulcer, asthma, pain in the loins and the back, etc.

32. [ci zhu liao fa] 磁 珠 疗 法 "Magnetic Bead Therapy"

A form of acutherapy in which magnetized steel beads taped to the points are used as substitutes for needles and left in place for prolonged stimulation, indicated in treating chronic diseases.

33. [zhi ya liao fa] 指 压 疗 法 "Finger-pressure Therapy"

A therapy performed by pressing and rubbing a given point with finger(s) for treating purpose. Indications are syncope, hysteria, epilepsy, toothache, etc.

34. [ti zhen liao fa] 体 针 疗 法 "Body Acupuncture"

A kind of acupuncture treatment generally referring to the acupuncture of the human body by puncturing the points along the channels, such as scalp-acupuncture, ear-acupuncture therapy, nose-acupuncture therapy, foot-acupuncture therapy, etc.

Chapter Seven

[cao yao] 草药"Herbal Medicine"

Of 5.767 currently described drugs in Chinese, fewer than 10 percent are commonly used. Most of these common used drugs are briefly described here. The drugs are listed alphabetically by their Latin names, or English names where more appropriate and Chinese pronunciation and names. Each entry is organized as follows: Chinese pronunciation/ Chinese names/ English Name/Latin

P: (Part used) **[bu wei]** 部位
T&N: (taste and nature) **[xing wei]** 性味(whether or not poisonous)
Act: (actions) **[gong neng]** 功能
Indi: (Indications) **[zhu zhi]** 主治
U&D: (Usage and dosage) **[yong fa yong liang]** 用法用量
C&C: (cautions and contraindications) **[xiao xin chen yong]** 小心慎用

The number in each of the drug shows the frequency of the medicine to be used 400 recipes of treating the diseases of urology, andrology and sexology. The most frequently used medicines are as follows:

[bai bian dou] 白扁豆White Hyacinth Bean (Semen Lablab Album) 8 times
[bai mao gen] 白茅根Lalang Grass Rhizome (Rhizoma Imperatae Tauntonii) 8 times
[bai shao] 白芍White Peony Root (Radix Paeoniae Albae) 45 times
[bai zhu] 白术Large head Atractylodes Rhizome (Rhizoma Atractylodes Macrocephalae) 48 times
[bai zi ren] 柏子仁Chinese Arborvitae Ker nel (Semen Platycladi) 15 times
[ba ji tian] 巴戟天Morinda Root (Radix Morindae Officinlis) 16 times
[ban xia] 半夏Pinellia Tuber (Rhizoma Pinelliae) 28 times
[bing lang] 槟榔Areca Seed (Semen Arecae) 8 times
[bo he] 薄荷Peppermint (Herba Menthae) 12 times
[bu gu zi] 补骨脂Malayter Scurpha Fruit (Fructus Psoraleae) 7 times
[cang zhu] 苍术Atractylodes Rhizome (Rhizoma Atractylodis) 16 times
[chai hu] 柴胡Chinese Thorowax Root (Radix Bupleuri) 34 times
[chan tui] 蝉蜕Cicada slough (Periostracum Serpentis) 8 times
[chen pi] 陈皮Dried Tangerine peel (Pericarpiun Citri Reticulatae) 45 times
[chen xiang] 沉香Chinese Eagewood Wood (Ligum Aquilariae Resinatum) 7 times
[chen qian zi] 车前子Plantian Seed (Semen Plantginis) 23 times
[chi shao] 少Red Peony Root (Radix Paeoniae Rubrae) 34 times
[chuan lian zi] 川楝子Szechwan Chinaberry Fruit (Fructus Toosendan) 14 times

[chuan mu tong] 川木通Sichuan Clematis Stem (Caulis Clematidis Armandii) also **[guan mu tong]** 广木通Manshuian Stem (Caulis Aristolochiae Manshuriensis) 20 times

[chuan shan jia] 穿山甲Pangolin Scale (Squama Manitis) 10 times

[chuan xiong] 川芎Szechwan Lovage（ Rhizoma Chuanxiong ）26 times

[da huang] 大黄Radix Rhei Rhubarb (Radix et Rhizoma Rhei) 35 times

[dang gui] 当归Chinese Angelica (Radix Angelicae Sinensis) 85 times

[dang shen] 党参Tangshen (Radix Codonopsis) 8 times

[dang shen] 党参Danshen Root (Radix Salviae Miltiorrhizae) 15 times

[di huang] 地黄Rehmannia Root （ Radix Rehmanniae ）45 times

[da zao] 大枣Chinese Date (Fructus Jujubae) 26 times

[di long] 地龙Ground Dragon（ Pheretima ）7 times

[du huo] 独活Deubleteeth Pubescent Angelica Root （ Radix Angelicae Pubescentis ）8 times

[du zhong] 杜仲Eucommia Bark (Cortex Eucommiae) 15 times

[fang feng] 防风Divaricate Saposhnikoviae Root (Radix Saposhnikoviae) 16 times

[feng mi] 蜂蜜Honey (Mel) 8 times

[fu ling] 茯苓Indian Bread (Proi) 90 times

[fu shen] 茯神Fu-shen (Poria cum Radice Pini) 10 times

[fu pen zi] 覆盆子Palm leaf Raspberry Fruit (Fructus Rubi) 7 times

[fu zi] 附子Prepared Common Monkshood Daughter Root

[shu fu zi] 熟附子Radix Aconiti Praeparata (Radix Aconiti Lateralis Praeparata) 30 times

[gan cao] 甘草Liquorice Root（ Radix Glycyrrhizae ）18 times

[gan jiang] 干姜Zingiber (processed) (Rhizoma Zingiberis) 24 times

[ge jie] 蛤蚧Tokay (Gecko) 6 times

[gou gu ye] 枸骨叶Chinese Holly Leaf (Folium Ilicis Cornutae) 8 times

[gou qi] 枸杞Cibot Rhizome (Rhizoma Cibotii) 16 times

[gou qi zi] 枸杞子Barbary Wolfberry Fruit (Fructus Lycii) 16 times

[gou teng] 钩藤Gambir Olant (Ramulus Uncariae cum Uncis) 9 times

[guan mu tong] 关木通 Manchurian Dutchmanspipe Stem（ Caulis Aristolochiae Manshuriensis) also **[chuan mu tong]** 川木通Sichuan Clematis Stem (Caulis Clematidis Armandii) 20 times

[gui jia] 甲(龟板Tortoise Shell Carapace et plastrum Testudinis 14 times

[gui zhi] 桂枝Cassia Twing (Ramulus Cinnamomi) 22 times

[he shou wu] 何首乌Fleeceflower Root（ Radix Polygoni Multiflori ）8 times

[hong hua] 红花Safflower (Flos Carthami) 10 times

[hou po] 厚朴Officinal Magnolia Bark (Cortex Magnoliae Officinalis) 22 times

[huang bo] 黄柏Amur Cork-tree (Cortex Phellodendri) 28 times

[huang lian] 黄莲Golden Thread (Rhizoma Coptidis) 26 times

[huangh qi] 黄芪Milkvetch Root (Radix Astragali) 36 times

[huang qin] 黄芩Baical Skullcap Root (Radix Scutellariae) 40 times

[hua shi] 滑石Talc (Talcum) 15 times

[jie zi] 芥子Mustard Seed (Semen Sinapis) 6 times

[jing jie] 荆芥Fineleaf Schizonepeta Herb (Herba Schizonepetaeis) 10 times
[jin yin hua] 金银花Honeysuckle Flower (Flos Lonicerae) 18 times
[ku xing ren] 苦杏仁Bitter Apricot Seed (Semen Armeniacae Amarum) 15 times
[lian qiao] 连翘Weeping Forsythia Capsule (Fructus Forsythiae) 17 times
[long dan] 龙胆Chinese Gentian (Radix Gentianae) 8 times
[long yan rou] 龙眼肉Longgra Aril (Arillus Longan) 6 times
[mo yao] 没药 Myrrh (Resina Myrrhae) 8 times
[mu dan pi] 牡丹皮Tree Peony Bark (Cortex Moutan) 9 times
[mu li] 牡蛎Oyster Shell (Concha Ostreae) 8 time
[mu xiang] 木香Costusroot (Radix Aucklandiae) 18 times
[niu bang zi] 牛蒡子Great Burdock Achene (Fructus Arctii) 9 times
[niu xi] 牛膝Twotooth Achyranthea Root (Radix Achyranthis Bidentatae) 10 times
[pu gong ying] 蒲公英Dandelion (Herba Taraxaci) 7 times
[qian hu] 前胡Hogfennel Root (Radix Peucedani) 7 times
[qian shi] 芡实Gordon Euryale Seed (Semen Euryales) 8 times
[rou gui] 肉桂Cassia Bark (Cortex Cinnamomi) 35 times
[shan yao] 山药Common Yam Rhizome (Rhizoma Dioscoreae) 24 times
[rou cong rong] 肉苁蓉 Desertliving Cistanche (Herba Cistanches) 16 times
[shan zhu yu] 山茱萸Asiatic Cornelian Cherry Fruit (Fructus Corni) 30 times
[she chuang zi] 蛇床子Common Cnidium Fruit (Fructus Cnidii) 10 times
[she xiang] 麝香Musk (Moschus) 10 times
[shi chang pu] 石菖蒲Grassleaf sweetflag Rhizome (Rhizoma Acori Tatarinow) 12 times
[shi gao] 石膏Gypsum (Gypsum Fibrosum) 16 times
[shi jue ming] 石决明Sea-ear Shell (Concha Haliotidis) 7 times
[suan zao ren] 酸枣仁Spine Date Seed (Semen Ziziphi Spinosae) 15 times
[tao ren] 桃仁Peach Seed (Semen Persicae) 19 times
[tian dong] [tian dong] 天冬 also **[tian men dong]** 天门冬Chinese Asparagus Root (Radix Asparagi) 10 times
[tu si zi] 菟丝子Dodder Seed (Semen Cuscutae) 22 times
[wu bei zi] 五倍子Chinese Gall (Galla Chinensis) 9 times
[wu wei zi] 五味子Chinese Magnoliavine Fruit (Fructus Schisandraeis) 30 times
[wu zhu yu] 吴茱萸Medicinal Evodia Fruit (Fructus Evodiae) 8 times
[xiang fu] 香附Nutgrass Galingale Rhizome (Rhizoma Cyperi) 9 times
[xian mao] 仙茅 Common Curculigo Rhizome (Rhizoma Curculiginis) 7 times
[xiao hui xiang] 小茴香Fennel (Fructuas Foeniculi) 9 times
[xiao ji] 小蓟 Field Thistle Herb (Herba Cirsii) 7 times
[xi xin] 细辛Manchurian Wildginger (Herba Asari) 8 times
[xuan shen] 玄参Figwort Root (Radix Scrophulariae) 12
[yuan zhi] 远志Thinleaf Milkwort Root (Radix Polygalae) 16 times
[zao jiao ci] 皂角刺Chinese Honeylocust Spine (Semen Gleditsiae) 6 times
[ze xie] 泽泻Oriental waterplantain Rhizome (Rhizoma Alismatis) 25 times

[zhi gan cao] 炙甘草 Liquorice Root (processed with honey) (Radix Glycyrrhizae Praeparata) 65 times
[zhi qiao] Orange Fruit (Fructus Aurantii) 13 times
[zhi shi] 志室Immature Orange Fruit (Fructus Aurantii Immaturus) 17 times
[zhi zi] 栀子Cape Jasmine Fruit (Fructus Gardeniae) 28 times
[zhu ling] 猪苓Chuling (Polyporus) 17 times
[zhu sha] 砂 Cinnabar (Cinnabaris) 15 times

INDEX **PLANTS, VEGETABLES AND MINERALS**	**INDEX** **PLANTS, VEGETABLES AND MINERALS**
[ai ye] 艾叶 Argy Wormwood Leaf (Folium Artemisiae Aregyi) **P:** dried leaf of Artemisia Aregyi **T&N:** pungent and bitter in flavor, warm in property. **Act:** to dispel cold, relieve pain and arrest bleeding. Folium Artemisiae Aregyi (carbonized and processed with vinegar) to arrest excessive menstrual discharge. **Indi:** pain in the lower abdomen with cold sensation; menstrual disorders of cold type; infertility; spitting of blood, epistaxis, uterine bleeding in pregnancy, excessive menstrual flow; external use for itching; Folium Artemisiae (carbonized and processed with vinegar), excessive menstrual flow of deficiency-cold-type. **U&D:** 3--9g, appropriate quantity for moxibustion or fuming and washing. **[an xi xiang] 安息香 Benzoin (Benzoinum)** **P:** the dried resin collected from the trunk of Styrax tonkinensis **T&N:** pungent and bitter in flavour, neutral in property. **Act:** to restore consciousness , to activate	• **[ai shu]** 艾 属 absinthium = Artemisia absinthium/A. santonica/A. pontica = wormwood, dysuria, stranguria and anuria (+ sil + nardus gallicus + vinegar) • **[chang pu shu] 菖蒲属** acorum = Iris pseudacorus / Acorus calamus = yellow flag iris/sweet flag, dysuria, stranguria and anuria • **[mo gu shu] 蘑菇属[shan jun]** 伞菌 agaricum = Boletus igniarius / B. laricis / B. flavus / B. hepaticus = a tree fungus, affections and pains of the bladder, stones in the bladder • **[ze xie]** 泽泻 alcima = alisma = Alisma plantago = water-plantain, dysuria, stranguria and anuria • **[suan jiang shu] 酸浆属** alicacabum/halicacabum (see also fysalis), stones in the bladder • **[cong shu] 葱属 [suan] 蒜 allium** = Allium sativum = garlic, stones in the

the flow of Qi and blood, and to relieve pain. **Indi:** loss of consciousness in stroke and attack of noxious factors; syncope due to violent excitement or postpartum anemia; pain in the chest and epigastrium; infantile convulsion. **U&D:** 0.6--1.5g, mostly used in making pills or powder. **[an you] 桉油Aucalyptus oil (Oleum Eucalypti)** **P:** the volatile oil obtained by steam distillation from the plants of Eucalyptus globulus. **Indi:** skin irritant, used in neural pain. **[ba dou] 巴豆Croton Fruit (Fructus Crotonis)** **P:** the dried ripe fruit of Croton Tillium. **T&N:** pungent in flavour, hot in property. **Act:** to cause cauterization by external use. **Indi:** malignant ulcer, scabies, and wart. **U&D:** appropriate quantity to be ground into powder for topical application or gauze for rubbing onto the affected skin. **[ba dou shuang] 巴豆霜 Defatted Croton Seed Powder (Semen Crotonis Pulveratum)** **P:** the processed product of Croton seed. **T&N:** pungent in flavour, hot in property. **Act:** to cause drastic purgation, to relieve edema, and to soothe the throat. **Indi:** constipation, and indigestion due to accumulation of cold; ascits and edema with oilguria and constipation; inflammation of the throat. **U&D:** 0.1--0,3g; mostly used for making pills or powder. **C&C:** contraindication in pregnancy.	bladder • **[xi la ming fan] 希腊明矾** Allium gallicum = Allium (but wild), affections and pains of the kidneys (here probably also = Synphyton tuberosum), affections and pains of the kidneys • **[tain xian zi] 天仙子 [lang dang zi] 莨菪子** altercum = Hyoscyamus niger = henbane, affections and pains of the bladder, dysuria, stranguria and anuria • **[dou kou shu] 豆蔻属** amomum = the product of one or more of the usual cardamom substitutes, such as Amomum subulatum, A. Cardamomum, A. Krevanh, affections and pains of the kidneys, affections and pains of the bladder • **[shen jiu de wan] 盛酒的碗** amulum, affections and pains of the kidneys, affections and pains of the bladder • **[ku xing ren] 苦杏仁** Amygdala amara, affections and pains of the kidneys (for the "reniculi" = adrenal glands), affections and pains of the kidneys • **[ku xing ren] 苦杏仁** Amygdala = Prunus amygdalus = almond, affections and pains of the kidneys, affections and pains of the bladder, dysuria, stranguria and anuria • **[tian xing ren] 甜杏仁** Amygdala dulcis, affections and pains of the kidneys, affections and pains of the bladder, dysuria, stranguria and anuria, haematuria

Incompatible with Semen Pharbitidis.

[bai bian dou] 白扁豆 White Hyacinth Bean (Semen Lablab Album)

P: the dried rope seed of Dolichos Lablab.
T&N: sweet in flavour, warm slightly in property.
Act: to invigorate the spleen and remove damp, particularly the summer- damp.
Indi: weakness of the spleen and stomach with loss of appetite and loss bowls; excessive leukorrhea; vomiting, diarrhea, distress in the chest and distension in the abdomen caused by summer-damp. Semen Lablab Ablbum (stie- fried); diarrhea and excessive leukorrhea in deficiency syndromes of the spleen.
U&D: 9--15g

[bai bu] 百部 Stemona Root (Radix Stemonae)

P: the dried root tuber of Stemona sessilifolia.
T&N: sweet and bitter in flavour, slightly warm in property.
Act: to moisten the lung and relieve cough, and to kill insects and worms.
Indi: acute and chronic cough, cough in phthisis, whooping cough, external use: for pediculosis capitis, pediculosis corporis, oxyriasis, pudendal itching.
U&D: 3--9g for external use, appropriate quantity to be decocted with water or infused in wine.

[bai fan] 白矾 Alum (Alumen)

P: a processed mineral of sulfates of Alum stone containing mainly potassium aluminium sulfate.
T&N: sour and astringent in flavour, cold in property.

- **[xing ren zi] 杏仁子** amygdalarum nuclei, affections and pains of the bladder
- **[dian fen] 淀粉** Amylum, affections and pains of the kidneys, affections and pains of the bladder, dysuria, stranguria and anuria
- **[yang hui qin gen] 洋茴芹根** Anagallis caerulea = Anagallis arvensis caerulea = pimpernel, dysuria, stranguria and anuria
- **[yang hui qin] 洋茴芹** Anagallis rubens = Anagallis arvensis phoenicea = pimpernel, dysuria, stranguria and anuria
- **[san zao shu] 伞藻属** Androsaces = Acetabularia mediterranea = sea-navel, dysuria, stranguria and anuria
- **[hui xiang] 茴香** Anesum = Pimpinella anisum = anise, affections and pains of the kidneys, affections and pains of the bladder, stones in the kidney, stones in the bladder
- **[shi luo]** 莳萝 Anethum = Anethum graveolens = dill, affections and pains of the kidneys, stones in the bladder
- **[man bing hua shu] 芒柄花属** Ononis = Ononis antiquorum = rest-harrow, stones in the bladder
- **[huang ju] 黄菊 [luo ma gan ju]** 罗马甘菊 Anthemis = Matricaria chamomilla / Anthemis chia = wild chamomile, stones in the bladder
- **[xi la qi shu] 希腊漆树** Anthillium = Cressa cretica = Cretan pitch-plant,

Act: to counteract toxicity, to kill parasites, to arrest discharges, and to relieve itching by external use, to arrest bleeding, to relieve diarrhea, and to dispel wind-phlegm by internal administration Alumen (calcined) Eczema.
Indi: discharge from ulcer otitis media with purulent discharge; excessive leukorrhea with pudendal itching; bleeding from the nose or gums; nasal polyp.
U&D: for external use, appropriate quantity to be ground into powder for topical application or dissolved in water for washing; 0.5--1.5g for oral administration.

[bai guo] 白果 Ginkgo Seed (Semen Ginkgo)
P: the dried ripe seed of Ginkgo Biloba
T&N: sweet, bitter and astringent in flavour, neutral in property.
Act: to arrest persistent cough and asthma, and to reduce leukorrhea and urination.
Indi: persistent cough and asthma with profuse expectoration; morbid leukorrhea with whitish discharge; enuresis, frequent urination.
U&D: 4.5--9g
C&C: Raw Semen Ginlco is toxic.

[bai mao gen] 白茅根 Lalang Grass Rhizome (Rhizoma Imperatae Tauntonii)
P: the dried rhizome of Imperata Cylindrica.
T&N: sweet in flavour., cold in property.
Act: to arrest bleeding by reducing heat in blood, to remove heat, and to cause diuresis.
Indi: spitting of blood, epistaxis and haematuria due to heat in blood; febrile

affections and pains of the bladder

- **[qin cai zi] 芹菜子** Apii semen, affections and pains of the kidneys, affections and pains of the bladder, stones in the bladder, haematuria (for the so-called "reniculi" = adrenal glands)

- **[qin cai] 芹菜** apium = Apium graveolens (in some cases also Petroselinum sativum) = celery / parsley, affections and pains of the kidneys, affections and pains of the bladder, dysuria, stranguria and anuria, stones in the kidney, stones in the bladder.

[ia **jue lei zhi wu] 蕨类植物** Arction = Inula candida = bear wort, dysuria, stranguria and anuria

- **[ma dou ling] 马兜铃** Aristolochia = Aristolochia rotunda / longa / clematitis / cretica = birthwort, dysuria, stranguria and anuria, stones in the bladder

- **[hai yu shu] 海芋属** Aron = Arum dracunculus = adderwort, dysuria, stranguria and anuria

- **[ai hao shu] 艾蒿属** Artemisia = Artemisia vulgaris = mugwort, affections and pains of the kidneys, stones in the bladder

- **[ou zhou xi xing] 欧洲细辛** Asarum = Asarum europaeum = hazelwort, affections and pains of the kidneys, affections and pains of the bladder, stones in the bladder

- **[tain men dong shu] 天门冬属 [lu sun] 芦笋** Asparagus = Asparagus officinalis/acutifolius/tenuifolius/albus/

diseases with thirst; jaundice, urinary infection with difficult painful urination; edema in acute nephritis.
U&D: 9--30g or 30--60g of the fresh rhizome.

[bai tou weng] 白头翁 Chinese Pulsatilla Root (Radix Pulsatillae)
P: the dried root of Pulsatilla Chinensis.
T&N: bitter in flavour, cold in property.
Act: to remove toxic heat and relieve blooding dysentery.
Indi: amoebae dysentery; pudendal itching with excessive leukorrhea.
U&D: 9--15g

[bai wei] Blackend Swallow Wort Root (Radix Cynanchi Atrati)
P: the dried root and rhizome of Cynancum atratum.
T&N: bitter and salty in flavour, cold in property.
Act: to remove heat from blood, to relieve dysuria, and to counteract toxicity and cure sores.
Indi: febrile diseases with invasion of the pathogenic factors into the blood; fever due to deficiency of Yin; in phthisis, or due to deficiency of blood after delivery; acute urinary infection; dysuria with ematuria; carbuncles and other subcutaneous pathogenic infections.
U&D: 4.5--9g

[bai xian pi] 皮 Dense fruit Pittany Root-bark (Cortex Dictamni)
P: the dried root bark of Dictamnus dasycarpus.
T&N: bitter in flavour; cold in property.
Act: to remove damp-heat detoxicating and dispel wind.
Indi: skin inflammation with yellowish watery discharge; eczema rubella, tinea, scabies, acute rheumatic arthritis,

aphyllus/verticillatus (Gr.) asparagus, affections and pains of the kidneys, affections and pains of the bladder, stones in the bladder

- **[mu er shu] 木耳属** Auricula marina: v. Auricula murina

- **[fu di cai] 附地菜** Auricula murina: v. Myosota, dysuria, stranguria and anuria, stones in the bladder (but someone call it "marina"!)

- **[zhen shu] 榛属** Avellana, affections and pains of the kidneys, affections and pains of the bladder, dysuria, stranguria and anuria, haematuria

- **[zhang guo qin]** 胀果芹 Cachrys = the white seed contained in the stone of the crethmos, affections and pains of the bladder, dysuria, stranguria and anuria

- **[xin feng lun shu] 新风轮属年 [jing jie shu]** 荆芥属 Calaminthe (sometimes = nepeta), stones in the bladder

- **[bo he] 薄荷**Calaminthe
  = probably Mentha silvestris
  = horse mint, affections and pains of the kidneys

- **[wu gong shu] 蜈蚣属** Calcifraga (also see Scolpendria) = perhaps = Ascleium scolopendrium = hartstongue, dysuria, stranguria and anuria, stones in the bladder

- **[tie xian jue]** 铁线蕨 **[jin fan xian shu] 金发藓属 C**allithrix = Asplenium thricomanes = maidenhair spleenwort, affections and pains of the bladder

jaundice with dark urine.
U&D: 4.5—9g for external use, appropriate quantity to be decocted for washing or ground into powder for topical application.

[bai zhu] 白术 Largehead Atractylodes Rhizome
(Rhizoma Tractylodis Macrocephalae)
P: the rhizome of Atractylodes Macrocephala Roidz.
T&N: bitter and sweet in flavour, warm in property.
Act: to invigorate the function of the spleen and replenish Qi, to eliminate damp by causing diuresis, to arrest excessive perspiration, and to prevent miscarriage. Rhizoma Atractylodis Macrocephalage (processed with Terra); to invigorate the function of the spleen and regulate the function of stomach, and to prevent miscarriage.
Indi: hypo function of the spleen with anorexia; abdominal distension and diarrhea; dizziness and palpitation due to the retention of phlegm and fluid; edema, spontaneous sweating, threatened abortion. Rhizoma of Atractylodis Macrocephlalae (processed with terra); hypo function of the spleen with anorexia and diarrhea, threatened abortion.
U&D: 6--12g

[ba jiao hui xiang] 八角茴香 Chinese Star Anise (Fructus Anisi Stellati)
P: the dried ripe fruit of Illicium verum Hook.
T&N: pungent in flavour, warm in property.
Act: to dispel cold, to regulate the flow of Qi and to relieve pain.
Indi: abdominal colic, lumbago due to deficiency in kidney; vomiting and

- **[shan gan shu] 山柑属** Capparis = Capparis spinosa = caper, stones in the bladder (root + panaces + radicula)

- **[fei lian shu] 飞廉属 [mi tou fei lian ju] 蜜透飞廉菊** Carduus = Scolymus hispanicus/Cynara cardunculus (wild and cultivated) = thistles, affections and pains of the bladder, dysuria, stranguria and anuria

- **[da zao] 大枣** Caryota = a kind of large date, affections and pains of the kidneys, affections and pains of the bladder

- **[rou gui] 肉桂 [jue ming shu] 决明属** Casia fistula, affections and pains of the bladder

- **[rou gui pi] 肉桂皮** Cassia = the bark of various species of Cinnamomum, especially C. iners, C. zeylanicum, C. tamala; sometimes it also indicates the Origanum vulgare, affections and pains of the kidneys, affections and pains of the bladder

- **[yue gui] 月桂** Cassia daphnitis, stones in the bladder

[you ya] 幼芽 [lun shu zhi] 嫩树枝 Cauliculus = a little stem or stalk, affections and pains of the bladder

- **[pu shu] 朴属** Celtica = perhaps = Celtis australis = nettle-tree, affections and pains of the kidneys, affections and pains of the bladder

- **[zi hua jing tian] 紫花景天** Cepaea = Sedum cepaea = an orpine, affections and pains of the bladder

epigastric pain due to cold in the stomach.
U&D: 3--6g

[ba ji tian] 巴戟天 Morinda Root (Radix Morindae Officinlis)
P: the dried root of Morinda Officinalis .
T&N: sweet and pungent in flavour, warm slightly in property.
Act: to reinforce the kidney Yang, to strengthen the tendons and the bones, and to relieve rheumatic conditions.
Indi: impotence, seminal emission, infertility, menstrual disorders; pain and cold feeling in the lower abdomen; rheumatic arthralgia, limpness of the legs.

U&D: 3--9g

[ban bian lian] Barbated Skullcap Herb (Herba Lobeliae Chinensis)
P: the dried herb of Lobelia Chinensis.
T&N: pungent in flavour, neutral in property.
Act: to cause diuresis, and to remove toxic heat.
Indi: anasarca and ascites; carbuncles, boils and snake or insect bite; ascites in late schistosomiasis.
U&D: 9--15g

[ban zhi lian] 蓝 Barbated Skullcup Herb (Herba Scutellariae Barbatae)
P: the dried whole plant of Scutellaria Barbata.
T&N: pungent and bitter in flavour, cold in property
Act: to remove toxic heat, and to cause diuresis.
Indi: boils, sores, swelling and pain of throat, venomous snakebite, traumatic injuries, edema, jaundice.

- **[yu gu ji] 鱼骨蓟** Chamaepeuce = Chmaepeuce mutica = fish bone thistle, dysuria, stranguria and anuria

- **[jin gu cao] 筋骨草** Chamaepitys = ground pine. Perhaps Ajuga chamaepitys = yellow bugle; Ajuga iva = herb ivy; Passerina hirsuta or Ajuga chia = chia bugle, affections and pains of the navel, affections and pains of the bladder, dysuria, stranguria and anuria, stones in the bladder

- **[hu er cao] 虎耳草** Crethmos = Crithmum maritimum = samphire, affections and pains of the bladder, dysuria, stranguria and anuria

- **[pan hong hua shu] 番红花属** Crocus = Crocus stivus/C. vernus = saffron, affections and pains of the kidneys, affections and pains of the bladder, dysuria, stranguria and anuria, stones in the bladder, haematuria

- **[tian gua shu] 甜瓜属** Cucumeris semen, stones in the bladder, affections and pains of the kidneys (both for “reniculi” = adrenal glands and kidneys), affections and pains of the bladder, stones in the bladder, haematuria

- **[xiang gua he] 香瓜核** Cucumis dulcis = either Cucumis sativus or the wild species = Ecballum elaterium = cucumber, affections and pains of the kidneys, affections and pains of the bladder

- **[xiang gua] 香瓜** Cucumis edulis: see Cucumis dulcis, affections and pains of the bladder, dysuria, stranguria and

U&D: 15--30g or 30--60g of fresh herb; for external use, appropriate quantity to be pounded into paste and applied topically.

[bian xu] 扁蓄 Common Knotgrass Herb (Herba Polygoni Avicularis)

P: the dried aerial part of Polygonum Aviculare.
T&N: bitter in flavour, slightly cold in property.
Act: to relieve dysuria, to kill parasites and alleviate itching.
Indi: urinary infection with difficult painful urination; passage of scanty reddened urine and dribbling of urine after urination, eczema; vulva itching with morbid leukorrhea.
U&D: 9--15g for external use, appropriate quantity to be decocted for irrigation.

[bi cheng qie] 茄 Mountain Spicy Fruit (Fructus Litseae)

P: the dried ripe fruit of Litsea cubeba.
T&N: pungent in flavour, warm in property.
Act: to warm the spleen and stomach,.
Indi: epigastric pain accompanied by feeling of cold; abdominal colic of cold type; turbid urine caused by cold damp.
U&D: 1.5--3g

[bi ma you] 油 Castor Oil (Oleum Ricini)

P: the fatty oil obtained by squeezing and purification from the ripe seed of Ricinus communis.
Act: purgative by stimulating intestinal peristalsis.
Indi: used for evacuation from the bowels.

- **[zi ran qin shu] 孜然芹属** cuminum = Cuminum cyminum = cummin, affections and pains of the bladder, dysuria, stranguria and anuria, stones in the bladder

- **[shu jiao] 树胶** Cummis = every kind of gum, dysuria, stranguria and anuria, haematuria

- **[bai ke bai mu shu] 柏科柏木属** Cupressi bacae, affections and pains of the kidneys

- **[bai shu ye] 柏树叶** Cupressi folia, affections and pains of the bladder, dysuria, stranguria and anuria

- **[bai shu] 柏树** Cupressus = Cupressus sempervirens = cypress, dysuria, stranguria and anuria

- **[fei zhou shi luo] 非洲莳萝 [zi ran qin shu] 孜然芹属** Cyminum africanum (see Cuminum), dysuria, stranguria and anuria, stones in the bladder

- **[sha cao shu] 莎草 属 [shui xian chang pu] 水仙菖蒲** Cyperos = a general term for the species Cyperus. In particular = Gladiolus segetum = gladiolus/ corn-flag, affections and pains of the kidneys, stones in the bladder

- **[hu luo bu shu] 胡萝卜属** Daucos = generally Daucus carota (subsp. Carota), but also various species of Athamanta; Malabaila aurea and Bupleurum fruticosum. In Pliny = wild carrot, affections and pains of the kidneys, affections and pains of the bladder, dysuria, stranguria and anuria, stones in

U&D: 10—20ml
C&C: incompatible with fat-soluble anthelmintics; contraindicated in pregnancy.

[bing lang] 槟榔Areca Seed (Semen Arecae)
P: the dried ripe seed of areca catechu.
T&N: bitter and pungent in flavour, warm in property.
Act: to kill worms, to remove undigested food, to promote the flow of Qi ,and to stop malaria attacks.
Indi: taeniasis, ascariasis, fasciolopsiasis, abdominal pain due to intestinal parasitosis; diarrhea and tenesmus due to accumulation of undigested food; edema and weakness of the legs, malaria.
U&D: 3--9g; for treatment of taeniasis and fasciolopsiasis, 30--50g.

[bo he nao] 薄荷脑Menthol (Mentholum)
P: a saturated, cyclic alcohol obtained from peppermint oil.
Indi: as described under peppermint oil。
U&D: 0.02--0.1g often in tablet; or for topical application in spirit or ointment.

[bo he you] 荷油 Peppermint Oil (Oleum Menthae)
P: the volatile oil obtained by steam distillation from the fresh stem leaf of Mentha haplocalyx.
Indi: aromatic flavouring agent, carminative, applies to the skin or mucous membrane to give cooling and to relieve pain or other uncomfortable symptoms.
U&D: 0.02—0.2ml; 0.06--0.6ml daily.

[bu gu zi] 补骨脂 Malayter Scurphea Fruit (Fructus Psoraleae)

the kidney, stones in the bladder

- **[xi la ye hu luo bu] 希腊野胡萝卜** Daucum creticum, affections and pains of the kidneys

- **[shiz hong bu ming shu jiao he cheng ruan gao] 十种不明树胶合成软膏** Dekamyron = an unguent compounded by ten unidentified gums, affections and pains of the kidneys

- **[dou zhong wu ming zhong zi he cheng wu] 多种无名种子合成物** diaspermaton = a compound of many unidentified seeds, affections and pains of the kidneys

- **[hai yu shu] 海芋属** Aron **[long xian chong shu] 龙线虫属** Dracunculus: see Aron

- **[jie gu mu shu] 接骨木属**Ebulum = Sambucus ebulus = dwarf elder, dysuria, stranguria and anuria, stones in the bladder

- **[guo shu shu guan] 果树树冠**Elate hortensia = Abies cephalonica (but probably it is a mistake of the manuscripts in Pliny, 26, 82) = silver-fir, affections and pains of the bladder, dysuria, stranguria and anuria

- **[shu wei cao shu] 鼠尾草属[sa er wei ya shu wei cao] 撒尔维亚鼠尾草** Elelisphacon = perhaps Salvia officinalis, S. Tribola, S. Calycina, S. Pomifera = sage, affections and pains of the kidneys

- **[tie xian cao] 铁线草** Empetros = Asplenium scolopendrium = hartstongue, dysuria, stranguria and anuria, stones in

P: the dried ripe fruit of Psoralea corylifolia. **T&N:** pungent and bitter in flavour, warm in property. **Act:** to invigorate the function of the kidney, to alleviate asthma, and to relieve diarrhea. **Indi:** impotence, seminal emission, enuresis, frequent urination, aching of the loins and knees with cold sensation; asthma in deficiency syndromes of the kidney; diarrhea occurring before dawn daily. External use for vitiligo and alopecia areata. **U&D:** 6--9g; for external use, tincture of Fructus Psoraleae of 20%--30% in concentration to be applied topically. **[cao wu] 草乌 Kusenezoff Monkshood Root (Radix Aconiti Kusenezoffii)** **P:** the dried root tuber of Aconitum Kusnezoffi. **T&N:** pungent and bitter in flavour, hot in property. **Act:** to relieve rheumatic conditions, to warm the channels and to alleviate pain. **Indi:** rheumatic and rheumatoid arthralgia. Precordial and abdominal pain with cold sensation, abdominal colic caused by cold. Anesthesia. **U&D:** usually used being processed. **C&C:** be caution when the unprocessed root is taken orally. Incompatible with Bulbus Fritillariae, Rhizoma Pinelliae, Rhizoma Bletillae, Radix Ampelopsis, Radix Ttichosanthis, Fructus Trichosanthis. **[chai hu] 柴胡 Chinese Thorowax Root (Radix Bupleuri)** **P:** the dried root of Bupleurum longiradiatum. **T&N:** bitter in flavour, slightly cold in property.	the bladder (sometimes = Calcifraga) • **[chao cai] 巢菜** Ervum = Ervum ervilia = bitter vetch, incontinence of urine • **[ci qin shu] 刺 芹 属** Eryngium = Eryngium campestre and perhaps also Eryngium maritimum = eryngo, dysuria, stranguria and anuria, stones in the bladder • **[xi yang qian cao] 西洋茜草** Erythrodanum = Rubia tinctorum = madder, dysuria, stranguria and anuria • **[da ji ke] 大 戟 科** Euforbium = Euphorbia antiquourm = milk-wort • **[yin du he hua] 印度荷花** Faba aegyptiaca = Nelumbo nucifera = Indian lotus, affections and pains of the kidneys • **[xia mai shu] 小 麦 属 shuang hui mai] 双惠 麦** Far = Triticum dicoccum = emmer or two-grained wheat, affections and pains of the kidneys • **[mian fen] 面粉** farina = wheat-meal, affections and pains of the bladder, stones in the bladder • **[xiong jue] 雄蕨** Felix = Pteris aquilina = bracken fern, or Aspidium felix mas = male fern, stones in the bladder • **[hui xiang zi] 茴 香 子** Foeniculi semen, affections and pains of the kidneys • **[hui xiang] 茴香** Foeniculum = Foeniculum vulgare = fennel, affections

Act: to relieve fever, to soothe the liver, and to cure dropping and ptosis.
Indi: influenza or common cold with fever; alternate chills and fever such as malaria; distending pain in the chest and hypochondriac regions; menstrual disorders, prolapse of uterus, prolapse of rectum.
U&D: 3--9g
C&C: the dried rhizome of Bupleurum longiradiatum Turoz, covered with numerous annular nodes externally is poisonous and cannot be used as Radix Bupleuri.

[cha you] Tea-Seed Oil (Oleum Camelliae)
P: the fatty oil obtained by squeeze from the ripe seed of Camellia oleifera .
U&D: used as the raw material of injectable Tea-seed oil and the ointment base.

[chen pi] 陈皮 Dried Tangerine peel (Pericarpiun Citri Reticulatae)
P: the dried pericarp of the ripe fruit of Citrus reticulata.
T&N: bitter and pungent in flavour, warm in property.
Act: to regulate the flow of Qi, to invigorate the spleen function, to eliminate damp and to resolve phlegm.
Indi: distension and fullness sensation in the chest and epigastrium with anorexia; vomiting and diarrhea, cough with copious phlegm.
U&D: 3--9g

[chen xiang] 沉香 Chinese Eagewood Wood (Lignum Aquilariae Resinatum)
P: the wood containing resin of Aquillaria sinensis.
T&N: pungent and bitter in flavour,

and pains of the kidneys, affections and pains of the bladder, dysuria, stranguria and anuria, incontinence of urine, stones in the bladder, haematuria

- **[xun yi cao shu] 熏衣草属[ju yuan ye] 枸橼叶** folium = leaves either of Lavandula officinalis = lavender or of Cymbopogon nardus = citronella, stones in the bladder

- **[an shu zhong] 桉树种** Fraxini semen = Fraxinus excelsior = ash-tree, stones in the bladder

- **[jie cao shu] 颉草属[gao jia suo jie cao] 高加索颉草** Fu (also see Phu) = Valeriana phu = Caucasian valerian, affections and pains of the kidneys, affections and pains of the bladder

- **[bu ke niao ge shu] 薄壳鸟蛤属** fulviana = Herba Fulviana = unidentified, stones in the bladder

- **[kang] 糠** Furfur = bran, affections and pains of the kidneys

- **[suan jiang shu] 酸浆属** Fysalis (= alicacabum/halicacabum) = Physalis alkekengi = strawberry tomato, stones in the bladder

- **[gu peng xiang zhi] 古蓬香脂[da hui xiang] 大茴香** Galbanum = the resin of the Ferula galbaniflua = giant fennel, affections and pains of the kidneys, affections and pains of the bladder

- **[jin que hua shu] 金雀花属** Genistae semen = Genista tinctoria/ G. pilosa = greenweed, dysuria, stranguria

slightly warm in property. **Act:** to promote the flow of Qi and relieve pain to arrest vomiting by warming the stomach and to relieve asthma. **Indi:** distension and pain in the chest and abdomen; vomiting or hiccup due to cold in the stomach; asthma in deficiency syndrome of the kidney. **U&D:** 1.5--4.5 to be added when the decoction is nearly done. **[che qian cao] 车前草 Plantain Herb (Herba Plantaginis)** **P:** the wood containing resin of Aquilaria sinensis. **T&N:** pungent and bitter in flavour, slightly warm in property. **Act:** to promote the flow of Qi and relieve pain; to arrest vomiting or hiccup due to cold in the stomach, asthma in deficiency syndrome of the kidney. **U&D:** 1.5--4.5g, to be added when the decoction is nearly done. **[chen qian zi] 车前子 Plantian Seed (Semen Plantaginis)** **P:** the dried ripe seed of Plantago asiatica. Or Plantago depressa. **T&N:** sweet in flavour., slightly cold in property. **Act:** to remove heat, to cause diuresis and eliminate damp, to relieve dysuria, to clear the eye, and to promote expectoration. **Indi:** edema, dysuria with difficult painful urination; diarrhea cause by summer damp;inflammation of the eye, cough cause by phlegm-heat. **U&D:** 9--15g to be wrapped for making decoction. **[chi shao] Red Peony Root (Radix Paeoniae Rubra)**	and anuria • **[ce jin zhan hua] 侧金盏花** Git = Nipitella sativa = Roman coriander, stones in the kidney • **[tang chang pu] 唐菖蒲** Gladiolus = Gladiolus segetum = corn flag, affections and pains of the bladder, dysuria, stranguria and anuria • **[gan cao] 甘草** Glycyrrhiza = Glycyrrhiza glabra/G. Echinata = liquorice, affections and pains of the kidneys, affections and pains of the bladder, dysuria, stranguria and anuria • **[suo yao] 芍药** Glycyside = Paeonia officinalis = peony, affections and pains of the kidneys, affections and pains of the bladder • **[gou chi cao] 狗齿草** gramen = grass in general; in particular = Cynodon dactylon = dog's tooth grass, affections and pains of the bladder (against ulcers of the bladder), affections and pains of the kidneys, affections and pains of the bladder, dysuria, stranguria and anuria, stones in the bladder • **[er shi liu jie cao] 二十六节草** Gramen nodorum XXVI = unidentified. Literally it means "grass of 26 nodes", dysuria, stranguria and anuria • **[lu wei] 芦苇** Harundo iudaea/Harundo syria = reed, the genus Arundo, dysuria, stranguria and anuria (with grass and seeds of apium) • **[chang chun teng shu] 长春藤属** Hedera (grown on an oak), stones in

P: the dried root of Paeonia lactiflora.
T&N: bitter in flavour, slightly cold in property.
Act: to remove heat from blood , to eliminate blood stasis, and to relieve pain.
Indi: maculation in epidemic diseases; spitting of blood, epistaxis, inflammation of eye, pain in the chest and costal regions amenorrhea dysmenorrhea; mass formation in the abdomen, traumatic injuries, boils and sores.
U&D: 6--12g
C&C: incompatible with Rhizoma et Radix Veratri.

[chi shi zhi] 脂 Red Halloysite (Halloysitum Rubrum)
P: a mineral of silicate salt of olyhydrate kaolinate group, containing mainly hydrate aluminium silicate.
T&N: sweet, sour and astringent in flavour, warm in property,
Act: to astringe the intestines, to arrest bleeding,and to promote the growth of new tissues.
Indi: chronic diarrhea, chronic dysentery, hematochezia, abnormal uterine bleeding, excessive leukorrhea,
external use for ulcers difficult to heal up, eczema with exudation.
U&D: 9--12g appropriate quantity to be ground into powder for topical application.

[chi xiao dou] Rice Bean (Semen Phaseoli)
P: the dried ripe seed of Phaseolus calcaratus.
T&N: sweet and soue in flavour Neutral in property.
Act: to cause diuresis, to counteract toxicity and to promote the drainge of pus
Indi: edema, jaundice with dark urine;

the bladder

- **[chang chun teng shu] 长春藤属**
- **[ye teng] 野藤** Hedera = Hedera helix = wild ivy, dysuria, stranguria and anuria

- **[hei teng] 黑藤**Hederae nigrae bacae, dysuria, stranguria and anuria, haematuria

- **[shui sheng suan mo cao] 水生酸模草** Herba britannica (= lapatium) = Rumex aquaticus = grainless dock, stones in the bladder

- **[shan dian cao] 山靛草 [shui yin] 水银** Herba mercurialis = Mercurialis annua/M. Perennis = annual mercury, affections and pains of the kidneys, affections and pains of the bladder

- **[sha bing cao] 萨宾草**Herba sabina = brathy, affections and pains of the kidneys

- **[sheng cao] 圣草** Herba sacra: see Hierobotane, stones in the bladder

- **[shan liu ju shu] 山柳菊属 [ying cao] 鹰草** Hierobotane = perhaps the Hieracion of Pliny = either Urospermum picroides (the large type), or Hymenonema graecum (the small type) = hawkweed, stones in the bladder

- **[da mai] 大麦** Hordeum = Hordeum ditichum / H. Vulgare / H. Hexastichum = barley, affections and pains of the kidneys, affections and pains of the bladder, dysuria, stranguria and anuria, incontinence of urine

acute rheumatic arthriitis, carbuncles, boils, appendicitis. **U&D:** 9--30g; for external use, appropriate quantity to be ground into powder and appplied topically after mixing with liquid. **[chong wei zi] 茺蔚子 Motherwort Fruit (Fructus Leonuri)** **P:** the dried ripe fruit of Leonurus heterophyllus 。 **T&N:** pungent and bitter in flavour, slightly cold in property. **Act:** to activate blood circulattion and regulate menstruation, to subdue hyperactivity of the liver, and to clear the eye of opacity. **Indi:** menstrual disorders amenorrhea; hysmenorrhea, inflammation of the eye with formation of corneal opacity; dizziness and headache. **U&D:** 4.5--9g **C&C:** used with caution for pupil dilation. **[chuan mu tong] ˜¨ 木通 Sichuan Clematis Stem (Caulis Clematidis Armandii) also [guan mu tong] Manshuian Stem (Caulis Aristolochiae manshuriensis)** **P:** the dried stem of Clematis armandii Franch, or Clematis montana Buch. **T&N:** tastless and bitter in flavour, cold in property. **Act:** to remove heat and induce diuresis, to stimulate menstrual discharge, and promote lactation. **Indi:** edema, stranguria oliguria; arthralgia, amenorrhea, lack of lactation. **U&D:** 3--9g **[chuan mu xiang] 香 Common Vladimiriae Root (Radix Vladimiriae)**	• **[tian xian zi] 天仙子** Hyoscyamus = Hyoscyamus niger = henbane, affections and pains of the kidneys, affections and pains of the bladder, dysuria, stranguria and anuria, haematuria • **[jin si tao shu] 金丝桃属[lian qiao]** 连翘 Hypericon [or Caro, or Corissus] = Hypericum crispum / H. Revolutum = St. John's wort, affections and pains of the bladder, dysuria, stranguria and anuria (if the bladder is not ulcerated) • **[mu jin shu] 木槿属** Ibiscus/Hibiscum/Hibiscus = Althaea officinalis = marsh-mallow, affections and pains of the kidneys • **[ma chi jian shu] 马齿苋属** Illecebra = Sedum stellatum = wild purslane (the Andrachle agria of the Greeks), stones in the bladder • **[ji yin shu shu] 蓟罂粟属** Inguinalis (or Argemonium) = Papaver argemone = wind-rose: a panacea for all urological diseases according to all the ancient authors • **[xuan fu hua shu] 旋覆花属** Inula = Inula helenium = elecampane, affections and pains of the kidneys • **[yuan wei shu] 鸢尾属** Iris ilirica = in Pliny it is generally either Iris germanica or Iris pallida = iris, in particular German iris, but – against the others - he does not suggest it for urological diseases, affections and pains of the bladder • **[ci bai shu] 刺柏属** Iuniperus = Juniperus = juniper tree, dysuria,

P: the dried root of Vladimiria souliei. **T&N:** pungent and bitter in flavour, warm in property. **Act:** to promote th flow of Qi and relieve pain. **Indi:** pain and distention in epigastrium and abdomen with borborygmi; diarrhea,and tenesmus; discomfort in the hypochondriac regions; pain in the liver and gall bladder diseases. **U&D:** 3--9g **[chuan wu] 川乌 Common Monkshood Mother Root (Radix Aconiti)** **P:** the dried partent root tuber of aconitum carmichaeli Debx. **T&N:** pungent and bitter in flavour, hot in property. **Act:** to relieve rheumatic conditions and alleviate pain by warming the channels. **Indi:** joint pain in rheumatic or rheumatoid arthritis, epigastric pain with cold sensation, or analgesic in anesthesis. **U&D:** usually used being processed. **C&C:** to be cautions when the unprocessed root is taken orally. Incmpatible with Bulbu Fritillariae, Rhizoma Ampelopsis, Radix Trichosanthis. **[chuan xin lian] 穿心莲 Common Andrographis Herb (Herba Andrograpgitis)** **P:** the dried aerial part of Andrographis paniculate. **T&N:** bitter in flavour, cold in property. **Act:** to remove heat, counteracte toxicity, and induce subsidence of swelling. **Indi:** influenza with fever, sore throat, ulcer in the mouth or on the tongue, acute or chronic cough, colitis, dysentery, urinary infection with difficult painful	stranguria and anuria • **[guo li qiao shu] 裹篱樵属** Iustiana, affections and pains of the kidneys • **[suan mo shu] 酸模属** Lapathium = species Rumex = dock and sorrel, affections and pains of the kidneys, affections and pains of the bladder, haematuria • **[niu pang] 牛 旁** Lappae radix = Arctium lappa = burdock, stones in the bladder • **[yue gui] 月桂** Lauri bacae = Laurus nobilis = bay, affections and pains of the kidneys, affections and pains of the bladder • **[shui qin] 水芹** Laver = Nasturtium officinale = water cress, stones in the bladder • **[ya ma zi] 亚 麻 子** Lini smen = Linum usitatissimum/L. Angustifolium = seed of flax, affections and pains of the kidneys, affections and pains of the bladder • **[zhang ke] 樟科 [cai gui] 柴桂 [gui pi] 桂 皮** Malabathrum/Malobatrum = (the leaves of a plant of the Extreme Orient, perhaps the Cinnamomum tamala), affections and pains of the kidneys • **[ping guo shu] 苹果属 [ping guo] 苹果 [hua hong] 花红 [hai tang guo] 海棠果** Malum erraticum = Malum terrae = apple tree, stones in the bladder • **[ping guo shu] 苹果属 [ping guo] 苹**

urination; carbuncles, sores venemous snake bite,
U&D: 6--9g appropriate quantity for external use.

[chui pen cao] 垂草 Stringy Stonecrop Herb (Herba Sedi)
P: the fresh or dried whole plant of Sedum sarmentosum.
T&N: sweet and tastless in flavour, cool in property.
Act: to remove damp-heat, and to counteracte toxicity.
Indi: jaundice with oliguria caused by damp-heat; acute and chronic hepatitis; carbuncles and sores.
U&D: 250g of fresh herb or 15--30g the dried herb.

[ci wu jia] 刺五加 Manyprickle Acanthopanax Root (Radix Acanthopanacia Senticosi)
P: the dried root and rhizome of Acanthopanax senticosus.
T&N: pungent and bitter in flavour, slightly cold in property.
Act: to reinforce Qi, to invigorate the function of the spleen and the kidney, and to calm the nerves.
Indi: hypofunction off the spleen and kindey marked by geaeral waekness; lassitude, anorexia, aching of the loins and knees; insomnia and dream-disturbed sleep.
U&D: 7--27g.

[da fu pi] 皮 Areca pee (Pericarpium Arecae)
P: the dried pericarp of Areca catechu L. The unripe fruit is collected in winter to the next spring, dried after boiled, cut longitudinally into two valves.

果 [hua hong] 花红[hai tang guo] 海棠果 Malum granatum = Punica granatum = pomegranate, affections and pains of the kidneys

- **[jing kui shu] 锦葵属** Malva = Malva silvestris = cheese flower (sometimes Althaea officinalis = marsh-mallow, or Lavatera arborea = tree-mallow), affections and pains of the bladder, dysuria, stranguria and anuria

- **[jing kui shu] 锦葵属[dong kui] 冬葵**Malva agrestis, affections and pains of the kidneys, affections and pains of the bladder, dysuria, stranguria and anuria

- **[jing kui shu] 锦葵属** Malva, affections and pains of the kidneys (for the "reniculi" = adrenal glands)

- **[ru xiang] 乳香** Mastix = Pistacia lentiscus = mastic tree, affections and pains of the kidneys

- **[ru xiang shu zhi] 乳香树脂**Mastix Chia, affections and pains of the bladder

- **[feng mi] 蜂蜜[gan yi] 甘饴**Mel = honey, affections and pains of the kidneys, stones in the kidney, stones in the bladder

- **[bo he shu] 薄荷属**Menta = Menta acquatica = water-mint (sometimes = Satureia calamintha and similar species), affections and pains of the bladder, dysuria, stranguria and anuria

- **[jue lei zhi wu] 蕨类植物**Meum = Meum athamanticum = bear-wort/spignel, affections and pains of the kidneys, affections and pains of the

The periarp is peeled. It is known as "Dafupi". The ripe fruit is collected from late spring to early autumn, dried after boiled the pericarp peeled, tapped to loosen and dried in the sun, known as "Dafumao".
T&N: pungent in flavour , warm slitghly in property.
Act: to promote the desending of Qi, to relieve abdominal distension,and to cause diuresis.
Indi: stagnation of Qi due to accumulation of damp marked by epigastric and abdominal distension; difficult evacuation of the faces, edems of the legs and oliguia.
U&D: 4.5--9g

[da ji] Japanese Thistle Herb/Japanese Thistle Root (Herba Cirsii Japonici)
P: the dried aerial part or root of Crisium japonicum DC.
T&N: sweet and bitter in flavour, cold in property.
Act: to arrest bleeding by reduceing heat in blood, to remove blood stasis, and to promote the subsidence of swelling.
Indi: epistaxis, spitting of blood, haematuria, hematochezia, abnormal uterine bleeding, traumatic bleeding, carbuncles and sores.
U&D: 9--15g for external use, appropriate quantity of the fresh herb to be punded into paste and applied topically.

[dang shen] 党参 Tangshen (Radix Codonopsis)
P: the dried root of Codonopsis pilosula.
T&N: sweet in flavour, neutral in property.
Act: to reinforce qi and invigorate the

bladder

- **[qi shu] 耆属** Millefolium = a secondary name of Achilleos = Achillea tomentosa / A. Millefolium A. Ptarmica / A. Magna = Achilles' wound-wort, dysuria, stranguria and anuria, stones in the bladder. When Millefolium is to be identified with the Herba sacra (or Hierobotane), dysuria, stranguria and anuria

- **[su mi cao shu] 粟米草属** Molligo / Mollugo = a kind of Lappago, = a sort of burdock (also see Lappa), affections and pains of the kidneys

[shu er cao shu] 鼠耳草属 myosota = Asperugo procumbens = mad-wort, stones in the bladder

- **[hu wei cao shu] 狐尾草属[gou wei ba cao] 狗尾巴草** Myriophyllon = Myriophyllum spicatum = water-milfoil (but also see Millefolium), affections and pains of the bladder, dysuria, stranguria and anuria

- **[ou zhou mo yao] 欧洲没药** Myrrha = either myrrh or the tree that produces it, that is the Balsamodendron myrrha, affections and pains of the kidneys, affections and pains of the bladder, dysuria, stranguria and anuria, stones in the bladder

- **[mo yao guo] 没药 果** Myrrahae stactes, affections and pains of the kidneys, stones in the bladder

- **[shan fan ke] 山矾科** Myrtus = Myrtus communis = myrtle tree, affections and pains of the bladder,

function of the spleen and the lung.
Indi: weakness of the spleen and thelung manifested by shortness of breath; cough, palpition, anorexia, loose stools; diabetes cauesd by intrenal heat.
U&D: 9--30g
C&C: incompatibles with Rhizoma et Radix Verayti.

[dan zhu ye] 淡竹叶 Lophatherum Herb (Herb Lophatheri)
P: the dried stem and leaf of Lophatherum gracile.
T&N: sweet and tastless in flavour Cold in property.
Act: to remove heat, ease the mind and cause diuresis.
Indi: fidgetness and thirst in febrile diseases; dysuria with reddened urine and painful urination; ulcer in the mouth and on the tongue.
U&D: 6--9g

[da zao] ´ó枣 Chinese Date (Fructus Jujubae)
P: the dried ripe fruit of Ziziphus jujuba Mill.
T&N: sweet in flavour and warm in property.
Act: to tonify the spleen and replenish Qi, to nourish blood, and to ease the mind, and also used to moderate the drug actions.
Indi: anorexia, lassitude and loose stools in deficiency syndromes of the spleen; hysteria in women.
U&D: 6--15g

[deng xin cao] 灯心草 Common Rush (Medulla Junci)
P: the dried stem pith of Juncus effusus.
T&N: sweet and tastless in flavour, slithly cold in property.
Act: to eliminate excess fire in the

dysuria, stranguria and anuria, stones in the bladder

- **[gan song shu] 甘松属[kuan ye gan song] 宽叶甘松** Nardus = Nardostachys Jatamansi = the rootstock of spikenard, stones in the bladder

- **[yin du gan song] 印度甘松** Nardus indica = Indian spikenard, affections and pains of the kidneys

- **[jia du xing cai shu] 家独行菜属** Nasturcium = Lepidium sativum = garden cress, affections and pains of the bladder

- **[jin jie shu] 荆芥属** Nepeta = generally Satureia calamintha, but particularly Satureia nepeta, affections and pains of the bladder, stones in the bladder

- **[bai shui lian] 白睡莲** Nymphaea heraclia = Nymphaea alba = white waterlily, affections and pains of the bladder, dysuria, stranguria and anuria

- **[luo le shu] 萝勒属** Ocimum = Ocymum basilicum = basil, affections and pains of the kidneys

- **[lu xi dou shu] 驴喜豆属** Oenobreches = Onobrychis vicaefolia = sainfoin, dysuria, stranguria and anuria

- **[ku you gao] 苦油膏** oleum amarum = bitter oil, not better identified, affections and pains of the kidneys

- **[ku you] 苦油** oleum = olive oil, affections and pains of the kidneys, dysuria, stranguria and anuria, stones in

heart, and to induce diuresis.
Indi: fidgentness and insomnia with oliguria and painful and difficult urination or with ceration in the mouth or onthe tongue.
U&D: 1--3g

[dian qie cao] 颠茄草 Belladonna Herb (Herba Belladonnae)
P: the dried herb of Atropa belladonna
Act: anticholinergics.

[di fu zi] 地肤子 Belvedere Fruit (Fructus Kochiae)
P: the dried ripe fruit of Kochia scoparia.
T&N: pungent and bitter in flavour, cold in property.
Act: to remove damp-heat, to dispel wind, and relieve itching.
Indi: painful and difficult urination, pruritus vulvae with leukorrhea, rubela, eczema, cutaneous pruritus.
U&D: 9--15g for external use, appropriate quantity to be decocted from fuming and washing.

[di jin cao] 地锦草Creeping Euphorbia (Herba Euphorbiae Humifusae)

P: the dried whole plant of Euphorbia humifusa.
T&N: pungent in flavour , neutral in property.
Act: to remove toxic heat and to arrest bleeding by reducing heat in blood.
Indi: dysentery, colitis; hemoptysis, haematuria, hematochezia, abdominal eterine bleeding, boils carbuncles.
U&D: 9--20g or 30--60g of the fresh herb, appropriate quantity for external use.

[ding gong teng] 丁公藤 Erycibe Stem (Caulis Erycibes)

the bladder

- **[gui hua you] 桂花油** oleum laurinum = laurel oil, affections and pains of the kidneys

- **[hu tu zi shu] 胡秃子属** Oliastri semen = seeds of Olea oleaster = oleaster, stones in the bladder

- **[ya pian] 鸦片** Opium, affections and pains of the kidneys, affections and pains of the bladder, dysuria, stranguria and anuria, haematuria

- **[xiang ye shu gao] 香液树膏** opobalsamum = balsam of Mecca = the juice of the Commifora opobalsamum = balsam tree, affections and pains of the kidneys, affections and pains of the bladder

- **[wan ling cao yao zhi] 万灵草药汁** opopanax = the juice of the Panaces, affections and pains of the kidneys

- **[jin que hua] 金雀花** Oxymyrsine (also see Ruscum) = Ruscus aculeatus = butcher's broom, dysuria, stranguria and anuria, stones in the bladder

- **[ma jia zi shu] 马甲子属**Paliurus = Zizyphus spina Cristi = Christ's thorn, stones in the bladder

- **[zong lu ke] 棕榈 科**Palmae cariota = Palma is chiefly the Phoenix dactilifera. Sometimes it is the Chamaerops humilis = dwarf palm, affections and pains of the bladder

- **[ai zong lu] 矮 棕榈** Palmulae = perhaps the Chamaerops humilis =

P: the dried stem of Erycibe obtusfolia Benth.or Erycibe schmidtii Vraib.
T&N: pungent in flavour,warm in property.
Act: to relieve rheumatic conditions, and to relieve swelling and pain.
Indi: rheumatic arthhralgia, hemiplegia, traumatic swelling and pain.
U&D: 3--6g used for making medicinal wines; orally or apply topically.
C&C: it exhibitions a strong diaphoretic activity; used with caution in week patients, contraindicated in pregnancy.

[ding xiang] 丁香 Clove (Flos Caryophlli)
P: the dried flower bud of Eugenia caryophyllata Thunb.
T&N: pungent in flavour, warm in propery.
Act: to warm the spleen and stomach, to ergulate the adverse flow of stomach Qi, and restore the kidney Yang.
Indi: hiccup, vomiting, anorexia, diarrhea and epigastric and abdominal pain with cold sensation in deficiency-cold syndromes of the spleen and stomach; impotence due to deficiency of the kidney Yang.
U&D: 1--3g

[ding xiang luo le you] 丁香罗勒油 Ocimum Oil (Oleum Ocimi Gratissimi)
P: the volatile oil obtained by steam distillation from the herb of Ocimum gratissimum L.
Act: local analgesic, antiseptic disinfectant.
Indi: toothache due to caries.

[di yu] 地榆 Garden Burnet Root

dwarf-palm, stones in the bladder

- **[a wei] 阿魏** Panaces = Ferula galbaniflua = all-heal, affections and pains of the bladder (if the bladder has no "scabies")

- **[ying su] 罂粟** Papaver = Papaver somniferum/P. Rhoeas/P. Hybridum/ P. Argemone = poppy, affections and pains of the kidneys, affections and pains of the bladder

- **[hei ying su] 黑罂粟** Papaver nigrum, affections and pains of the kidneys, affections and pains of the bladder

- **[qiang cao shu] 墙草属** Parietaria = Parietaria officinalis = wall pellitory, dysuria, stranguria and anuria

- **[ye hu luo bu shu] 野胡萝卜属** Pastinaca = a generic term for Daucus carota = carrot and other plants similiar to carrot, like Althaea officinalis/Athamanta cretensis/ A. Cervaria/ Seseli ammoides/ Malabaila aurea, incontinence of urine, stones in the bladder

- **[ren dong shu] 忍冬属** Periclymenon = perhaps Lonicera etrusca or L. Caprifolium = honeysuckle, dysuria, stranguria and anuria, haematuria

- **[xi xin shu] 细辛属** Perpressa = baccar = Asarum europaeum = hazelwort, stones in the bladder

- **[he lan qin] 荷兰芹** Petroselinum = Petroselinum sativum = parsley,

(Radix Sanguisorbae) **P:** the dried root of Sanguisorba officinalis. **T&N:** bitter sour and astringent in flavour. **Act:** to arrest bleeding by dispelling heat for blood, and to conteract toxicity and cure sores. **Indi:** hematochezia, haemorrhoidal blooding, bloody dysentery, abnormal uterine bleeding, scalds and burns, carbuncles, boils and sores. **U&D:** 9--15g for external use, appropriate quantity to be ground into powder and applied topically. **ɔng xia cao] 冬虫夏草 Chinese Caterpill (Fungus Cordyceps)** **P:** a composile consisting of the stroma of the Fungus Cordyceps sinensis, parasitzed on the larva of some species of insects and the dead caterpills. **T&N:** sweet in flavour, natural in property. **Act:** to tonify the lung and the kidney, arrest bleeding, and dispel phlegm. **Indi:** chronic cough and asthma; hemoptysis in phthisis; impotence and seminal emissions with aching of loins and knees. **U&D:** 3--9g **[dong gua pi] 冬瓜皮 Chinese Waxgourd peel (Exocarpium Benincasae)** **P :** he dried exoarp of Benincasa hispida. **T&N:** sweet in flavour Coolin property. **Act:** to cause diuriesis. **Indi:** edema with oliguria, thirst and oliguria duc to summer-heat. **U&D:** 9--30g **[dong kui guo] 冬葵果 Cluster Mallow Fruit (Fructus Malvae)** **P:** the dried ripe fruit of Malua	affections and pains of the kidneys, affections and pains of the bladder, dysuria, stranguria and anuria, stones in the kidney, stones in the bladder • **[ma qi dun he lan qin] 马其顿荷兰芹** Petroselinum Macedonicum, affections and pains of the kidneys, stones in the bladder (for the "renunculi") • **[qian hu] 前 胡** Peucedanum = Peucedanum officinale = sulphur-wort, affections and pains of the bladder • **[huang nie shu] 黄 孽 属** Phelandrium = unidentified plant, affections and pains of the bladder, stones in the bladder • **[jie cao shu] 颉 草 属** Phu = Valeriana phu = Valeriana caucasica = Caucasian valerian, affections and pains of the kidneys, affections and pains of the bladder • **[song zi] 松 子** pinei nuclei = the stones of the pinus, a term which generally indicates the Pinus sylvestris = Scotch pine; but in sometimes it indicates probably the Pinus pinea = stone pine, affections and pains of the kidneys, affections and pains of the bladder, dysuria, stranguria and anuria, stones in the bladder, haematuria • **[bai hu jiao] 白胡椒** Piper album = white pepper, affections and pains of the kidneys, dysuria, stranguria and anuria, stones in the bladder • **[hu jiao] 胡 椒** Piper =generally Piper longum = long pepper, affections and pains of the kidneys, stones in the

verticillata, commonly used by the Mongol nationality. **T&N:** sweet and astringent in flavour, cool in property. **Act:** to remove heat and induce diuresis, to relieve edema. **Indi:** urinary infection with oliguria, edema and thirst. **U&D:** 3--9g **[rou dou kou] 肉豆蔻 Round Cardamon Fruit (Fructus Amomi Rotundus)** **P:** the dried ripe fruit of Amonum kravanh. **T&N:** pungent in flavour, warm in property. **Act:** to resolve damop, to remove stagnancy of food, and to promote digestion. **Indi:** loss of appetite due to accumulation of turbid damp in the spleen and stomach; feeling of suffocation in the chest with anorexia at the early stage of damp-warm syndromes; nausea, vomiting; distension and pain in the chest and abdomen caused by cold-damp; indigestion with retention of food **U&D:** 3--6g to be added when the decoction is nearly done. **[duan shi gao] 煅石 Gypsum (calcined) (Gypsum Fibrosum Praeparata)** **P:** the processed Gypsum. **T&N:** sweet, pungent, and astringent in flavour, cold in property. **Act:** to check exudation, promove the growth of new tissue, and arrest bleeding. **U&D:** external use for ulcers difficulte to heal up, eczema with itching, scalds into powder and applied topically. **[duan xue liu] 断血流 Clinopodium Herb (Herba Clinopodii)** **P:** the dried aerial part of Clinopodium	bladder (both for kidneys and "reniculi" = adrenal glands) affections and pains of the bladder, dysuria, stranguria and anuria, stones in the bladder, affections and pains of the kidneys • **[hei hu jiao] 黑胡椒** Piper nigrum = perhaps Xylopia aethiopica = African pepper, affections and pains of the kidneys • **[che qian cao] 车前草** Plantago = Plantago major / P. Lagopus = large plantain, affections and pains of the kidneys, affections and pains of the bladder, dysuria, stranguria and anuria, stones in the bladder • **[xi lan jie cao] 希腊颉草** Polemonia = either hypericum olympicum = Olympic St. John's wort, or Polemonium ceruleum = Greek valerian, affections and pains of the bladder, stones in the bladder • **[xiang ke shu] 香科属** Polium = Teucrium polium = hulwort, stones in the bladder • **[ying gao ji] 硬膏剂** Polyarchion emplastrum = an unidentified poultice, literally "invented by the physician Polyarchos", affections and pains of the kidneys • **[liang er cao] 两耳草** Plygonum = Polygonum aviculae = knotgrass, affections and pains of the bladder, dysuria, stranguria and anuria • **[bai yang] 白杨** Populus alba (berries) = abele berries, dysuria, stranguria and anuria

polycephalum. **T&N:** bitter slitghly and pungent in flavour, cool in property. **Act:** to arrest bleeding. **Indi:** excessive menstrual discharge, haemorrhoea from hysteromyoma, haematuria, epistaxis gingival bleeding, traumatic bleeding. **U&D:** 9--15g for external use, approriate quantity to be ground into powder or the fresh herb to be pounded into paste for topical application. **[du huo] 独活 Deubleteeth Pubescent Angelica Root （Radix Angelicae Pubescentis）** **P:** the dried root of Angelica pubescens. **T&N:** pungent and bitter in flavour, slightly warm in property. **Act:** to relieve rheumatic conditions and to remove obstruction from the channels and relieve pain. **Indi:** rheumatic arthritis with pain in the lower back and knees; headach due to attack of cold on the Shaoyin channel characterized by association of headache with precordial pain and cold legs. **U&D:** 3--6g **[du zhong] 杜仲 Eucommia Bark (Cortex Eucommiae)** **P:** the dried stem bark of Eucommia ulmoides. **T&N:** sweet in flavour, warm in property. **Act:** to tonify the liver and the kidney, to strengthen the tendons and bones, and to prevent miscarrige. **Indi:** deficinency condition of the kidney and lack of strength, threatened abortion, hypertension . **U&D:** 6--9g	• **[cong] 葱** Porrum = Allium porrum = leek, affections and pains of the kidneys • **[shui chu] 水 醋** Posca = water and vinegar, affections and pains of the kidneys (for the "reniculi" = adrenal glands) • **[hei ci li] 黑 刺 李** pruna silvestria (nucleoli) = stones of Prunus spinosa = blackthorn, affections and pains of the bladder, stones in the bladder • **[hui qin shu] 茴芹属** Pseudobunion = Pimpinella cretica = Cretan pimpinella, dysuria, stranguria and anuria • **[ou zhou che qian] 欧 洲 车 前** Psyllion = Plantago psyllium = fleawort, fleabana, affections and pains of the kidneys, affections and pains of the bladder • **[bo he lei xiang cao] 薄荷类香草** Puleium = Mentha pulegium = pennyroyal, affections and pains of the kidneys, affections and pains of the bladder, dysuria, stranguria and anuria, stones in the bladder • **[luo ma huang ju]** 罗 马 **黄 菊** Pyrethrum = Anthemis pyrethrum, but on the basis of the habitat described by Pliny, perhaps it is Anthemis tinctoria, var. Pallida, dysuria, stranguria and anuria, stones in the bladder • **[pu tao wei ling cai] 葡萄委陵菜** Quinquefolium = Potentilla reptans / P. Rupestris / Tormentilla reptans = cinquefoil, dysuria, stranguria and anuria

[Eer cha] 儿茶 Cutch Black Catechu (Catechu) **P:** the dried concentrated decoction prepared from the peeled branch and stem of Acacia catechu (L) Willd. **T&N:** bitter and astringent in flavour, slightly cold in property. **Act:** to arrest exudation, promote the growth of new tissue, and cure wounds. **Indi:** festering wound difficult to heal up, skin diseases with watery discharge, ulcers in mouth, tranmatic injury with pain and bleeding. **U&D:** 1--3g wrapped on making decoction, used frequently for making pills or powder, appropriate quantity for external use. **[fa ban xia] 法半夏 Pinellia Tuber (Processed with Radix Glycyrrhizae and lime)** **Rhizoma Pinelliae Praeparata)** **P:** the processed Rhizoma Pinelliae. **T&N:** pungent in flavour, warm in property. **Act:** to remove damp and phlegm. **Indi:** cough and palpitation due to retentation of phlegm and fluid; vertigo causedby wind-phlegm; headach with cold extremities due to attack of phlegm. **U&D:** as described under Pinellia Tuber. **[fang feng] 防风Divaricate Saposhnikovia Root (Radix Saposhnikoviae)** **P:** the dried root of Saposhnikovia divericata. **T&N:** pungent and sweet in flavour, warm in property. **Act:** to induce diaphoresis, to dispel wind, to alleviate rheumatic conditions and to relieve spasm.	• **[fei zao cao] 肥皂草** Radicula = Saponaria officinalis = soapwort, or Reseda luteola = dyers's wed, or Gypsophila struthium = Egyptian soapwort, dysuria, stranguria and anuria, stones in the bladder (+ panaces + capparis radix) • **[ku gen] 苦根**radix amara = perhaps black or white salsify, affections and pains of the kidneys • **[du nou xiang shu zhi] 笃耨香树脂** resina terebinthina = the resin of the terebinthus = Pistacia terebinthus = terebinth, affections and pains of the kidneys • **[da huang] 大黄**Rhecoma = the root of a kind of rhubarb, perhaps Rheum ribes, affections and pains of the kidneys • **[lu shui] 露水** ros = dew, stones in the bladder • **[qiang wei] 蔷薇** Rosa = Rosa centifolia and oter species = rose, affections and pains of the kidneys • **[ou zhou ye qiang wei] 欧洲野蔷薇** Rosae agrestis spongia = rose-gall, stones in the bladder • **[fu pei zi gen] 覆盆子根** Rubi radices = roots of rubus, dysuria, stranguria and anuria, stones in the bladder • **[jia ye shu] 假叶树**Ruscus (also see Oxymyrsine) = Ruscus aculeatus = butcher's broom, dysuria, stranguria and anuria, stones in the bladder

Indi: headache in colds, urticaria rheumatic arthralgia, tentanus. **U&D:** 4.5 - 9g **[fang ji] 防己 Fourstamen Stephania Root (Radix Stephaniae Tetrandrae)** **P:** the dried root of Stephanina tetrandria. **T&N:** bitter in flavour, cold in property. **Act:** to cause diuresis and to relieve rheumatic conditions. **Indi:** edema with oilguria; eczema, rheumatic arthritis, hypertension. **U&D:** 4.5--5g **[fan xie ye] 番泄叶Senna Leaf (Folium Sennae)** **P:** the dried leaflet of Cassia angustifolia. **T&N:** sweet and bitter in flavour, cold in property. **Act:** to purge away heat, relax the bowels and induce diuresis. **Indi:** accumulation of heat marked by constipaton and abdominal pain; edema. **U&D:** 3--9g **C&C:** used with caution in pregnancy. **[fei zi] Grand Torreye Seed (Semen Torreyae)** **P:** the dried ripe seed of Torreya grandis. **T&N:** sweet in flavour, neutral in property. **Act:** to kill worms and relax bowels. **Indi:** ankylostomiasis, ascariasis, taeniasis, abdominal pain and malnutrition caused by intestial parasitosis in children; constipation. **U&D:** 9--15g **[fen bi xie] 粉萆Hypoglaucous Collett Yam (Rhizoma Dioscoreae Hypoglaucae)** **P:** the dried rhizome of Dioscorea hypoglauca. **T&N:** bitter in flavour, neutral in	• **[jia ye shu] 假 叶 树** Ruscus hypophyllon = double tongue or Vinca herbacea = perwinkle, dysuria, stranguria and anuria, stones in the bladder • **[yun xiang ye] 云 香叶**Ruta = Ruta greveolens = rue, affections and pains of the kidneys, affections and pains of the bladder, dysuria, stranguria and anuria • **[liu shu ye] 柳 树 叶** Salicis folia = the leaves of many kinds of Salix = salice, stones in the bladder • **[fa guo gan song] 法 国 甘 松** Saliunca = Valeriana celtica = French spikenard, affections and pains of the bladder, dysuria, stranguria and anuria, stones in the bladder • **[mo qiao luan na shu] 茉荞栾那属** Sampsuchum = Origanum marjorana = sweet marjoram, affections and pains of the kidneys, dysuria, stranguria and anuria • **[bei mu shu] 贝 母 属** Satyrum (or Satyrion / Satyrios) = probably the Aristolochia polyrrhizos, but sometimes also Acera Anthropohora, or a species of Orchis, or Tritillaria graeca = fritillary, affections and pains of the kidneys • **[tie xian jie] 铁 线 蕨** Saxifraga = adiantum = Adiantum capillus Veneris = black maidenhair / Asplenium thrichomanes or maidenhair speenwort, affections and pains of the kidneys, dysuria, stranguria and anuria, stones in the bladder (= Scolopendrios for the "reniculi" = adrenal glands) • **[xiang mao shu] 香茅属** Schoenum

property.
Act: to remove turbid damp, and to relieve rheumatic conditions.
Indi: chyluria, turbid urine mixed with whitish subtance or whitish discharge from urethra; excessive leukorrhea, rheumatic arthralgia with limitation of motion and pain in the loins and knees.
U&D: 9--15g

[feng xiang zhi] 风香子 Beautiful Sweetgum Fruit (Resina Liquidambris)
P: the dried resin of Liquidambar formosana;
T&N: pungent and slitghly, bitter in flavour, neutral in property.
Act: to promote blood circulation and relieve pain, to counteracte toxicity, to stimulate tissue regeneration, and to reduce heat from blood.
Indi: traumatic injuries, swelling and pain of carbuncle and boil, spitting of blood, epistaxis and traumatic haemorrhea.
U&D: 1.5--3g used in making pills or powder, appropriate quantity for external.

[fu ling] 茯苓 Indian Bread (Proi)
P: the dried sclerotium of the fungus, Poria coco.
T&N: sweet and tastless in flavour, neutral in property.
Act: to cause diuresis, to invigorate the spleen function and to calm the mind.
Indi: edema with oliguria, dizziness and palpitation caused by retained fluid; diminished function of the spleen marked by anorexia; loose stools or diarrhea, restlessness and insomnia.
U&D: 9--15g

= Cymbopogon schoenanthus = camel-hay, affections and pains of the kidneys

- **[wu gong ke] 蜈蚣科** Scolpendria (see Callithrix) = Asplenium thricomanes = maidenhair spleenwort, stones in the bladder

- **[di fu] 地肤** Scopa regia = Chenopodium scoparia, dysuria, stranguria and anuria, stones in the bladder (= Oxymyrsine)

- **[shi can] 石蚕** Scordion = Teucrum scordium = germander, dysuria, stranguria and anuria

- **[hu jiao hu er cao] 胡椒虎耳草** Silaus = a water tree such as the Apium graveolens (= Celery), but not identified, for certain affections and pains of the bladder

- **[bai jie zi] 白芥子** Sinapis = Brassica alba = white mustard/B. Nigra or black mustard, dysuria, stranguria and anuria

- **[da suan jie shu] 大蒜芥属** Sisymbrium= Mentha aquatica = bergamot mint, affections and pains of the bladder, dysuria, stranguria and anuria

- **[yin du kuan ye gansong] 印度宽叶甘松** Spica indica = unidentified but perhaps = Spica nardi (Nardostachys Jatamansi), affections and pains of the kidneys, affections and pains of the bladder

- **[kuan ye gan song] 宽叶甘松** Spica nardi = Nardostachys Jatamansi =

[fu shen] 茯神 Fu-shen
(Poria cum Radice Pini)
P: the drug consists of Fu Ling (Proi) with a piece of pine root embeded, used as a sedative for palpitation and insomnia.

[fu pen zi] 覆盆子 Palmleaf RaspberryFruit (Fructus Rubi)
P: the dried fruit of arubus chinigii.
T&N: sweet and soue in flavour and warm in property.
Act: to benefit the kidney, and arrest seminal discharge and excessive urination.
Indi: enuesis, frequent urination, impotence, premature ejaculation, seminal emission and spermatorrhea in deficiency syndromw of the kidney.
U&D: 6--12g

[fu ping] 浮萍 Common Ducksmeat Herb (Herba Spirodelae)
P: the dried whole plant of Spirodela polyrrhiza.
T&N: pungent in flavour, cold in property.
Act: to dispel wind-heat, to promote eruption,and to cause diuresis.
Indi: measles without adequate eruption, urticaria with itching, edema with oliguria.
U&D: 3--9g for external use, appropriate quantity to be decocted for washing or immersion.

[fu zi] 附子 Prepared Common Monkshood Daughter Root (Radix Aconiti Lateralis Praeparata)
P: the processed daughter root of Aconitum carmichacli.
T&: pungent and sweet in flavour, hot in property.

spikenard, affections and pains of the kidneys, stones in the bladder

- **[an xi xiang] 安息香** Storax = both the resin and the tree which produces it = Storax officinalis = officinal storax, affections and pains of the kidneys, affections and pains of the bladder

- **[cheng liu] 柽柳** Tamarice = Tamarix articulata = myrice, tamarisk, dysuria, stranguria and anuria

- **[bai li xiang] 百里香 [she xiang cao] 麝香草** Thymum = Thymus vulgaris, garden thyme, stones in the bladder

- **[zi yun ying shu] 紫云英属** Tragacanthum = Astragalus tragacantha = tragacanth / goat's thorn, affections and pains of the kidneys, affections and pains of the bladder, stones in the bladder, haematuria

- **[che zhu cao] 车轴草** Tribolum = Tribulus terrestris = land caltrop, but also Fagonia celtica (= caltrop) and also Trapa natans = water chestnut, stones in the bladder

- **[ji li shu] 蒺藜属** Trifolium = Trifolium fragiferum = strawberry-headed trifoil, dysuria, stranguria and anuria, stones in the bladder

- **[ru xiang shu] 乳香属** Tus = in particular Boswellia Carteri = frankincense-tree, stones in the kidney, stones in the bladder, hematuria

- **[xun ma shu] 寻麻属** Urtica = Urtica urens/ U. Dioica/ U. Pilulifera/ U.

Act: to cause restoration from collapse, to supplement body fire and reinforce Yang, and to dispel wind, cold and damp. **Indi:** collapse with cold limbs and faint pulse; impotence, frigidity, precordial and abdominal pain with cold sensation , vomiting and diarrhea or edema accompanied by aversion to cold and cold extremities, cold in patients with Yang deficiency, chronic arthritis due to attack of cold and damp (marked by persitent severe joint pain, fixed in place and accompanied by heaviness sensation and numbness) **U&D:** 3--15g **C&C:** contraindicated in pregnancy, Incompatible with rhizoma Pinelliae, Fructus Trichosanthis, Bulbus Fritillariae and Rhizome Bletillae. **[gan cao] 甘草 Liquorice Root (Radix Glycyrrhizae)** **P:** the dried root and rhizome of Glycryrhiza uralensis Fisch, Glyctrrhiza inflata bat. Or Glycyrrhiza glabra L. **T&N:** sweet in flavour, neutral in property. **Act:** to reinforce the function of the spleen and replenish Qi, to remove heat and counteract toxicity, to dispel phlegm and relieve cough, to alleviate spaamodic pain, and to moderate drug actions. **Indi:** weakness of the spleen and the stomach marked by lassitude and weakness; cardiac palpitation and shortness of breath; cough with much phlegm; spasmodic pain in the epigastrium. Abdomen and limbs; carbuncles and sores. It is often used for reducing the toxic or drastic actions of other drugs. **U&D:** 1.5--9g **C&C:** incompatible with Radix Euphorbia Pekinensis, Flos Genkwa and	Membranacea/ U. Rupestris/ U. Atravirens = nettle, affections and pains of the kidneys, dysuria, stranguria and anuria • **[xun ma shu] 寻麻属** Urtica marina = sea-nettle, stones in the bladder • **[pu tao gan] 葡萄干** Uva passa = raisins, affections and pains of the kidneys • **[ma bian cao] 马鞭草** Verbena = Verbena officinalis = vervain, dysuria, stranguria and anuria, stones in the bladder • **[ma bian cao] 马鞭草** Verbenaca = Verbena officinalis = vervain, stones in the bladder (= Hierobotane) • **[yao shui su shu] 药水 苏属** Vettonica = Betonica officinalis = betony, affections and pains of the bladder, dysuria, stranguria and anuria, stones in the bladder, affections and pains of the kidneys (for the adrenal glands) • **[jin cai shu] 堇菜属[zi luo lan] 紫萝兰** Viola coronaria = Mathiola incana / Viola odorata = stock / sweet violet, affections and pains of the bladder • **[jin cai shu] 堇菜属** Viola erratica rustica, affections and pains of the bladder • **[tang chang pu] 唐菖蒲** Xiphion = Gladiolus segetum = corn-flag, dysuria, stranguria and anuria • **[sheng jiang] 生 姜** Zinziber = zingiber officinalis = ginger, affections

Radix Kansui. **[gan jiang] 干姜Zingiber (processed) (Rhizoma Zingiberis)** **P:** the dried rhizome of Zingiber officinale (Willd) Rossc. **T&N:** pungent in flavour, hot in property. **Act:** to dispel cold from the spleen and the stomach; to promote recovery from collapse; and to eliminate damp and phlegm. **Indi:** epigastric pain with cold feeling, vomiting and diarrhea accompanied by cold extremities and faint pulse; dyspnea and cough with copious frothy expectoration. **U&D:** 3--9g **[gan sui] Gansui Root (Radix kansui)** **P:** the deired tuber root of Euphorbia Kansui. **T&N:** bitter in flavour; cold in property. **Act:** to cause drastic purgation and expel the retained water. **Indi:** anasarca, hydrothorax or ascites with dyspnea, consiption, and oliguria. **U&D:** 0.5--1.5g mostlyused for makingpills or powder after processing. **C&C:** contraindicated in prenancy, incimpatible with Radix Glycyrrhizae. **[ge gen] Kudzuvine Root (Radix Puerariae)** **P:** the dried root of Pueraria lobate. **T&N:** sweet in flavour and cool in property. **Act:** to relieve fever topromote the production of body fluid, to facilirate eruption, and to arrest diarrhea. **Indi:** fever, headache and affections thirst; diabetes, measles within adequate eruption, acute dysentery or diarrhea, stiff	and pains of the kidneys, stones in the bladder

and painful nape in hypertension.
U&D: 9--15g

[gou qi zi] 子 Barbary Wolfberry Fruit (Fructus Lycii)
P: the dried ripe fruit of Lycium barbarum.
T&N: sweet in flavour, neutral in property.
Act: to benefit the liver and the kidney, to replenish vital essnce and to improve eyesight.
Indi: general debility with deficiency of vital essence manifested by aching of the loins and knees, dizziness and tinnitus, diabetes caused by internal heat, and anemia, impaired vision.
U&D: 6—12g

[gua lou] 瓜蒌 Snakeground Fruit (Fructus Trichosanthis)
P: the dried ripe fruit of Trichosanthes kirilowii.
T&N: sweet and slighhly bitter in flavour, and cold in property.
Act: to remove heat and eliminate phlegm, to alleviate chest pain, and to facilitate bowel movement.
Indi: cough with thick purulent sputum; angina pectoris and stuffiness sensation in the chest; mastitis, lung abscess, appendicitis; constipation.
U&D: 9--15g
C&C: incompatible with Radix Aconiti and allied drugs.

[guang fang ji] 广防己 Southern Fangchi Root (Radix Aristolochiae Fangchi)
P: the dried root of Aristolochia fangchia.
T&N: bitter and pungent in flavour, cold in property.
Act: to dispel wind, relieve pain, reduce heat and induce diuresis.
Indi: general aching caused by damp-

heat; rheumatic arthralgia; edema of the lower extremities with oliguria.
U&D: 4.5--9g

[guang huo xiang] 广藿香 Cablin Patchouli herb (Herba Pogostemonis)
P: the dried aerial part of Pogostemon cablin.
T&N: pungent un flavour, warm slitghly in property.
Act: to resolve turbid damp, improve appetite, arrest vomiting and diepel summer-heat or summer-damp.
Indi: lingering of turbid damp in the spleen and stomach manifested by summer-damp affection marked by abdominal pain, vomiting and diarrhea, sinusitis with headache
U&D: 3—9g

[guang jin qian cao] 广金钱草 Snowbelleaf Tickclover Herb (Herba Desmodii Styracifolii)
P: the dried aerial part of Desmodium styracifolium.
T&N: sweet and tastless in flavour, cool in property.
Act: to remove damp-heat, induce diuesis and relieve dysuria.
Indi: urination disturbance caused by damp-heat or urolithiasis accompanied by difficult painful urination; edema with oliguria, jaudice with dark urine.
U&D: 15--30g

[guang zao] 广枣 Axillary Choerospondias Fruit (Fructus Choerospondiatis)
P: the dried ripe fruit of Choerospondias axillaris.
T&N: sweet and sour in flavour, neutral in property.
Act: to promote the flow of qi and blood, to replenish the heat and allay

excitement. **Indi:** stagnation of qi and blood with pectoral pain, palpitation and shortness of breath; uneasiness in mind. **U&D:** 1.5--2.5g **[guan mu tong] 关木通 Manchurian Dutchmanspipe Stem (Caulis Aristolochiae Manshuriensis) also [chuan mu tong] 川木通 Sichuan Clematis Stem (Caulis Clematidis Armandii)** **P:** the dried stem of Aristolochia manshuriensis. **T&N:** bitter in flavour, cold in property. **Act:** to remove heat from the heart, to relieve dysuria and promote diuresis, to stimulate menstrual discharge. **Indi:** ulcers in the mouth and on the tongue accompanied by fidgets and dark urine, edema; painful difficult urination; excessive leukorrhea amenorrhea; lack of lactation; acute arthritis due to damp heat. **U&D:** 3--6g **C&C:** used with caution in pregnancy. **[gui zhi] 桂枝Cassia Twing (Ramulus Cinnamomi)** **P:** the dried young stem of Cinnamomum cassia. **T&N:** pungent and sweet in flavour, warm in property. **Act:** to induce perspiration, to warm the channels and stimulate menstrual discharge, to reinforce Yang, to relieve palpitation and to promote the descending of Qi. **Indi:** common cold, eprgastric pain with cold feeling; amenorhea due to cold in blood, aethralgia, edema, cardiac palpitation;gastro-intestinal neurrosis with a feeling of masses of gas	

rushing up through the chest to the throat from the lower abdomen.
U&D: 3--9g

[gu jing cao] 谷精草 Pipewort Flower (Flos Eriocauli)
P: the dried capitulum with peduncle of Ericaulon buergerianum.
T&N: pungent and sweet in flavour, neutral in property.
Act: to expel wind and heat and to clear the eye of corneal opacity.
Indi: inflammation of the eye with photohobia and headache caused by wind heat, nebula.
U&D: 4.5--9g

[gu sui bu] 骨 Fortune's Drynaria Rhizome (Rhizoma Drynariae)
P: the dried rhizome of Drynaria fortunei.
T&N: bitter in flavour, warm in property.
Act: to reprenish the kidney, to strengthen the bones, to promote the healing of fracture, and to relieve pain
Indi: deficiency syndrome of the kidney marked by back pain; tinnitus, impairment injury, bone fracture; external use for alopecia areata, vitiligo.
U&D: 3—9g or 6--15g of the fresh rhizome. For external use, appropriate quantity of the fresh rhizome.

[hai zao] 海藻Seaweed (Sargassum)
P: the dried alga of Sargassum pallidum.
T&N: bitter and salty in flavour, cold in property.
Act: to soften indurated mass, to eliminate phlegm and dissipte nodulation and to induce diuresis.
Indi: goiter; scrofuld, swelling and pain of the testis, edema.

U&D: 6--12g **C&C:** incompatible with Radix Glycyrrizate. **[hei zhi ma] 黑芝麻 Black Sesame (Semen Sesami Nigrum)** **P:** the dried ripe seed of Sesamum indicum. **T&N:** sweet in flavour, neutral in property. **Act:** to tonify the liver and the kidney; to replenish vital essence and blood, and to relax the bowels. **Indi:** dizziness, blurred vision, tinnitus, impaired hearing, premature greying of the hair and beard, loss of hair after a serious disease; constipation. **U&D:** 9--15g **[hei zhong cao zi] 黑种草子 Fennelflower Seed (Semen Nigellae)** **P:** the dried seed of Nigella glandulifera. **T&N:** sweet and pungent in flavour, warm in property. **Act:** to replenish the kidney and benfit the brain, to stimulate menstruation, to promote the flow of milk, and to induce disuresis. **Indi:** tinnitus and forgetfulness, amenorrhea, inadequate secretion of milk, urinary infection, urolithiasis. **U&D:** 1.5--6g **C&C:** contraindicated in pregnancy and in patients with febrile diseases. **[he shou wu] 何首乌 Fleeceflower Root (Radix Polygoni Multiflori)** **P:** the root tuber of Polygonum multiflorum. **T&N:** bitter, sweet, and astringent in flavour, warm in property. **Act:** to counteract toxicity, to cure carbuncles, and to relax bowels.	

Indi: lymphadentitis, carbuncles, urticaria with itching, constipation, hyperlipemia. **U&D:** 6 - 12g **[he tao ren] 核桃仁 English Walnut Seed (Semen Juglandis)** **P:** the dried ripe seed of Juglans regia. **T&N:** sweet in flavour, warm in property. **Act:** to tonify the kidney, to warm the lung, and to relax the bowels. **Indi:** aching and weakness of the loins and knees, asthma and cough of deficiency-cold type, seminal emission, impotence. **U&D:** 6--9g **[he ye] 荷叶 Lotus Leaf (Folium Nelumbinis)** **P:** the dried leaf of Nelumbo nucifera. **T&N:** bitter in flavour, neutral in property. **Act:** to relieve summew-heat, to invigorate the hypofunction of the spleen; and to arrest bleeding by reducing heat in blood. Folium Nelumbinis (caebonized), to arrest bleeding, to remove blood stasis. **Indi:** summer-heat with dire thirst; diarrhea caused by summer-damp or hypofunction of spleen; spitting of blood, epistaxis, haematochezia and abbnormal uterine bleeding caused by heat in blood. Folium Nelumbinis (carboniza), various kinds of bleeding and massive postpartion haemorrhage. **U&D:** 3--9g **[hong da ji] Knoxia Root (Radix Knoxiae)** **P:** the dried root of Knoxia valerianoides. **T&N:** bitter in flavour,cold in property. **Act:** to cause drastic purgation and	

expel the retained water, and to conteract toxcity and induce subsidence of swelling and nodulation. **Indi:** hydrothorax and ascites with constipation and oliguria, carbuncles, sores scrofula. **U&D:** 1.5—3g **[hong hua] Safflower (Flos Carthami)** **P:** the dried flower of Carthamus tinctirius. **T&N:** pungent in flavour, warm in property. **Act:** to activate blood circulation and stimulate menstrual discharge; and to remove blood stasis and relieve pain. **Indi:** amenorrhea, dysmenorrhea retention of lochia; formation of mass in the abdomen; traumatic injuries or sores with swelling and pain. **U&D:** 3--9g **C&C:** used with caution in pregnancy. **[hong qi] Manyinflorescenced Sweetvetch Root (Radix Hedysari)** **P:** the dried root of Hedysarum polybotrys. **T&N:** sweet in flavour, warm in property. **Act:** to reinforce Qi and strengthen the superficial resistance, to cause diuriesis and to promote the drainage of pus and the growth of new tissue. **Indi:** deficiency of Qi with lack of strength; anorexia and loose stools; sinking of the spleen Qi marked by protracted diarrhea and prolaps of the rectum; haematochezia and abnormal uterine bleeding spontaneous sweating due to weakened superficial resistance; edema due to deficiency of Qi; abscess or boil difficult to burst; anemia diabetes mllitus; albuminuria in chronic	

nephritis.
U&D: 9—30g

[huang bo] 黄柏Amur Cork-tree (Cortex Phellodendri)

P: the dried bark of Phellodendron chinensis

T&N: bitter inflavour Cold in property.

Act: to remove damo-heat, quench fire, counteract toxicity, and to relieve consumptive fever. Cortex phellodendrri (processed with salt); to nourish Yin and reduce fire.

Indi: dysentery, jaundice and morbid leukorrhea caused by damp-heat. urinary infection; weakness and edema of legs; consumptive fever and night sweat; seminal emission; sores and skin infection with local redness and swelling; eczema with itching. Cortex Pgellidenri (processed with salt); Night sweating and consumptive fever due to exberant fire secondary to deficiency of Yin.

U&D: 3—12g appropriate quantity for external use.

[huang jing] 黄精Solomonseal Rhizome (Rhizoma Polygonati)

P: the dried rhizome of Polygonatum kinganum.

T&N: sweet in flavour, neutral in property.

Act: to reinforce Qi and nourish Yin, to invigorate the function of the spleen, to moisten the lung and to benefit the kidney.

Indi: weakness of the spleen and the stomach marked by lassitude; dryness in mouth and anorexia; dry cough due to deficiency of Yin of the lung; deficiency of vital essence and blood, diabetes caused by internal heat

U&D: 9—15g

[huangh qi] 黄芪 Milkvetch Root (Radix Astragali)

P: the dried root of Astragalus membranabeus.

T&N: sweet in flavour, warm in property.

Act: to reinforce qi and strengthen the superfical resistance, and to promote the discharge of pus and the growth of new tissue. Radix Astragali (processed with honey), to reinforce Qi and invigorate the function of the spleen.

Indi: deficiency of Qi with lack of strength; anorexia and stools, sinking of the spleen Qi manifesed by chronic diarrhea; prolapse of the rectum, haematochezia and abnormal uterine bleeding; spontaneous sweating due to weakneed superficial resistance; edema due to deficiency of Qi, abscess difficult to burst or healing; anemia, diabetes caused by internal heat, albuminuria in chronic nephritis; diabetes mellitus. Radix Astragali (processed with honey), deficiency of Qi with lack of strength, anorexia and loose stools.

U&D: 9—30g

[hu po] 琥珀Amber (Succinum)

P: a yellowish or brownish fossil resin.

Act: to calm mental state, activate blood circulation, remove blood stasis, promote diuresis, relieve stranguria.

Indi: insomnia, dreamfulness, infantile convulsion, epilepsy, abdominal pain due to blood stasis; haematuria due to acute urinary infection and urinary calculus; dysuria, straguria complicated by haematuria.

[hu lu ba] Common Fenugreek Seed (Semen Trigonellae)

P: the dried ripe seed of Trigonella foenum-graecum. **T&N:** bitter in flavour, warm in property. **Act:** to warm the kidney, dispel cold, and relieve pain. **Indi:** cold syndrome of the kidney due to Yang deficiency marked by pain and coldness in the lower abdomen, hernia; waekness and edema of the legs caused by cold-damp. **U&D:** 4.5--9g **[jiang huang] 姜黄 Turmeric** **(Rhizoma Curcumae Longae)** **P:** the dried rhizoma of Curcuma longa. **T&N:** pungent and bitter in flavour, warm in property. **Act:** to eliminate blood stasis, pronote the flow of Qi, stimulate menstrual discharge and relieve pain. **Indi:** pricking pain in the chest and hypochondriac regions; amenorrhea, mass formation in the abdomen, rheumatic pain of shoulders and arms, traumatic swelling and pain. **U&D:** 3—9g appropriate quantity for external. **[jin deng long] 锦灯笼 Franchet Groundcherry Fruit** **(Calyx seu Fructus Physalis)** **P:** the dried persistent calyx or the persistent calyx with fruit of Physalis alkekengi. **T&N:** bitter in flavour, cold in property. **Act:** to remove toxic heat, to soothe the sore throat, to resolve phlrgm, and to relieve dysuria. **Indi:** sore throat and hoarseness of voice; cough with yellow sticy sputum; dysuria, external use for pemphigus and eczema,.	

U&D: 4.5--9g for external use, appropriate quantity to be pounded into paste and applied topically. **[ji nei jin] 鸡内金 Chicken's Gizzard-skin (Endothelium Corneum Gigeriae Galli)** **P:** the dried inner wall of gizzard of Gallus gallus domesicus. **T&N:** sweet in flavour, neutral in property. **Act:** to promote digestion, to arrest seminal emission, and to cure enuresis. **Indi:** vomiting and diarrhea due to ingegestion; malnutrition due to improper feeding, and enuesis in children, seminal emission. **U&D:** 3—9g **[jing da ji] Peking Euphorbia Root (Radix Euphorbiae Pekinenisis)** **P:** the dired root of euphorbia pekinensis. **T&N:** bitter in flavour, cold in property. **Act:** to cause drastic purgation **Indi:** anasarca, hydrothroax and ascites with dyspnea, constipation and oliguria. **U&D:** 1.5—3g **C&C:** contraindicated in pregnancy, incompatible with Radix glycyrrhizae. **[jin qian cao] 金钱草 Chriatina Loosestrife (Herba Lysimachiae)** **P:** the drie herb of Lysimachia christinae. **T&N:** sweet and salty in flavour, slightly cold in property. **Act:** to remove damp-heat, relieve dysuria, to promote subsidence of swelling. **Indi:** acute urinary infection or urolithiasis with difficult painful urination; jaudice with dark urine, hepatite or biliary calculus; carbuncles,	

sores, venomous snake bite.
U&D: 15—60g of the dried hern or 30--120g of the fresh herb.

[jin ying zi] 金樱子 Cherokee Rose Fruit (Fructus Rosae Laevigatae)
P: the dried ripe fruit of Rosa laevigata.
T&N: sour, sweet and astringent in flavour, neutral in property.
Act: to arrest seminal emission, to restrain urination, and to chsk diarrhea.
Indi: nocturnal emission, spermatorrhea, enuresis, frequent urination, abnormal uterine bleeding, excessive leukorrhea, protracted diarrhea; chronic dysentery.
U&D: 6—12g

[jiu cai zi] 韭菜子 Tuber Onion Seed (Semen Allii Tuberosi)
P: the dried ripe seed of Allium tuberosum.
T&N: pungent and sweet in flavour, warm in property.
Act: to tonify the liver and kidney, to promote virility,and to arrest spontaneous emissiom.
Indi: mpotence. Seminal emission; aching of loins and knee; enuresis, frequent urination; morbid leukorrhea.
U&D: 3—9g

[ju he] Tangerine Seed (Semen Citri Reticulatae)
P: the dried ripe seed of Citrus reticulata.
T&N: bitter in flavour, neutral in property.
Act: o regulate the flow of Qi, cause subsidence of nodulation, and relieve pain.
Indi: hernia, painful swelling of the testis, mastitis with formation of painful nodules.
U&D: 3--9g

[ju ju] 菊苣 Chicory Herb (Herba Cichorii)
P: the aerial part of Cihorium glandulosum.
T&N: slightly bitter and salty in flavour, cool in property.
Act: to remove heat from the liver, to stimulate the discharge of bile, to promote digestion and increase appetite, and to cause diuresis.
Indi: jaudice caused by damp-heat; epigastric pain with impairment of appetite, edema with oliguria.
U&D: 9--18g

[kun bu] 昆布 Kelp or Tangle (Thallus Echloniae)
P: the dried thalline of Laminaria japonica.
T&N: salty in flavour, cold in property.
Act: to eliminate phlegm, soften hard masses and dissolve lump, and to cause diuresis.
Indi: goiter, scrofula, swelling and pain of the tentis, edema.
U&D: 6--12g

[ku shen] Lightyellow Sophora Root (Radix Sophirae Flavescentis)
P: the dried root of Sophora flavescens.
T&N: bitter in flavour, cold in property
Act: to remove heat and damp, to kill parasites, and to cause diuresis.
Indi: acute dysnetery with bloody stools; jaudice with oliguria; bloody and purulent leukorrhea, pudendal swelling and itching, eczema. sores with Exudation; itching of skin, scales and leprosy, external use for trichomonas vaginitis.
U&D: 4.5--9g for external use, appropriate quantity to be decocted for washing.

C&C: incompatible with ehizoma et Radix Veratri.

[lian fang] 莲房 Lotus Receptacle (Receptaculum Nelumbinis)

P: the dried receptacle of Nelumbo nucifera.

T&N: bitter and astringent in flavour, warm in property.

Act: to remove blood stasis and arrest bleeding.

Indi: abnormal uterine bleeding, haematyria, haemorrhoidal bleeding, postpartum blood stasis; ochiorrhea.

U&D: 4.5--9g

[lian qian cao] 连钱草 Longtube Ground Ivy Herb (Herba Glechomae)

P: the dried aerial part of Glechoma longituba.

T&N: pungent, and slightly bitter in flavour, cold slitghly in property.

Act: to relieve dysuria, to remove toxic heat, to eliminate blood stasis, and to cause subsidence of swelling.

Indi: acute urinary infection, urolithiasis, acute jaundice, painful swelling in sores and carbuncles, traumatic injuries,

U&D: 15--30g for external use, appropriate quantity of the dried herb to be decocted for washing or the fresh herb to be poundede into paste for topical application.

[lian qiao] 连翘 Weeping Forsythia Capsule (Fructus Forsythiae)

P: the dried fruit of Forsythia suspnsa.

T&N: bitter in flavour bitter in flavour, slightly cold in property

Act: to remove toxic heat , to cause subsidence of swelling, and to eliminate nodulation.

Indi: carbuncles. boils, lymphadenitis,

mastitis, erysipelas, upper respiratory infection, febrile disease at the early stage and at the stage with high fever, dry thirst, delirium and maculation, acute urinary infection with oliguria. **U&D:** 6—15g **[lian xu] 连须 Lotus Stamen (Stamen Nelumbinis)** **P:** the dried syamen of Nelumbo nucifera. **T&N:** sweet and astringent in flavour, neutral in property. **Act:** to astringe the kidney and arrest spontaneous emission. **Indi:** seminal emssion, spermatorrhea, excessive leukorrhea, frequent urination. **U&D:** 3—4.5g **[lian zi] 莲子 Lotus Seed (Semen Nelumbinis)** **P:** the dried root seed of Nelumbo nucifera. **T&N:** sweet and astringent in flavour, neutral in property. **Act:** to tonify the spleen, to relieve diarrhea, to replenish the kidney, to arrest seminal emission, and to nourish the heart, to induce tranquillization, **Indi:** protracted diarrhea due to hypofunction of the spleen; seminal emission, leukorrhea, palpition, insomnia. **U&D:** 6—15g **[lian zi xin] 莲子心 Lotus Plumule (Plumula Nelumbinis)** **P:** the dried young cotyledon and radicle of ripeseed of Nelumbo nucifera. **T&N:** bitter in flavour, cold in property. **Act:** to remove heatfrom the heart to calm the nerves, to restore the coordination between the heart and	

the kidney, to check emission, and to arrest bleeding.
Indi: delirium due to heat, insomnia and seminal emission due to breakdown of coordination between the heart and the kidney, haemoptysis due to heat in blood.
U&D: 1.5--3g

[li zhi he] Lychee Seed (Semen Litch)
P: the dried ripe seed of Litchi chinensis.
T&N: sweet and slitghly bitter in flavour, warm in property.
Act: to promote the flow of Qi and the subsidence of induration, and to dispel cold and relieve pain.
Indi: hernial pain of cold type, swellijng and pain of the testis,
U&D: 4.5--9g

[long dan] Chinese Gentain (Radix Gentianae)
P: the dried root and rhzime of Gentiana manshurica or Gentiana regescens.
T&N: bitter in flavour, cold in property.
Act: to eliminate damp-heat and quench the fire of the liver and gall bladder.
Indi: jaundice caused by damp-heat; swelling and itching of the vulva with excessive leukorrhea; prolonged erection; eczema accompanied by itching; blood-shot eye; impairment of hearing, pain in the mouth; convulsion.
U&D: 3—6g

[lu gen] Reed Rhizome (Rhizoma Phragmitis)
P: the fresh or dried rhizoma of Phragmites communis.
T&N: sweet in flavour, cold in property.
Act: to remove heat, to promote the production of body fluid, to relieve emesis and to alleviate dysuria,
Indi: dire thirst in febrile diseases; vomiting or retching due to heat in the

stomach; heat in the lung with cough, lung abscess, urinary infection with difficult painful urination.
U&D: 15--30g or 30--60g of the fresh rhizome to be decocted or pounded for juice.

[luo bu ma ye] 罗布麻叶 Dogbane Leaf (Folium Apocyni Veneti)
P: the dried leaf of Apocynum venetum.
T&N: sweet and bitter in flavour, cool in property.
Act: to subdue hyperactivity of the liver and soothe the nerves, to remove heat and to induce diuresis.
Indi: dizziness, palpitation and insomnia due to hyperactivity of the liver; edema with oliguria, hypertension, neurasthenia, nephritic edema.
U&D: 6--12g

[luo shi teng] 络石藤 Chinese Starjasmine Stem (Caulis Trachelospermi)
P: the dried viny stem with leaf of Trachelospermum jasminoides.
T&N: bitter in flavour, slightly cold in property.
Act: to dispel wind andd remove obstruction from the channls and to remove heat from blood and cause Subsidence of swelling,
Indi: rheumatic arthritis with muscular contracture; aching of throat, carbuncles and boils, traumatic injuries,
U&D: 6--12g for external use, thefresh drug of appropriate quantity to be pounded in to paste for topical application.

[ma dou ling] 铃 Dutchmanspipe Fruit (Fructus Aristolochiae)
P: the dried ripe fruit of Aristolochia

contorta or Aristolochia debilis.
T&N: bitter in flavour, slightly cold in property.
Act: to remove heat from the lung and relieve cough and asthma, and to remove heat from the large intestine (rectum) for the treatment of haemorrhoids.
Indi: asthma, cough and bloody stutum due to heat in the lung; bleeding, swollen and painful haemorrhoids due to heat in the large intestine.
U&D: 3--9g

[ma huang] 黄 Ephedra (Herba Ephedrae)
P: the dried herbaceous stem of Ephedra sinica.
T&N: pungent and slightly bitter in flavour, warm in property.
Act: to induce perspiratin for dispeling cold, to relieve sthma, and to cause diuresis.
Indi: common cold with wind-cold syndrome (marked by hilliness and mild fever, headache, stuffed and runing nose, general aching, but no sweating); edma in acute nephritis, bronchial asthma. Herba Ephedrae (processed with honey), cough in common cold at ater stage when chilliness has been absent.
U&D: 1.5—9g.

[mian bi xie] 萆榍 Sevenlobed Yam (Rhizoma Rhizoma dioscoreae Septemlobae)
P: the dried rhizome of Dioscorea spetemloba.
T&N: bitter in flavou, neutral in property.
Act: to remove turbid damp and to relieve rheumatic conditions.
Indi: gonorrhea with whtitish discharge from the urethra; xcessive leukorrhea,

ulcers caused by damp-heat; arthralgia of lumbar spine and knees. **U&D:** 9--15g **[mo yao] 没药Myrrh (Resina Myrrhae)** **P:** a gum-resin obtained from the stem of Commiphora molmol Engler. **T&N:** bitter in flavour, neither warm nor cool in porperty. **Act:** o disperse blood and dissolve effusion, to suppress swelling and stop pain. **U&D:** 3-9g as decoction, pill, powder; external use, paste from the powder. **[mo han lian] 墨旱莲 Yerbadetajo Herb (Herba Ecliptae)** **P:** the dried aerial part of Eclipta prostrata. **T&N:** sweet and sour in flavour, cold in property. **Act:** to relenish the liver and the kidney and to arrest bleeding by removing heat from blood. **Indi:** looseness of teeth; premature greying of hair and earb; dizziness, tinnitus, achingand weakness of loins and knees; spittingof blood; epitaxias, haematuria and diarrhea with bloody stools due to heat in blood; abnormal uterine bleeding, traumatic bleeding. **U&D:** 6--12g appropriate quantity of the fresh herb for external use. **[mu bie zi] Cochinchina Momordica Seed (Semen Momordicae)** **P:** the dried ripe seed of Momor dica cochinchinensis. **T&N:** bitter and slightly sweet in flavour, warm in property. **Act:** to promote the subsidence of nodulation and swelling, combat poisons	

and cure sores. **Indi:** sores and inflammatory swelling; mastitis, scrofula, aemorrhoids, anal fistula, chronic eczema, neurodermatitis, scald. **U&D:** 0.9--1.2g for oral administration; appropriate uantity to be grouned into powder and mixed with oil or vinegar for topical application. **[mu xiang] 木香 Costusroot (Radix Aucklandiae)** **P:** the dried root of Aucklandia lappa. **T&N:** pungent and sweet in flavour, warm in property. **Act:** to relieve pain by promoting the flow of Qi, and to improte digestion by reinforcing the spleen function. Radix Aucklandia (roasted); to check diarrhea. **Indi:** distending pain in the chest and epigastrium, tenesmus in dysentery, indigestion with anorexia. Radix Aucklandia (roaste), diarrhea with abdominal pain. **[nao yang hua] 闹羊花 Yellow Azalea Flower (Flos rhododendri Mollis)** **P:** the dried flower of Rhododendron molle. **T&N:** pungent in flavour, warm in property. **Act:** to relieve rheumatic, and to eliminalte blood stasis and alleviate pain. **Indi:** rheumatic arthralgia, traumatic injuries, wingworm. **U&D:** 0.5--1.5g to be made into infuson with wine or into pills or powder; for external use, appropriate quantity to be decocted for washing or the fresh flower to be pounded into paste for topical application.	

[nu zhen zi] Glossy Privert Fruit (Fructus Ligustri lucidi)

P: the dried ripe fruit of Ligusyrum lucidum.

T&N: sweet and bitter in flavour, cool in property.

Act: to relenish the liver and kidney, improve eyesight and promote the growth of black hair.

Indi: vertigo, tinnitus weakness in the loins and knees, premature whitening of hair and impair eyesight due to deficiency of Yin of the liver and kidney.

U&D: 6—12g.

[ou jie] 藕节 Lotus Rhizome Node (Nodus Nelumbinis Rhizomatis)

P: the dried node of Nelumbo nucifera.

T&N: sweet and astringent in flavour, neutral in property.

Act: to arrest bleeding and remove blood stasis.

Indi: haematemsis, haemoptysis, haematuria, abnormal uterine bleedintg.

U&D: 9—15g

[pu gong ying] 蒲公英 Dandelion (Herba Taraxaci)

P: the dried herb of Taraxacum mongolicum.

T&N: bitter and sweet in flavour, cold in property.

Act: to remove toxic heat, to cause subsidence of swelling and nodulation and to relieve dysuria.

Indi: boils and sores, mastitis, lymphadenitis, inflammation of the eye, sore throat, lung abscess, appendicitis, jaudice caused by damo-heat; urinary infection with difficult paimful urination.

U&D: 9--15g for external use; appropriate quantity of the fresh herb to be poundedinto paste for topical application or made into hot decoction for fumigation and irrigation. **[pu huang] 蒲黄 Cattail Pollen (Pollen Typhae)** **P:** the dried polllen of Typha angustifolia. **T&N:** sweet in flavour, neutral in property. **Act:** to arrest bleeding, to remove blood stasis, and to relieve dysuria. **Indi:** haematemisis, epistaxis, haemoptysis, abnormal uterine bleeding, traumatic bleeding, amenorrhea, dysmenorrhea; picking pain in the epigastrium; traumatic swelling and pain; dysuria with difficult pain passage of bloody urine. **U&D:** 4.5--9g for external use; appropriate quantity to be applied topically. **C&C:** used with caution in pregnancy. **[qian cao] 茜草 Indian Madder Root (Radix Rubiae)** **P:** the dried root and rhizome of Rubia cordifolia. **T&N:** bitter in flavour, cold in property. **Act:** to remove heat from blood and arrest bleeding; to eliminate blood stasis and to situmilate menstrual discharge. **Indi:** spitting of blood, epistaxis, abnormal uterine bleeding, traumatic bleeding; amenorrhea with blood stasis; arthralgia; traumatic swelling and pain. **U&D:** 6--9g **[qian jin zi] 千金子 Caper Euphoribia Seed (Semen Euphorbiae)** **P:** the dried ripe seed of Euphorbia	

lathyris L.

T&N: pungent in flavour and warm in property.

Act: to cause drastic purgation for treating edema, and eliminate blood stasis for treating masses.

Indi: edema or retaines fluid with abdominal distension,oliguria and constipation; amenorrhea due to blood stasis; external use for ringworm and verrucous vegetations.

U&D: 1--2g without shell and oil, usually made into pills or powder; for external use, approprite quantity to be pounded into paste and applied topically.

C&C: contraindicated in pregnancy or debility with loose bowels.

[qian niu zi] 牵牛子 Pharbitis Seed (Semen Pharbitidis)

P: the dried ripe seed of Pharbitis nil.

T&N: bitter in flavour, cold in property.

Act: to cause drastic purgation for clearing away retained fluid, and to kill worms.

Indi: anasarca with constipation and oliguria; dyspnea and cough causedby retained fluid; abdominal pain due to intestinal parasitosis, ascariasis, taniasis.

U&D: 3--6g

C&C: contraindicated in pregnancy, incomtible with Fructus Cortonis.

[qian shi] 芡实 Gordon Euryale Seed (Semen Euryales)

P: the dried kernel of ripe seed of Euryale ferox.

T&N: sweet and astringent in flavour, neutral in property.

Act: to benfefit the kidney and arrest seminal discharge, to invigorate the function of the spleen and relieve diarrhea, and toremoev damp and check

excessive leukorrhea.
Indi: nocturnal emission, spermatorrhea, enuresis, frequent urination, chronic diarrhea due to hypofunction of the spleen; turbid discharge mixed with urine, excessive leukorrhea.
U&D: 9—15g

[qing fen] 轻粉 Calomel (Calomelae)
P: a mercurous chloride.
T&N: pungent in flavour, cold in property.
Act: to external use: to kill parasites, to counteracte toxicity, and to promote the healing of ulcers; internal use: to remove phlegm and cause drastic purgation.
Indi: for external use: scabies, ringworm, ulcers cruris, syphilis, ulcers, eczema; for oral adminatration; edema and abdominal distension with pliguria and constipation.
U&D: for external use: appropriate quantity to be ground into powder and apply topically; for oral use: 0.1--0.2g 1--2 times a day. Mostly to be made into pills or capsules, hargle after taking the drug.
C&C: because of its toxicity, overdosage should be avoided; caution should be used when it is taken orally, and it is contraindicated in pregnancy.

[qing feng teng] 青风藤Orientvine Stem (Caulis Sinomenii)
P: the dried lianoid stem of Sinomenium acutum.
T&N: bitter and pungent in flavour, neutral in property.
Act: to relieve rheumatic conditions to remove obstruction of channles and collaterals, and to cause diuresis.
U&D: 6—12g.

[qing ye dan] Mile Swertia Herb (Herba Swertiae Mileensis)
P: the dried whole plant of Swertia mileensis.
T&N: bitter and sweet in flavour, cold in property.
Act: to increase the flow of bile, and to remove heat and damp.
Indi: jaudice with dark urine; acute urinary infection with difficult painful urination.
U&D: 10--15g
C&C: used with caution to patients with deficiency-cold.

[qu mai] Lilac Pink Herb (Herba Dianthi)
P: the dried aerial part of Dianthus superbus.
T&N: bitter in flavour and cold in property.
Act: to relieve dysuria and to stimulate menstrual discgarge.
Indi: urinary infection and urolithiasis with difficult painful urination or haematuria, amenorrhea.
U&D: 9--15g
C&C: contraindicated in pregnancy.

[ren dong teng] 忍冬藤 Honeysuckle Stem (Caulis Lonicerae)
P: the dried stem and branch of Lonicera japonica.
T&N: sweet in flavour, cold in property.
Act: to remove toxic heat and to dispel wind from the channels and collaterals.
Indi: epidemic febrile diseases, acute dysentery, carbuncles, sores, acute arthritis with redness, swelling and pain of joint.
U&D: 9--30g

[ren shen] 人参 Ginseng
(Radix Ginseng)

P: the dried root of panax ginseng C.A.Mey. The drug derived from the cultivated form is known as [yuan shen] 园参 "Yuanshen" (Garden Ginseng) and the drug derived from the wild origin is known as [shan shen] 山参 "Shansheng" (Wild Ginseng).the drug is collected in autumn and washed clean. sun-dried or bake dried.

T&N: sweet and slightly bitter in flavour, neutral in property.

Act: to reinforce the vital energy, to remedy collapse and restore the normal pulse, to benefit the spleen and lung, to promote the production of body fluid, and to calm the nerves.

Indi: prostration with impending collapse marked by cold limbs and faint puls; diminished functuin of spleen with loss of appetite; cough and dyspnea due to disminished function of lung thirst due to impairment of body fluid and of diabetes caused by internal heat; general weakness with irritability and insomnia in chronic diseases; impotence or frigidity; heart failure,cardiogenic shock.

U&D: 3--9g

C&C: incompatible with Rhozoma et Radix Veratri.

[rou cong rong] 肉从蓉Desertliving Cistanche
(Herba Cistanches)

P: the dried fleshy stem with scales of Cistanche deserticola.

T&N: sweet and salty in flavour, warm in property.

Act: to reinforce the kidney, replenish vital essence and blood, and induce laxation.

Indi: impotence, infertility; general weakness with aching of the loins and kness, constipation. **U&D:** 6--9g **[rou gui] 肉桂 Cassia Bark (Cortex Cinnamomi)** **P:** the dried stem bark of Cinnamomum cassia. **T&N:** pungent and sweet in flavour, hot in property. **Act:** to supplement boddy fire, reinforce Yang and lead the fire back to the kidney, to dispel cold and relieve pain, and to activite blood circulation and stimulate menstrual discharge. **Indi:** impotence, frigidity, feeling of coldness and pain in the loins and knees; dyspnea in deficiency syndrome of the kidney, dizziness, inflammation of the eye and sore throat due to Yang deficiency; precordial and abdominal pain with cold sensation, vomiting and diarrhea in deficiency-cold syndrome; neurosis with a feeling of gas rushing up through the chest to the throat from the lower abdomen; amenorrhea, dysmenorrhea. **U&D:** 1--4.5g **C&C:** used with caution in patients with bleeding tendency or pregnancy; incompatible with Halloysitum Rubrum. **[san bai cao] Chinese Lizardtail Rhizome or Herb (Herba Saurur)** **P:** the died rhizome or herb of Saururus chinensis (lour).Baill (fam, Saururaceae). **T&N:** pungent and sweet in flavour, cold in property. **Act:** to remove toxic heat, and chase diuresis. **Indi:** dysuria with painful and difficult	

urination; urinary infection, nephritic edema, morbid leukorrhea; external use for boils,sores and eczema. **U&D:** 15--30g for external use, appropriate quantity to be pounded into paste for topical application. **[sang bai pi] White Mulberry Root-bark (Cortex M)** **P:** the drid root bark of Morus alba. **T&N:** bitter in flavour, cold in property. **Act:** to remove heat from the lung, to relieve asthma, and to induce diuresis. **Indi:** cough and astma caused by heat in the lung; anasarca with oliguria. **U&D:** 3--9g **[sang piao xiao] Egg Capsule of mantid (Ootheca Mantidis)** **P:** the dried gee capsule of Tenodera sinensis. **T&N:** sweet and salty in flavour, neutral in property. **Act:** to tonify the kidney, arrest spontaneous emission, reduce excessive urination and cure turbid discharge from the urethra. **Indi:** nocturnal emission, frequent urination, turbid discharge with urine. **U&D:** 4.5--9g **[san qi] 三七Sanchi (Radix Notoginseng)** **P:** the dried rot of Panax notoginseng (Burk).F.H.Chen (Fam.Araliaceae). **T&N:** sweet, bitter slightly in flavour, warm in property. **Act:** to eliminate blood stasis, arrest bleeding, cause subsidence of swelling and alleviate pain.. **Indi:** haemoptysis, haematemesis, epistaxis, haematochezia, abdomal uterine bleeding, traumatic bleeding,	

pricking pain, in the chest and abdomen, traumatic swelling and pain. **U&D:** 3--9g to be grund into powder and taken with water; appropriate quantity for external use. **C&C:** used with caution in pregnancy. **[sha ji] 沙棘 Seabuckthorn Fruit (Fructus Hippophae)** **P:** the dried ripe fruit of Hippophae rhammnoides. **T&N:** sour and astringent in flavour,warm in property. **Act:** to relieve cough and promote expectoration, to promote indigestion and remove stagnancy of food and to promote blood circulation and remove blood stasis. **Indi:** cough with profuse expectoration; indigestion, stagnancy of food with abdominal pain; traumatic swelling and ecchymoses. Amenorrhea due to blood stasis. **[shang lu] 商陆 Pokeberry Root (Radix Phytolaccae)** **P:** the dried root of Phytolacca acinosa. **T&N:** bitter in flavour, cold in property. **Act:** to cause drastic purgation and alsodiuresis, to counteract toxicity, and to reduce nodulation. **Indi:** anasarca with oliguria and constipation; external use for carbuncles and sores. **U&D:** 3--9g for external use appropriate quantity of the fresh root to be pounded into paste or the dried root to be grounded into powder, and applied topically. **C&C:** contraindicated in pregnancy. **[shan yao] 山药Common Yam Rhizome (Rhizoma Dioscoreae)** **P:** the dried rhiaome of Dioscorea	

opposita Thunb.
T&N: sweet in flavour, neutral in property.
Act: to replenish the spleen and stomach, to promote fluid secretion and benefit the lung, and to strengthen the kidney and restrain seminal discharge; Rhizoma Dioscoreae (stir-fried with bran), to replenish the spleen and promote the stomach function.
Indi: anorexia and chronic diarrhea due to diminish function of the spleen; cough and dyspnea due to diminish function of the lung; seminal emossion, excessive leukorrhea; frequency of urination or
diabetes due to deficiency condition of the kidney; Rhizoma Dioscoreae (stir-fried with bran); diminish function of the spleen with anoexia, diarrhea and excessive leukorrhea.
U&D: 15--30g

[shan zhu yu] 山茱萸 Asiatic Cornelian Cherry Fruit (Fructus Corni)
P: the dried ripe scarcocarp of Cornus officinalis Sieb.et Zucc.
T&N: sour and astringent in flavour, slightly warm in property.
Act: to replenish the liver and kidney, restrain seminal discharge and relieve collapse.
Indi: dizziness, tinnitus, soreness in the loins and knees, impotence, seminal emission, enuresis, frequency of urination, excessive uterine bleeding and leukorrhea; collapse with profuse sweating diabetes.
U&D: 6--12g

[sha yuan zi] 沙苑子 Flatstem Milkvetch Seed (Semen Astragali Complanati)
P: the dried ripe seed of Astagalus

complanatus.
T&N: sweet in flavour, warm in property.
Act: to benefit the liver and the kidney, arrest seminal discharge, restrain urination and improve eyesight.
Indi: back pain, nocturnal emission and premature ejaulation in deficiency syndromes of the kidney; turbid discharge with urination; excessive leukorrhea; dribbling of urine after urination; dizziness and blurred vision.
U&D: 9--15g

[she chuang zi] 蛇床子 Common Cnidium Fruit (Fructus Cnidii)
P: the dried ripe fruit of Cnidium monnieri.
T&N: pungent and bitter in flavour, warm in property.
Act: to warm the kidney and promote virility, to remove damp, to dispel wind and to kill worms.
Indi: impotence, frigidity, excessive leukorrhea caused by cold-damp; extenal use for eczema of external genitalia, vulval itching trichomonas vaginitis.
U&D: 3--9g appropriate quantity to be made into hot decoction for fuming and washing, or to be ground into powder for topicalapplication after mix with liquid.

[shi wei] 石苇 Shearer's Pyrrosia Leaf (Folium Pyrrosiae)
P: the dried leaf of Pyrrosia shearei or Ptrrosia petiolosa.
T&N: sweet and bitter in flavour, slightly cold in property.
Act: to Induce diuresis, relieve dysuria, remove heat and arrest bleeding.
Indi: urinary infection and urolithiasis

with difficult painful urination; spitting of blood, epistaxis, haematuria, abnormal uterine bleeding; cough and asthma due to heat in the lung. **U&D:** 6--12g **[shu di huang] 黄Rehmannia Root (Processed)** **(Radix Rehmanniae Praeparata)** **P:** the processed Rehmanniae. **T&N:** sweet in flavour, slightly warm in property. **Act:** to nourish Yin tonify blood and reprenish essence. **Indi:** defficiency of Yin of the liver and the kidney marked by aching and limpness of the loin and knee, consumptive fever; night eating and eminal emssion; diabete caused by internal heat, anemia; cardiac palpitation; menstrual disorder, abnormal uterine bleeding; dizziness, tinnitus; premature greying of beard and hair. **U&D:** 9--15g. **[su mu]苏木 Sappan Wood** **(Lignum Sappan)** **P:** is the dried heart wood of Caesalpinia sappan. **T&N:** sweet and salty in flavour, neutral in property. **Act:** to promote blood circulation and remove blood stasis, and to cause subsidence of swelling and relieve pain. **Indi:** amenorrhea, dysmenorrhea, blood stasis after delivery; prickking pain in the chest and abdomen, traumatic swelling and pain. **U&D:** 3--9g **C&C:** used with caution in pregnancy.	

[suo yang] 锁阳 Songaria Cynomorium Herb (Herba Cynomorii)

P: the dried fleshly stem of Cynomorium songaricum.

T&N: sweet in flavour, warm in property.

Act: to reinforce the kidney Yang, to replenish vital essence and blood, and to relax bowels.

Indi: aching and weakness of the loins and knees; impotence, spermatorrhea, constipation.

U&D: 4.5--9g

[ting li zi]葶苈子 Pepperweed Seed or Tansymustard Seed (Semen Descurainiae/Semen Lepidii)

P: the dried ripe seed of Lepidium apetalum.

T&N: pungent and bitter in flavour, cold in property.

Act: to quench fire in the lung, to relieve dyspnea, and to cause diuresis.

Indi: dyspnea or orthopnea; cough with profuse expectoration and fullness sensation in the chest; accompanied by hydrothorax; ascities and oliguria, edema in pulmonary heart disease.

U&D: 3--9g

[tong cao] Ricepaperplant Pith (Medulla Tetrapanacis)

P: the dried stem pith of Tetrapanax papyriferus.

Act: to remove heat, induce diuresis and stimulate the flow of milk.

Indi: dysuria with difficult painful urination, edema and oliguria, lack of milk secretion.

U&D: 3--4.5g

[tu fu ling] 土茯苓 Glabrius Greenbrier Rhizome (Rhizoma Smilacia Glabrae) **P:** the dried rhizome of Smilax glabra Roxb. **T&N:** sweet and tastless in flavour, neutral in property. **Act:** to remove damp, to counteract toxicity, and to improve the mobility of joints. **Indi:** dysuria with turbid discharge, morbid leukorrhea, chronic eczema; contracture of limbs and muscle pain in syphilis with mercury poisoning. **U&D:** 15--60g **[tu si zi] 菟丝子 Dodder Seed (Semen Cuscutae)** **P:** the dried ripe seed of Cuscuta chinensis **T&N:** sweet in flavour, warm in property. **Act:** to arrest seminal discharge and abnormal urination, prevent abortion; to improve eyesight and relieve diarrhea by rplenishing and tonifying the liver and the kidney. **Indi:** impotence, seminal emission; dripping of urine after urination, enuresis, frequent urination; aching and weakness of loins and knees; blurred vision and tinnitus; threatend abortion due to hypofunction of the kidney; diarrhea due to hypofunction of the spleen and thekidney; external use for vitiligo. **U&D:** 6—12g appropriate quantity for external use. **[wu wei zi] 五味子 Chinese Magnoliavine Fruit (Fructus Schisandraeis)** **P:** the dried ripe fruit of Schisandra chinensis or Schisandra sphenanthera.	

T&N: sour and sweet in flavour, warm in property. **Act:** to arrest discharge, relenish Qi, promote fluid secretion, tonify the kidney, and induce sedation. **Indi:** chronic cough and asthma; nocturnal emission, spermatorrhea; enuresis, frequent urination; protracted diarrhea, spontaneous sweating, night sweating; impairment of body fluid with thirst; shortness of breath and feeble pulse; diabetes caused by internal heat; palpitation and insomnia. **U&D:** 1.5--6g **[wu yao]乌药Combined Spicebush Root** **(Radix Linderae)** **P:** the dried root tuber of Lindera aggregata. **T&N:** pungent in flavour, warm in property. **Act:** to smooth the flow of Qi and relieve pain and to warm and tonify the kidney and the urinary bladder. **Indi:** distending pain in the chest, and abdomen accompanied by dyspnea; enuresis and frequency of urination due to hypo function of the urinary bladder; hernia, dysmenorrhea. **U&D:** 3--9g **[xian he cao] 仙鹤草 Hairyvein Agrimonia Herb** **(Herba Agrimoniae)** **P:** the dried aerial part of Agrimonia pilosa. **T&N:** bitter and astringent in flavour, neutral in property. **Act:** to arrest bleeding, to stop malarial attacks, to relieve dysentery, and to counteract toxicity. **Indi:** haemoptysis, hematemesis,	

abnormal uterine bleeding; malaria; dysentery with bloody stools; overstrain; boils and sores; pudental itching with excessive leukorrhea. **U&D:** 6—12g appropriate quantity for external use. **[xian mao] 仙茅 Common Curculigo Rhizome (Rhizoma Curculiginis)** **P:** the dried rhizome of Gurculigo orchioides. **T&N:** pungent in flavour, hot in property. **Act:** to reinforce the kidney Yang, to strengthen the tendons and bones, and to dispel cold - damp. **Indi:** impotence, limpness of the limbs, arthritis of the lumbar and knee joints due to affection of cold-damp; watery diarrhea with aversion to cold. **U&D:** 3--9g **[xiao hui xiang] 小茴香 Fennel (Fructuas Foeniculi)** **P:** the dried ripe fruit of Foeniculum vulgare Mill. **T&N:** pungent in flavour, warm in property. **Act:** to dispel cold and relive pain, to regulate the stomach function; Fructus Foeniculi (processed with salt), to dispel cold from the interior and relieve pain. **Indi:** scrotal hernia with pain and cold extremities; dysmenorrhea with lower abdominal pain and cold sensation; distending pain in epigastrium with anorexia, vomiting and diarrhea, hydroceles of tunica vaginalis; Fructus Foeniculi (processed with salt), scrotal hernia with pain and cold extremities; dysmenorrhea with abdominal pain cause by cold. **U&D:** 3--6g	

[xiao ji] 小蓟 Field Thistle Herb (Herba Cirsii) **P:** the dried aerial part of Cirsium setosum. **T&N:** sweet and bitter in flavour, cool in property. **Act:** to arrest bleeding by reducing heat in blood, and to remove blood stasis and induce the subsidence of swelling. **Indi:** epistaxis, spitting of blood, haematuria, haematochezia, abdominal uttering bleeding, traumatic bleeding; carbuncles and sores. **U&D:** 4.5--9g for oral administration, appropriate quantity of the fresh herb to be pounded for topical application. **[xiao tong cao] 小通草 Stachyurus or Japanese Helwingia Pith (Medulla Helwingiae/Medulla Stachyuri)** **P:** the dried stem pith of Stachyurus himalaicus Hook or Helwingia japonica. **T&N:** sweet and tasteless in flavour, cold in property. **Act:** to remove heat, to cause diuresis, and to promote lactation. **Indi:** oliguria, galactostasis, urinary infection. **U&D:** 2.5--4.5g **[xie bai] Longstamen Onion Bullb (Bulbus Allii Macrostemi)** **P:** the dried bulb of Allium macrostemon. **T&N:** pungent and bitter in flavour, warm in property. **Act:** to remove the retained phlegm from the chest, promote the flow of Qi and relieve its stagnation. **Indi:** angina pectoris, cough and dyspnea caused by retained phlegm, tenesmus in dysentery.	

U&D: 4.5--9g

[xue jie] 血竭Dragon's Blood (Sanguis Draconis)

P: a red resin secreted from the fruit of Daemonops draco BL.

Act: to eliminate blood stasis, to relieve pains and to promote the healing of wounds.

Indi:

[ya hu nu] 亚乎奴 (锡生藤) Common Cissampelos Herb (Herba Cissampelotis)

P: the dried whole plant of Cissampelos pareira.

T&N: sweet bitter in flavour, warm in property.

Act: to cause the subsidence of swelling, and relieve pain, to arrest bleeding, and to promote the growth of new tissues.

Indi: traumatic swelling, pain and bleeding.

U&D: for traumatic swelling and pain; appropriate quantity of the dried powder to be applied after mixing with egg white; for traumatic bleeding, appropriate quantity of dry powder to be applied externally, 1--2 times daily.

[yi mu cao] 益母草 Mothwort Herb (Herba Leonuri)

P: the dried aerial part of Leonurus heterophyllus.

T&N: bitter and pungent in flavour, slightly in property.

Act: to regulate menstruation by activating blood circulation, and induce diuresis.

Indi: menstrual disorders, dysmenorrhea, amenorrhea, incessant dripping of lochia edema and oliguia such as edema in acute nephritis.

U&D: 9--30g
C&C: contraindicated in pregnancy.

[ying su qiao] Poppy Capsule
(Pericarpium Papaveris)
P: the dried pericarp of ripe fruit of Papaver somniferum.
T&N: sour and astringent in flavour, neutral in property.
Act: to relieve cough, to arrest diarrhea and to alleviate pain.
Indi: chronic cough; chronic diarrhea with prolapse of rectum; epigastric and abdominal pain.
U&D: 3--6g
C&C: long-term administration is prohibited for prevention of addiction.

[yin yang huo] 淫羊藿 also [xian ling pi] 仙灵脾 Epimedium Herb
(Herba Epimedi)
P: the dried aerial part of Epimedium breviconum.
T&N: pungent and sweet in flavour, warm in property.
Act: to reinforce the kidney Yang, strengthen the tendons and bones, and relieve rheumatic conditions.
Indi: impotence, seminal emission, weakness of the limbs; rheumatic or rheumatoid arthralgia with numbness and muscle contracture, climacteric hypertension.
U&D: 3--9g

[yi yi ren] 薏苡仁 Coix Seed
(Semen Coici)
P: the dried ripe kernel of Coix lacrymajobi.
T&N: sweet and tasteless in flavour, cool in property.
Act: to invigorate the spleen function and promote diuresis, to alleviate arthritis, to arrest diarrhea, to remove

heat and facilitate the drainage of pus.
Indi: edema, oliguria, arthritis with contracture of joints; diarrhea due to diminished function of the spleen; lung abscess, appenndicitis; verruca plana.
U&D: 9--30g

[yi zhi] 益智 also [yi zhi ren] 益智仁 Sharpleaf Glangal Fruit (Fructus Alpiniae Oxyphyllae)
P: the dried ripe fruit of Alpinia oxyphylla.
T&N: pungent in flavour, warm in property.
Act: to warm the spleen, relieve diarrhea, and arrest excessive discharge of saliva, and to warm the kidney, and arrest seminal discharge and abnormal urination.
Indi: cold syndrome of the spleen characterized by diarrhea; abdominal pain with cold sensation and salivation; cold syndrome of kidney characterized by enuresis; frequent urination, seminal emission and whitish discharge from urethra.
U&D: 3--9g

[yuan hua] Lilac Daphne Flower Bud (Flos Genkwa)
P: the dried flower bud of Daphne genkwa.
T&N: bitter and pungent in flavour, cold in property
Act: to cause drastic purgation and expel the retained water, and to kill parasites.
Indi: anasarca, hydrothorax and ascitc with dyspnea, constipation and oliguria, external use for scabies, tinea and frostbite.
U&D: 1.5--3g Flos Genkwa (processed with vinegar), to be ground into powder

0.6--0.9g, once daily.
C&C: contraindicated in pregnancy. Incompatible with Radix Glycyrrhizae.

[yu li ren] 郁李仁 Chinese Dwarf Cherry Seed (Semen Pruni)

P: the dried ripe seed of Prunus humilis.
T&N: pungent and bitter and sweet in flavour, neutral in property.
Act: to relax the bowels and to cause diuesis.
Indi: stagnancy of undigested food with abdominal distension and constipation; weakness and edema of the legs with oliguria.
U&D: 3--9g
C&C: used with caution in pregnancy.

[yu xing cao] 鱼腥草 Heartleaf Houttuynia herb (Herba Houttuyniae)

P : the dried aerial part of Houttuynia cordata.
T&N: pungent in flavour, slightly cold in property.
Act: to remove toxic heat, to promote the drainage of pus, and relieve dysuria.
Indi: lung abscess with purulent expectoration; heat in the lung with cough and dyspnea; acute dysentery; acute urinary infection; carbuncles and sores.
U&D: 15--25g to be boiled briefly. 30-50g of the fresh herb to be decocted or pounded to make juice for oral administration. For external use, appropriate quantity to be pounded into paste for topical application or made into hot decoction for fuming and washing of the lesion.

[yu zhi zi] Akebia Fruit
(Fructus Akebiae)

P: the dried nearly ripe fruit of Akebia quinata.
T&N: bitter in flavour, cold in property.
Act: to regulate the flow of the liver Qi, to promote blood circulation and relieve pain, and to cause diuresis.
Indi: epigastric and hypochondriac distension and pain; amenorrhea, dysmenorrhea, oliguria, snake and insect bite.
U&D: 3--9g

[ze xie] Oriental water-plantain Rhizome
(Rhizoma Alismatis)

P: the dried tuber of Alisma orientalis.
T&N: sweet in flavour, cold in property
Act: to cause diuresis, and to remove damp-heat.
Indi: edema with oliguria; diarrhea with diminished discharge of urine; vertigo due to retention of fluid; acute urinary infection with difficult painful urination; hyperlipemia.
U&D: 6--9g

[zhi zhi] Cape Jasmine Fruit
(Fructus Gardeniae)

P: the dried ripe fruit of Gardenia jasminoides.
T&N: bitter in flavour, cold in property.
Act: to reduce fire and ease the mind, to eliminate damp-heat, and to remove heat from blood and counteract toxicity; Fructus Gardeniae (charred), to arrest bleeding by remove heat from blood.
Indi: febrile diseases with restlessness; jaundice with dark urine; haematuria with difficult painful urination; hemoptysis and epistaxis caused by heat in the blood;

inflammation of the eye, boils and sores; external use for sprains and burses. Fructus Gardeniae (charred), hemophthisis, epistaxis, haematuria and abnormal uterine bleeding caused by heat in the blood. **U&D:** 6--9g for external use, appropriate quantity of unprocessed fruit to be ground into powder and applies topically after mixing with a liquid. **[zhu ling] Chuling (Polyporus)** **P:** the dried sclerotium of Polyporus umbrellatus. **T&N:** sweet and tasteless in flavour and neutral in property. **Act:** to induce diuresis and remove damp. **Indi:** oliguria, edema, diarrhea, dysuria, excessive leukorrhea. **U&D:** 6--12g **[zi he che] 紫河车 Human Placenta (Placenta Hominis)** **P:** the dried placenta of a healthy woman. **T&N:** sweet and salty in flavour, warm in property. **Act:** to warm the kidney, replenish vital essence Qi and blood. **Indi:** emaciation, hectic fever, night sweating, cough, breath and anorexia in consumptive diseases; impotence, seminal emission; shortness of infertility; lack of lactation. **U&D:** 1.5--3g. to be ground into powder for oral administration.	
MINERALS	**MINERALS**
[hua rui shi] 花蕊石 Ophicalcite (Ophicalcitum) **P:** a marble containing green serpentine.	• **[ming fan] 明矾 alumen** = alum, affections and pains of the kidneys, incontinence of urine

T&N: acid and astringent in flavour, neither warm nor cool in property.
Act: to eliminate blood stasis, to dissolve clots and effusion, to stop bleeding.
Indi: haemoptysis, haematemesis, externally used as haemostatic for incised wounds.
U&D: 3-9g as powder.
C&C: used with caution for pregnancy.

[hua shi] 滑石 Talc (Talcum)
P: a silicates mineral of Talcum group, containing mainly hydrate magnesium silicate.
T&N: sweet and tasteless in flavour, cold in property.
Act: to relieve dysuria, to eliminate summer heat and damp, and to arrest discharges.
Indi: urinary infection, urolithiasis with difficult urination accompanied by burning pain; fidgetiness and thirst caused by summer damp, diarrhea caused by damp-heat; external use for eczema, sores with marked exudation, miliaria.
U&D: 9--24g appropriate quantity for external use.

[hu po] 琥珀 Amber (Succinum)
P: a yellowish or brownish fossil resin.
Act: to calm mental state, activate blood circulation, remove blood stasis, promote diuresis, and relieve stranguria.
Indi: insomnia, dreamfulness, infantile convulsion, epilepsy, abdominal pain due to blood stasis; haematuria due to acute urinary infection and urinary calculus; dysuria, stranguria complicated by haematuria.

[liu huang] Sulphur (Sulphur)
P: obtained from the natural sulphur of the natural elemental mineral group.

- **[ming fan] 明矾** alumen fissum (broken alum), haematuria
- **[ming fan] 明矾** alumen scistum (cut out alum), incontinence of urine
- **[han tie shui] 含铁水** aqua ferrata = ferruginous water, affections and pains of the bladder
- **[li qing] 沥青** bitumen, affections and pains of the kidneys

[bai e] 白垩 cimolia creta, affections and pains of the bladder, stones in the bladder

- **xiao hua] 硝花** nitri flos = flower of saltpetre or of nitre, affections and pains of the bladder
- **[xiao shi] 硝石** nitrum = saltpetre or nitre, affections and pains of the kidneys, affections and pains of the bladder
- **[li qing] 沥青** pix = pitch, affections and pains of the kidneys
- **[yan] 盐** sal = salt, dysuria, stranguria and anuria, stones in the bladder
- **[ze shi] 赭石** sil pictorium = ochre of the painters (probably red or yellow ochre), stones in the bladder
- **[fu shi] 浮石** spongites = an unidentified spongy stone, dysuria, stranguria and anuria
- **[hu bo] 琥珀** sucinum = amber, dysuria, stranguria and anuria, stones in

The drug is collected and melted to free from foreign matter, or obtained by processing the minerals containing sulphur. **T&N:** sour in flavour, warm in property **Act:** to counteract poisons, kill parasites, and sores when used externally, to reinforce Yang and relax the bowels when taken orally. **Indi:** external use for scabies, favus, chronic sores and malignant ulcers oral administration for impotence with cold lower extremities; asthma or constipation of deficiency -cold type. **U&D:** for external use, appropriate quantity to be applied topically after being ground into powder and mixed with oil for oral administration 1.5--3g being used in making pills or powder after being processed. **C&C:** used with caution in pregnancy. **[zi ran tong] 自然铜 Pyrite (Pyritum)** **P:** a mineral of sulfide of Pyrite group, containing mainly iron sulfide. **T&N:** pungent in flavour, neutral in property. **Act:** to eliminate blood stasis, promote healing of fracture and relieve pain. **Indi:** traumatic swelling and pain, bone fracture. **U&D:** 3--9g mostly used in making pills or powder, appropriate quantity for external use. **[zi shi ying] 紫石英 Fluorite (Fluoritum)** **P:** a fluoride mineral of fluorite group, containing mainly calcium fluoride. **T&N:** sweet in flavour, warm in property. **Act:** to induce sedation and to warm the lung and the uterus. **Indi:** insomnia, dream-disturbed sleep and cardiac palpitation; cough and	the bladder • **[zi ran liu] 自然硫** sulphur = sulphur, affections and pains of the kidneys, stones in the bladder • **[bu li fen] 玻璃粉** vitrum tritum = glass powder, affections and pains of the kidneys

asthma in deficiency syndrome of the lung; infertility. **U&D:** 9--15g	
ANIMALS, THEIR PARTS AND SPELLS	**ANIMALS, THEIR PARTS AND SPELLS**
[ban mao] Blister Beetle (Mylabris) **P:** the dried body of mylabris phalerata. **T&N:** pungent in flavour, hot in property. **Act:** to eliminate blood stasis and masses, to induce blisters and to cauterize ulcers. **Indi:** mass in the abdomen, cancer, chronic tinea, scrofula, vegetation, abscess difficult to burst, malignant sore and slough. **U&D:** 0.03--0.06g, decocted after processing or used for making pills or powders, for external use, appropriate quantity to be ground into powder or seeped into wine or vinegar or preparing for ointment for topical application in limited areas. **C&C:** very toxic, caution for oral administration, contraindicated in pregnancy. **[chan su] Toad Venom (Venenum Bufonis)** **P:** the dried secretion of Bufobufo gargarizans. **T&N:** pungent in flavour, warm in property. **Act:** to counteract toxicity, to relieve pain, and to restore consciousness . **Indi:** carbuncles, boils sore throat; vomiting, diarrhea, abdominal pain and impaired consciousness in heatstroke;	• **[lu shen]** 驴肾 ass (kidneys), affections and pains of the bladder, dysuria, stranguria and anuria, incontinence of urine • **[wu ming yu]** 无名鱼 bacchus (an unidentified fish) (the stone of the head), stones in the bladder • **[kao xi shuai]** 烤蟋蟀 balm crichets (toasted), affections and pains of the bladder, dysuria, stranguria and anuria • **[bian fu nao]** 蝙蝠脑 bat (brain), affections and pains of the kidneys • **[feng la]** 蜂蜡 bees wax, affections and pains of the kidneys • **[wu ming dong wu]** 无名动物 bestiolae adhaerentes saxis in lapidicinis (unidentified “little animals that adhere to the walls of stone quarries”), stones in the bladder • **[gong yang xue]** 公羊血 billy goat (blood), stones in the kidney, stones in the bladder • **[mu gou ru]** 母狗乳 bitch (milk), affections and pains of the kidneys, incontinence of urine • **[huang you]** 黄油 butter, affections

anesthesia for surgical operations.
U&D: 0.015--0.03g almost used in making pills or powder, appropriate quantity for external use.
C&C: used with caution in pregnancy.

[chan tui] 蝉蜕 Cicada Slough (Periostracum Serpentis)
P: the slough of Cryptotympana pustulata Fabricii.
Act: to dispel wind-heat ,to soothe sore throat, to promote eruption, to clear the eye of corneal opacity, and to arrest spasm.
Indi: upper respiratory infection with sore throat; hoarseness of voice, measles with inadequate eruption; urticaria with itching, inflammation of eye.
U&D: 3--6g

[chong bai la] 腊 Insect Wax (Cera Chinensis)
P: the purified wax secreted by male insect of Ericerus pela, which dwelling gregariously at the stem and branch of Frasxinus chinensis.
Indi: excipient and lubricant for making pills and tablets.

[di long] 地龙 Ground Dragon (Pheretima)
P: the dried body of Pheretima aspergillum.
T&N: salty in flavour, cold in property.
Act: to remove heat, to arrest convulsions to remove obstruction from the collaterals, to relieve asthma, and cause diuresis.
Indi: high fever with impaired consciousness; convulsions, arthralgia, numbness of limbs, hemiplegia, cough and asthma due to heat in the lung, edema and oliguria, hypertension.
U&D: 4.5--9g

and pains of the kidneys, dysuria, stranguria and anuria

- **[xiao niu] 小 牛** calf (tallow) affections and pains of the kidneys, dysuria, stranguria and anuria

- **[hai li] 海 狸** castoreum, affections and pains of the kidneys

- **[ji pang guang jie shi] 鸡膀胱结石** chicken (little stones in the bladder), dysuria, stranguria and anuria, stones in the kidney, stones in the bladder

- **[ji wei mo] 鸡胃膜** chicken (membrane of the stomach), stones in the bladder

- **[chou chong] 臭虫** cimex (smeared on the glans), affections and pains of the bladder

- **[xie tou] 蟹头** crab (head), stones in the bladder

- **[wu ze luan] 乌贼卵** cuttle-fish (eggs), affections and pains of the kidneys

- **[lu jiao] 鹿角** deer (horns), affections and pains of the kidneys

- **[gou wuo] 狗 窝** dog's bed (with the spell: "May I not urinate in my bed as does the dog in its!"), incontinence of urine

- **[gou rou] 狗肉** dog (fat), incontinence of urine

- **[ge fen] 鸽粪** dove (excrements), affections and pains of the kidneys,

[e jiao] 阿胶 Donkey-hide Gelatin (Ass-hide Glue Colla Corii Asini) **P:** solid glue prepared from the skin of ass, Equus asinus L. **T&N:** sweet in flavour, light in property. **Act:** to nourish the blood for anemia, to nourish the vital essence, to arrest bleeding. **Indi:** general weakness, all kinds of bleeding, insomnia, dry cough, haemoptysis, haematemesis, haematuria, and excessive menstrual discharge. **feng fang] 蜂房 Wasp's nest (Nidus Vespae)** **P:** the nest of wasps or hornets, Polistes olivaceus (Degeer), Polistes japonicus Sauss. or parapolybia varia Fabricii. **T&N:** sweet in flavour, neutral in property. **Indi:** used externally for suppurative skin diseases; as gargles for pain and swelling of gums; internally for convulsions, urticaria, tumor and chronic cough. **[feng mi] 蜂蜜 Honey (Mel)** **P:** a saccharine fluid deposited by Apis mellifica. **T&N:** sweet in flavour, neutral in property **Act:** to replenish the spleen and stomach, to relieve dryness, to alleviate pain, and to counteract toxicity. **Indi:** epigastric pain alleviatc after meal or by pressing, dry cough, constipation, external use for sore, scalds and burns **U&D:** 15--30g	affections and pains of the bladder, dysuria, stranguria and anuria, stones in the kidney, stones in the bladder • **[ge wei zhong sui shi] 鸽胃中碎石** dove (little stones in the stomach), dysuria, stranguria and anuria, stones in the bladder • **[ge wei mo] 鸽胃膜**dove (membrane of the stomach), stones in the bladder • **[ge wei] 鸽胃** dove (stomach), dysuria, stranguria and anuria, stones in the kidney, stones in the bladder • **[dan bai] 蛋白** eggs (albumen), affections and pains of the kidneys • **[xian dan] 鲜蛋** eggs (fresh), dysuria, stranguria and anuria • **[ge zhong dan] 各种蛋**eggs (of all kinds), affections and pains of the kidneys, affections and pains of the bladder • **[ge zhong zhi fang] 各种脂肪**fat (of all kinds), affections and pains of the kidneys • **[da hai niao] 大海鸟 [hai yan] 海燕** giant petrel (dried stomach), dysuria, stranguria and anuria, stones in the bladder • **[shan yang] 山羊**goat **[yang mao hui] 羊毛灰**(ashes of the hair), dysuria, stranguria and anuria, stones in the bladder • **[shan yang niao pao] 山羊尿泡**goat (bladder), incontinence of urine

[ge qiao] Clam Shell
(Concha Meretricis seu Cyclinae)

P: the shell of meretrix meretrix.

T&N: bitter and salty in flavour, cold in property

Act: to remove heat and resolve phlegm, to soften hard masses and eliminate nodulations, and to alleviate Epigastric pain by inhibiting acid secretion.

Indi: cough, chest pain and bloody sputum caused by heat in the lung scrofula; goitre; epigastric pain associated with acid regurgitation; external use for eczema and scalds.

U&D: 6--15g to be decocted before other ingredients, and wrapped for making decoction if powdered concha is used; for external use. Appropriate quantity to be ground into extremely fine powder and separated on the lesions or applied topically after mixing with oil.

[gui jia] 甲(龟板) Tortoise Shell Carapax (Plastrum Testudinis)

P: the carapace and plastron of Chinemys Revesii.

T&N: salty and sweet in flavour, slightly cold in property.

Act: to nourish yin and subdue the overflowing of Yang, to replenish the kidney and strengthen the bones, and to enrich blood and benefit the mentality.

Indi: consumptive fever and night sweating due to deficiency of Yin; vertigo, tremors, weakness of leg; forgetfulness.

U&D: 9--24g to be decocted before other ingredients.

- **[shan yang ru] 山羊乳** goat (milk), affections and pains of the kidneys
- **[jia yang shan yang fenbian] 家养山羊粪便** goat (mostly domestic) (excrements), stones in the bladder
- **[shan yang niao] 山羊尿** goat **(urine),** dysuria, stranguria and anuria, stones in the bladder
- **[e nao] 鹅脑** goose (brain), affections and pains of the kidneys
- **[e zhi fang] 鹅脂肪** goose (fat), affections and pains of the kidneys, incontinence of urine
- **[e se] 鹅舌** goose (tongue), incontinence of urine
- **[ye tu] 野兔** hare **[sheng huo zhu shi] 生活煮食**(boiled while still alive), stones in the bladder, haematuria
- **[ye tu nao] 野兔脑** hare (brain), affections and pains of the bladder, incontinence of urine
- **[ye tu shen] 野兔肾** hare (kidneys), affections and pains of the kidneys, dysuria, stranguria and anuria, stones in the bladder
- **[ye tu] 野兔**hare **[gan wei mo] 干胃膜**(rennet), incontinence of urine
- **[ye tu mao pi] 野兔毛皮** hare (skin and hair), affections and pains of the bladder, stones in the bladder
- **[ye tu gao wan] 野兔睾丸** hare (testicles), affections and pains of the

[hai long] 海Pipe Fish (Syngnathus)
P: the dried body of Soenognathus Hardwickii.
T&N: sweet in flavour, warm in property.
Act: to warm the kidney and promote virility, to reduce nodulation, and to induce subsidence of swelling.
Indi: impotence and seminal emission, mass in the abdomen, scrofula; traumatic injuries; external use for carbuncles and boils.
U&D: 3--9g for external use, appropriate quantity to be ground into powder and applied topically.

[hai ma] 海 Sea-Horse (Hippocampus)
P: the dried body of Hippocampus Kelloggi.
T&N: sweet in flavour, warm in property.
Act: to warm the kidney and promote virility, to reduce nodulation, and to induce subsidence of swelling.
Indi: impotence, enuresis, dyspnea in deficiency syndrome of the kidney; mass in abdomen; traumatic injuries; external use for carbuncles and boils.
U&D: 3--9g for external use, appropriate quantity to be ground into powder and applied topically.

[hai piao xiao] 海 Cuttlebone (Os Sepiae)
P: the internal shell of Spiella Maindroni.
T&N: salty and astringent in flavour, warm in property.
Act: to stop bleeding arrest seminal discharge or leukorrhea, to inhibit gastric secretion, and to promote the healing of wound.
Indi: peptic ulcer with hyperacidity; spitting of blood, epistaxis; abnormal bladder, incontinence of urine

- **[ci wei dan zhi] 刺猬胆汁** hedgehog (bile), affections and pains of the kidneys

- **[ci wei rou] 刺猬肉** hedgehog (flesh, not touched by its urine, otherwise it causes dysuria), dysuria, stranguria and anuria, stones in the bladder

- **[ma ti hui] 马蹄灰** horse (powder or ashes of its hoof), stones in the bladder

- **[ma qian xi gai gu] 马前膝盖骨** horse (the bony outgrowth under the front knees and on the fetlock), stones in the bladder

- **[zhi shen zhang teng tong de zhou yu] 治肾脏疼痛的咒语** karabrath (magic word against pains of the kidneys), affections and pains of the kidneys

- **[xiao er pang guang] 小儿膀胱**kid (bladder), incontinence of urine

- **[xiao er fei] 小儿肺** kid (lung), incontinence of urine

- **[yang ti] 羊蹄** lamb (hoofs), affections and pains of the bladder, dysuria, stranguria and anuria, stones in the bladder

- **[qian zu chong] 千足虫(蜈蚣)** millepede (the so-called "oniscus" that in Pliny seems to be the wood-louse), affections and pains of the bladder

- **[lao shu fen] 老鼠粪** mouse (excrements), affections and pains of the kidneys, dysuria, stranguria and anuria, stones in the bladder uterine bleeding, haematochezia; seminal emission, spermatorrhea, morbid leukorrhea; gastric pain with acid regurgitation; external use for traumatic bleeding and wound with purulent discharge.

U&D: 4.5--9g for external use, appropriate quantity to be ground into powder and applied topically.

[jiu xiang chong] 九香虫 Jiuxiang Bug (Aspongopus)

P: the dried body of Aspongopus chinesis Dallas (Fam. Pentatomidae).
T&N: salty in flavour, warm in property.
Act: to regulate the flow of Qi and relieve pain, to warm the stomach, and to restore the kidney Yang.
Indi: epigastric pain with distention due to cold in the stomach , or due to stagnation of Qi in the liver and stomach; impotence and aching of the loins and knees in deficiency syndromes of kidney.
U&D: 3--9g

[long gu] 龙骨 Dragon's Bone (Os Draconis)

P: fossil bone of ancient large mammals, such as Stegodon orientalis and Rhinocerus sinensis,
T&N: odorless and tasteless.
Act: to calm mental states, suppressing sthenic Yang and astringing.
Indi: palpitation, frightened, insomnia, dreamfullness, headache and dizziness, spontaneous, perspiration, night sweat, emission and leucorrhagia. Calcined Os Draconis is applied for spontaneous perspiration and night sweat, emission, chronic diarrhea and dysentery.

[lu jiao] 鹿角 Deerhorn (Antler)

- **[luo (xi gai gu)] 骡(膝盖骨)** mule (the bony ourgrowth under the front knees and on the ferlock), dysuria, stranguria and anuria

- **[liu yu (tou ji gu)] 留鱼(头脊骨)** mullet (the spine on of the head), affections and pains of the kidneys, stones in the bladder

- **[zhu (ti hui)] 猪(蹄灰)** pig (ashes of the hoof), incontinence of urine

- **[zhu(niao pao)] 猪(尿泡)** pig (bladder), incontinence of urine

- **[zhu(you)] 猪(油)** pig (fat), affections and pains of the kidneys

- **[zhu da tui ti uang] 猪(大腿 蹄膀)** pig (head of the femur), dysuria, stranguria and anuria

- **[zhu bian]猪(猪鞭)** pig (penis), incontinence of urine

- **[shuan hu chong hong kao] 珊瑚虫(烘 烤)** polyp (toasted), stones in the bladder

- **[xie zi fen] 蝎子(粉)** scorpions (ashes), stones in the bladder

- **[hai xie wei bu shi kuai] 海蝎(尾部石块)** sea scorpion (stone of its tail), affections and pains of the bladder, dysuria, stranguria and anuria, stones in the bladder

(Cornu Cervi)

P: the ossified antler, or antler base, which dropped off in, the next spring after the pilose antler of Cervus elaphus is cut.
T&N: salty in flavour, warm in property.
Act: to warm the kidney and strengthen the tendons and bones; and to promote blood circulation and cause subsidence of swelling.
Indi: impotence, seminal emission, back pain with cold sensation; chronic ulcers mastitis at early stage marking by congestion, swelling and pain.
U&D: 6--15g

[lu jiao jiao] 鹿角胶 Deerhorn Gelatin (Colla Cornus Cervi ; Antler Glue)

P: prepared part by decocting the antler repeatedly in water, the filtrate is concentrated to a certain consistency and left to coagulate, cut into flattened cubes and dried.
T&N: sweet in flavour, light in odor, bland and sticky in property.
Act: to nourish the kidney, to tonify the liver, enrich essence and blood with the effect superior to that of Lu Jiao.
Indi: impotence, spermatorrhea, aching and coldness in the loin and knees and metrorrhagia.

[lu jiao shuang] 鹿角霜 Degelatinated Deer horn (Cornu Cervi Degelatinatum)

P: the piece of antler removed off gelatin.
T&N: salty in flavour, warm in property.
Act: to reinforce the kidney Yang and to arrest bleeding.
Indi: Yang deficiency of the spleen and the kidney characterized by anorexia, vomiting, diarrhea, excessive leukorrhea, enuresis or frequent urine, abnormal

- **[hai ci wei lai pici]** 海刺猬(獭 皮刺) sea urchin (with its prickles), dysuria, stranguria and anuria, stones in the bladder

- **[mian yang]** sheep 绵羊 (grease of its unwashed wool), affections and pains of the kidneys

- **[mian yang (pi)]** sheep 绵羊皮 (skin), affections and pains of the kidneys

- **[wo niu (fei zhou)]** snail 非洲蜗牛 (African), incontinence of urine

- **[wo niu(lian ke zhu)]** snails 蜗牛(连壳煮 (boiled with their shells), affections and pains of the kidneys

- **[wo niu(qu ke zhu)]** snails 蜗牛(去壳煮) (boiled without their shells), dysuria, stranguria and anuria, stones in the bladder

- **[wo niu (sheng rou)]** snails 蜗牛生肉(raw flesh), stones in the bladder

- **[mu zhu(niao pao)]** sow 母猪(尿泡) (bladder), incontinence of urine

- **[hai mian]** sponge 海绵 (seasoned), affections and pains of the kidneys

- **[ren ti puang guang jie shi]**stone 人体膀胱结石 (powder of a human bladder stone), stones in the bladder

- **[yan wo ni]** swallow 燕窝泥 (bits of the mud of its nest), dysuria, stranguria and anuria, stones in the bladder

uterine bleeding, subcutaneous infections and nodulations. **U&D:** 9--15g **[lu jiao] 鹿角 Deerhorn (Antler) (Cornu Cervi)** **P:** the ossified antler, or antler base, which dropped off in, the next spring after the pilose antler of Cervus elaphus is cut. **T&N:** salty in flavour, warm in property. **Act:** to warm the kidney and strengthen the tendons and bones; and to promote blood circulation and cause subsidence of swelling. **Indi:** impotence, seminal emission, back pain with cold sensation; chronic ulcers mastitis at early stage marking by congestion, swelling and pain. **U&D:** 6--15g **[lu jiao jiao] 鹿角胶Deerhorn Gelatin (Colla Cornus Cervi ; Antler Glue)** **P:** prepared part by decocting the antler repeatedly in water, the filtrate is concentrated to a certain consistency and left to coagulate, cut into flattened cubes and dried. **T&N:** sweet in flavour, light in odor, bland and sticky in property. **Act:** to nourish the kidney, to tonify the liver, enrich essence and blood with the effect superior to that of Lu Jiao. **Indi:** impotence, spermatorrhea, aching and coldness in the loin and knees and metrorrhagia. **[lu jiao shuang] 鹿角霜 Degelatianed Deer hron (Cornu Cervi Degelatinatum)** **P:** the piece of antler removed off gelatin. **T&N:** salty in flavour, warm in property. **Act:** to reinforce the kidney Yang and	• **[dong wu zhi]** 动物脂 tallow, affections and pains of the kidneys • **[dong]thrush** 鸫 affections and pains of the bladder, dysuria, stranguria and anuria • **[ban jiu tang]** turtle-dove 斑鸣汤 (broth), stones in the bladder • **[ban jiu fen]** turtle-dove 斑鸣粪 (excrements), affections and pains of the kidneys, dysuria, stranguria and anuria, stones in the bladder • **[huan zhe xiao bian]** urine of the patient **患者小便**(with all the materials contained in it), incontinence of urine • **[huan zhe xiao bian]** urine of the patient **患者小便** incontinence of urine • **[shui she gan]** water snake **水蛇肝** (liver), stones in the bladder • **[ye zhu (ti hui)]** wild boar **野猪(蹄灰** (ashes of the hoof), dysuria, stranguria and anuria, incontinence of urine • **[ye zhu(niao pao)]** wild boar **野猪(尿泡) (bladder)**, affections and pains of the bladder, dysuria, stranguria and anuria, incontinence of urine, stones in the bladder • **[ye zhu (gao wan fen)]** wild boar **野猪(睾丸粉** (ashes of the testicles), incontinence of urine

to arrest bleeding.

Indi: Yang deficiency of the spleen and the kidney characterized by anorexia, vomiting, diarrhea, excessive leukorrhea, enuresis or frequent urination, abnormal uterine bleeding, subcutaneous infections and nodulations.

U&D: 9--15g

[lu rong] 鹿茸 Lurong (Pilose Antler) (Cornu Cervi Pantotritum)

P: the young pilose antler of male Cervus, Nippon Temminck or Cervus elaphus L.

T&N: sweet and salty in flavour warm in property.

Act: to promote virility, replenish vital essence and blood, and strengthen the tendons and bones, to regulate the meridians related to the uterus and conception, and promote the bursting of abscess and drainage of pus.

Indi: impotence, spermatorrhea, or frigidity and infertility, emaciation, lassitude, aversion to cold, dizziness, tinnitus, impairment of hearing, back pain accompanied by cold sensation, and weakness of the limbs, abnormal uterine bleeding and leukorrhea, chronic cores difficult to heal.

U&D: 1--2g to be ground into powder and taken liquid with it.

[mu li] Oyster Shell (Concha Ostreae)

P: the shell of Ostrea talienwhanensis.

T&N: salty in flavour, slightly cold in property.

Act: to nourish Yin and subdue the overflowing of Yang, to induce sedation, to soften hard masses and eliminate nodulation, and to arrest discharge;
Concha ostreae (calcined), to arrest discharge.

- **[ye zhu(gan jie shi)]** wild boar **野猪(肝结石)** (stones in the liver), stones in the bladder

- **[ye zhu (niao)]** wild boar **野猪(尿)** (urine), affections and pains of the bladder, dysuria, stranguria and anuria, stones in the bladder

- **[ye shan yang fen]** wild goat **野山羊粪**(excrements), stones in the bladder

- **[ye e she]** wild goose **野鹅舌** (tongue), incontinence of urine, stones in the bladder

- **[shuang tai fu nu]** woman who has had a twin birth **双胎**妇 **女** (she must jump on the aching kidneys), affections and pains of the kidneys

- **[mu ge (fen hui)]** wood pigeon **木鸽(粪灰** (ashes of the bowels), stones in the bladder

- **[mu ge (yu mao hui)]** wood pigeon **木鸽(羽毛灰** (ashes of the feathers), dysuria, stranguria and anuria, stones in the bladder

- **[chong]** worms **虫** affections and pains of the kidneys, affections and pains of the bladder, stones in the bladder

Indi: palpitation, insomnia, dizziness and tinnitus, scrofula, mall formation in abdomen; spontaneous sweating, seminal emission, abnormal uterine bleeding, excessive leukorrhea, epigastric pain with acid regurgitation; Concha Ostreae (calcined). Spontaneous sweating, night sweating, seminal Emission; abnormal uterine bleeding, excessive leukorrhea, epigastric pain with acid regurgitation.
U&D: 9--30g to be decocted before other ingredients.

[shui zhi] Leech
(Hirudo)
P: the dried body of Whitmania pigra or Whitmania acranulata.
T&N: satly and bitter in flavour, neutral in property.
Act: to eliminate blood stasis and stimulate menstrual discharge.
Indi: mass formation in the abdomen, amenorrhea due to blood stasis; traumatic injuries.
U&D: 1.5--3g
C&C: contraindicated in pregnancy.

[shui zhi] Leech
(Hirudo)
P: the dried body of Whitmania pigra or Whitmania acranulata.
T&N: salty and bitter in flavour, neutral in property.
Act: to eliminate blood stasis and stimulate menstrual discharge.
Indi: mass formation in the abdomen, amenorrhea due to blood stasis; traumatic injuries.
U&D: 1.5--3g
C&C: contraindicated in pregnancy

[xie yu tan] **Carbonized Hair (Crinis Carbonisatus)** **P:** the carbonized human hair. **T&N:** bitter in flavour, neutral in property. **Act:** to arrest bleeding and remove blood stasis. **Indi:** haematemesis, epistaxis, haematuria, abnormal uterine bleeding, traumatic bleeding. **U&D:** 4.5--9g	

Table of Apothecaries' Weights Equivalents

Ancient Market System (旧市称)	Meritic System (公制)	Modern Market System (市制)	Meritic System (公制)
1 Jin (斤)	500 g (克)	1 Jin ((斤)	500g (克)
1 Liang (两)	31.25 g (克)	1 Liang (两)	50g (克)
1 Qian (钱)	3.125 g (克)	1 Qian (钱)	5g (克)
1 Fen ((分)	0.3125 g (克)	1 Fen (分)	0.5g (克)

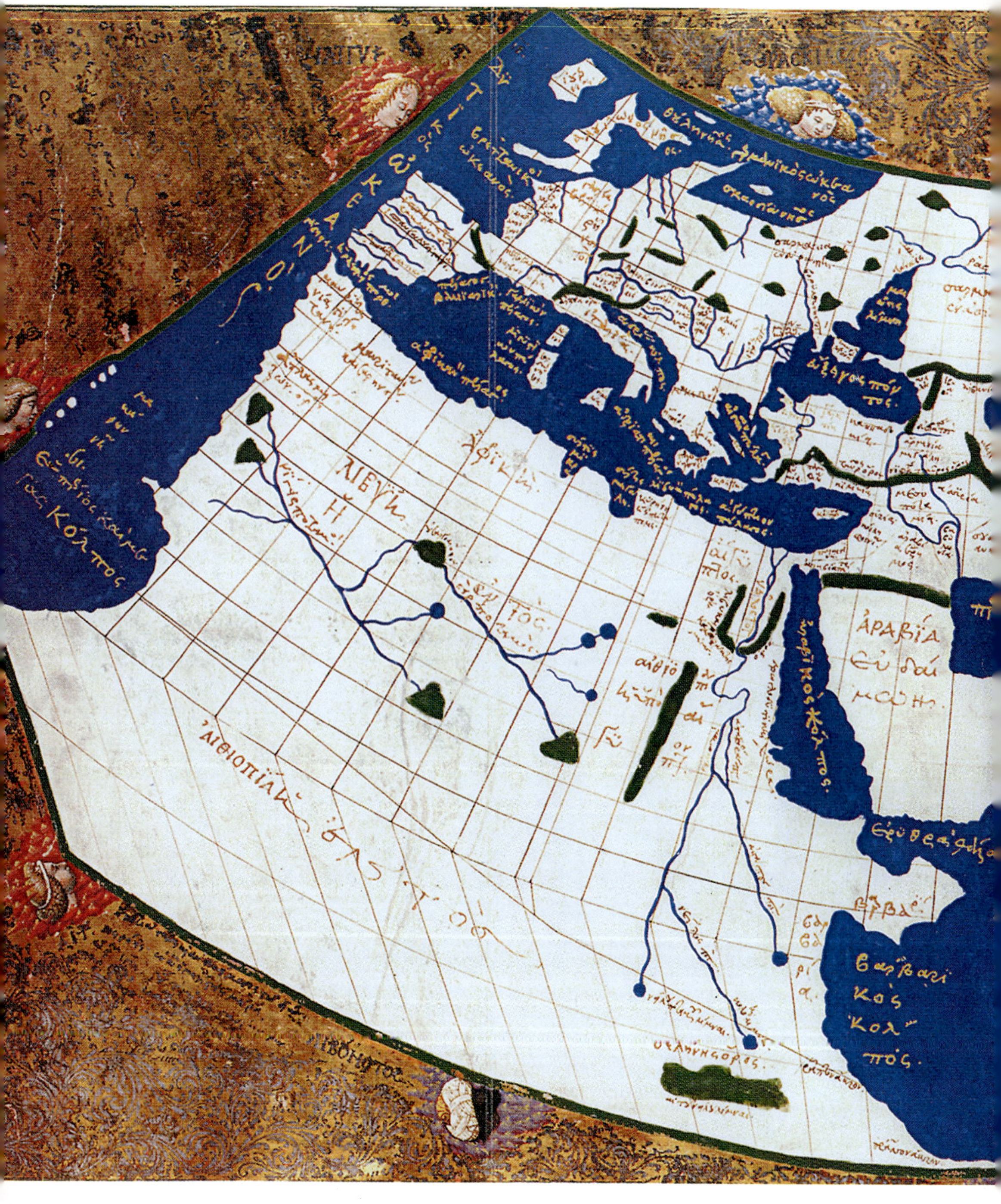